Cardiovascular Disease in AIDS

Second Edition

Giuseppe Barbaro • Franck Boccara (Eds)

Cardiovascular Disease in AIDS

Second Edition

In cooperation with
Giorgio Barbarini

Foreword by
Paul R. Skolnik

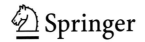 Springer

GIUSEPPE BARBARO
Department of Medical Pathophysiology
"Sapienza" University of Rome
Rome, Italy

FRANCK BOCCARA
Department of Cardiology
Saint Antoine University Hospital
Assistance Publique -
Hôpitaux de Paris and
Université Pierre et Marie Curie
Paris, France

In cooperation with
GIORGIO BARBARINI
Department of Infectious and Tropical Diseases
Policlinico "San Matteo"
University of Pavia
Pavia, Italy

Library of Congress Control Number: 2007941073

ISBN   978-88-470-0760-4 Springer Milan Berlin Heidelberg New York
e-ISBN 978-88-470-0761-1

Springer is a part of Springer Science+Business Media
springer.com
© Springer-Verlag Italia 2009

Cover design: Simona Colombo, Milan, Italy
Typesetting: Graphostudio, Milan, Italy
Printing: Grafiche Porpora, Segrate (MI), Italy

Printed in Italy
Springer-Verlag Italia S.r.l., Via Decembrio 28, I-20137 Milan

Foreword to the Second Edition

Highly active antiretroviral therapy (HAART) has changed the face of HIV infection and AIDS into a treatable, chronic illness in resource-rich areas of the world. The hope is that we will overcome availability and distribution issues in resource-poor settings so the same is true in these regions of the world in the future. When available, HAART has dramatically decreased the incidence of opportunistic infections, which were frequently the direct cause of mortality during HIV infection. The paradox of this situation is that morbidities that were never relevant previously, because of truncated longevity before HAART, have now come to the fore as important aspects of HIV-related management. Diseases that shorten life in patients without HIV infection must now be attended to with particular rigor in caring for patients with HIV infection. This is especially true since the manifestations of these co-morbidities are often worsened by HIV infection, and special considerations, including drug interactions, must be taken into account.

Cardiovascular diseases are especially important in this regard because of their prevalence in the population and their frequent relationship to morbidity and mortality. Whether the heart and vascular system are affected by HIV infection is in little doubt, although the extent of these effects in different populations, and the relative contribution of HIV infection compared to classical risk factors, is a matter of some controversy. Much data has accumulated to suggest that there are significant effects of HIV, and concomitant therapy, on the cardiovascular system.

The chapters in this book describe what is clearly understood, and what is not. They go on to present the data upon which these opinions are based, and to make practical suggestions for proper diagnosis and management. They make important reading for researchers and clinicians in this field, both to provide the clinical basis for basic research that will inform new diagnostic and treatment paradigms, and to suggest the best, current therapies for these maladies.

Perhaps the most urgent area for research, leading to a more concise, mechanism-based understanding of pathogenesis, is

HIV-associated lipodystrophy. This catch-all phrase actually subsumes several areas that may have distinct pathophysiologic etiologies. Lipoatrophy has in some ways become the new "scarlet letter" of HIV infection, a distinction previously held by cutaneous Kaposi's sarcoma. The cause of this manifestation, characterized by thinning of the face, arms, legs, and buttocks, remains unclear, as does the relative contribution of HAART and HIV infection to these changes. Fat redistribution syndrome, characterized by fatty deposits of the neck and abdomen ("buffalo hump" and "protease paunch") most often occurs during HAART, but whether fat redistribution is associated with an increased risk of cardiovascular disease, and whether lipoatrophy engenders similar risk, remains uncertain.

HAART may lead to changes in serum lipids, and it is likely that these changes increase the risk of atherosclerotic heart disease, myocardial infarction, and stroke. Whether or not these lipid changes during HIV infection carry the same, or greater, risk compared to the general population without HIV infection, it is clear that clinicians should measure these changes and treat them accordingly. In this context, it is often necessary to know the relative magnitude of lipid changes with various antiretroviral agents so that treatment regimens can be modified appropriately if standard lipid-lowering therapy does not suffice. It is also crucial for clinicians to know the many drug–drug interactions that can occur and that modify the efficacy and tolerability of antiretroviral drugs and lipid-lowering agents. Newer diagnostic modalities, that have both clinical and research applications, are currently being assessed, as are the best drugs to use in these situations.

Other metabolic changes that occur during HIV infection, or are modified by HIV infection, also affect cardiovascular risk and optimal treatment of these disorders. Diabetes mellitus, associated with insulin resistance and the metabolic syndromes mentioned above, may have exaggerated effects on the cardiovascular system during HIV infection. Antiretroviral drugs may also be associated with lactic acidosis and acute, life-threatening illness, or may cause life-threatening pancreatitis through drug-induced hypertriglyceridemia or direct toxicity.

Other HIV-related effects may occur directly on the myocardium or pulmonary tissues, and lead to cardiomyopathy or HIV-associated pulmonary arterial hypertension. As longevity increases for those with HIV infection, a fuller understanding of these disorders becomes important for proper diagnosis and treatment. It is likely that the immune activation that occurs during HIV infection, even with effective HAART, is related to the expression of these diseases during HIV infection. Once again, it is difficult to determine the relative contribution of HIV infection and risk factors such as amphetamine, tobacco, or cocaine use, but it is clear that HIV infection alone can lead to cardiomyopathy and HIV-associated pulmonary hypertension. There is an important need to understand the natural history of these disorders to better plan when certain diagnostic and therapeutic interventions should be initiated.

This book should be read by all those interested in the cardiovascular complications that occur during HIV infection. The gold mine of information contained herein will stimulate new ideas about pathogenesis, inform in vitro and animal model research to test these hypotheses, and lead to patient-oriented research and clinical trials to test practical interventions that might improve diagnosis and treatment of cardiovascular comorbidities. In this context, the combined knowledge and expertise of scientists and clinicians in the fields of infectious diseases, lipid metabolism, endocrinology, cardiology, and other relevant subspecialties must be brought to bear to unravel the mysteries that still exist, so that we may optimally prevent illness and care for those who suffer from the sometimes devastating effects of cardiovascular disease.

Paul R. Skolnik, MD
Professor of Medicine
Boston University School of Medicine
Boston, Massachusetts, USA

Foreword to the First Edition

Never in the history of humanity has knowledge progressed as quickly as in the field of AIDS. Over a period of 15 years, successive discoveries of the disease, its viral origin, the virus responsible, its physiopathology and highly effective therapies have led to spectacular improvement in life expectancy and in the quality of life of people who have access to these treatments.

However, this progress in therapy has been accompanied by initially unforeseeable anomalies, such as abnormalities in lipid and glucose metabolism and modifications in fat distribution, particularly in perivisceral and trunkal accumulation as well as pseudo-obesity usually accompanied by peripheral atrophy.

Several of these anomalies constitute risk factors for cardiovascular diseases and may be predictors of these diseases. Over time, most investigators have come to accept that HIV-infected patients are at an increased risk for cardiovascular complications.

However, several issues remain unclear:

- Does the increased risk merely reflect modification of the usual factors: metabolic disorders, tobacco consumption, infectious context related to HIV infection or opportunistic infections, inappropriate immune and cytokine response, or genetic background?
- The physiopathology of disorders in glucose or lipid metabolism remains to be clarified. It is unclear whether they result from treatment, use of a specific medication, use of a therapeutic class of medication, or an association of treatments. Here, too, genetic background may well be a factor, along with the history of the individual's HIV infection.

It is particularly difficult to devise a therapeutic strategy under these conditions, especially since the efficacy of the usual lipid- or glucose-modifying medication is not established, and the benefit of any eventual correction of such biological anomalies in this population is unclear. The issue is further complicated by the many drug interactions between antiretroviral medications and medications likely to act on the lipid metabolism, which renders their usage complex.

In this atmosphere of uncertainty, the simple measure of

diminishing tobacco usage is itself difficult, and overconsumption of tobacco is regularly observed in this population.

The medical management of HIV-infected patients is mostly carried out by infectious disease specialists, and the field of cardiovascular diseases is not usually familiar to them.

The history of AIDS has taught us that phenomena are most quickly and effectively understood when light is cast on them from a variety of angles, using a variety of tools. The dynamism which has always characterized AIDS research will doubtless benefit from greater comprehension of the mechanisms of these poorly understood metabolic disorders.

The present volume contributes to disseminating knowledge in the field so that the various actors can pool their expertise towards a successful management of cardiovascular disease in HIV-infected patients.

Willy Rozenbaum, MD
Professor of Infectious Diseases
Université Pierre et Marie Curie
Paris, France

Contents

Contributors

Sabrina Audagnotto
Department of Infectious Diseases, University of Turin,
Amedeo di Savoia Hospital, Turin, Italy

Giorgio Barbarini
Department of Infectious and Tropical Diseases,
Policlinico San Matteo, University of Pavia, Pavia, Italy

Giuseppe Barbaro
Department of Medical Pathophysiology,
"Sapienza" University of Rome, Rome, Italy

Franck Boccara
Département de Cardiologie,
Centre Hospitalier Universitaire Saint-Antoine,
Assistance Publique - Hôpitaux de Paris and
Université Pierre et Marie Curie, Paris, France

Damien Bonnet
Service de Cardiologie Pédiatrique,
Hôpital Necker-Enfants Malades, Paris, France

Nicolas Bonnet
Service de Chirurgie Cardio-vasculaire et Thoracique,
Institut de Cardiologie, Groupe Hospitalier Pitié-Salpêtrière,
Paris, France

Stefano Bonora
Department of Infectious Diseases, University of Turin,
Amedeo di Savoia Hospital, Turin, Italy

Andrea Calcagno
Department of Infectious Diseases, University of Turin,
Amedeo di Savoia Hospital, Turin, Italy

Jaqueline Capeau
INSERM U402, Faculté de Médecine Saint-Antoine,
Département de Biochimie, Hôpital Tenon,
Université Pierre et Marie Curie, Paris, France

Martine Caron
INSERM UMRS680, Faculté de Médecine Saint-Antoine,
Paris, France

Claire Cipriano
Service de Médecine Interne et Maladies Infectieuses,
Hôpital Haut-Lévêque, Centre Hospitalier Universitaire
de Bordeaux, Pessac, France

Ariel Cohen
Département de Cardiologie, Assistance Publique-Hôpitaux
de Paris et Université Pierre et Marie Curie, Centre
Hospitalier Universitaire Saint-Antoine, Paris, France

Dominique Costagliola
INSERM U720, Epidémiologie Clinique et Traitement de
l'Infection à VIH, Université Pierre et Marie Curie,
Paris, France

Giovanni Di Perri
Department of Infectious Diseases, University of Turin,
Amedeo di Savoia Hospital, Turin, Italy

Ludovic Drouet
Laboratoire de Thrombose et d'Athérosclérose,
Hôpital Lariboisière, Paris, France

Ghislaine Dufaitre
Département de Cardiologie, Assistance Publique-Hôpitaux
de Paris et Université Pierre et Marie Curie, Centre
Hospitalier Universitaire Saint-Antoine, Paris, France

Stéphane Ederhy
Département de Cardiologie, Assistance Publique-Hôpitaux
de Paris et Université Pierre et Marie Curie, Centre
Hospitalier Universitaire Saint-Antoine, Paris, France

Iradj Gandjbakhch
Service de Chirurgie Cardio-vasculaire et Thoracique,
Institut de Cardiologie, Groupe Hospitalier Pitié-Salpêtrière,
Paris, France

Jérôme Garot
Fédération de Cardiologie, Hôpital Henri Mondor, Créteil,
France

Federico Gobbi
Department of Infectious Diseases, University of Turin,
Amedeo di Savoia Hospital, Turin, Italy

Nabila Haddour
Département de Cardiologie, Assistance Publique-Hôpitaux
de Paris et Université Pierre et Marie Curie, Centre
Hospitalier Universitaire Saint-Antoine, Paris, France

Sandra Janower
Département de Cardiologie, Assistance Publique-Hôpitaux
de Paris et Université Pierre et Marie Curie, Centre
Hospitalier Universitaire Saint-Antoine, Paris, France

Sylvie Lang
Département de Cardiologie, Assistance Publique-Hôpitaux
de Paris et Université Pierre et Marie Curie, Centre
Hospitalier Universitaire Saint-Antoine, Paris, France

Brigitte Le Bail
Laboratoire d'Anatomophatologie, Hôpital Pellegrin, Centre
Hospitalier Universitaire de Bordeaux, Bordeaux, France

Pascal Leprince
Service de Chirurgie Cardio-vasculair Thoracique,
Institut de Cardiologie, Groupe Hospitalier Pitié-Salpêtrière,
Paris, France

Robert Loire
Institut de Médecine Légale, Lyon, France

Murielle Mary-Krause
INSERM U720, Epidémiologie Clinique et Traitement de
l'Infection à VIH, Université Pierre et Marie Curie,
Paris, France

Patrick Mercié
Service de Médecine Interne, Hôpital Saint-André,
Centre Hospitalier Universitaire de Bordeaux et INSERM U593,
Université Victor Segalen Bordeaux 2, Bordeaux, France

Catherine Meuleman
Département de Cardiologie, Assistance Publique-Hôpitaux
de Paris et Université Pierre et Marie Curie, Centre
Hospitalier Universitaire Saint-Antoine, Paris, France

Antoine Moulignier
Fondation Adolphe de Rothschild, Service de Neurologie,
Paris, France

Letizia Oberto
Department of Infectious Diseases,
Policlinico San Matteo, University of Pavia, Pavia, Italy

François Raoux
Département de Cardiologie, Assistance Publique-Hôpitaux
de Paris et Université Pierre et Marie Curie, Centre
Hospitalier Universitaire Saint-Antoine, Paris, France

Daniele Scevola
Department of Infectious and Tropical Diseases,
Policlinico San Matteo, University of Pavia, Pavia, Italy

Alain Tabib
Institut de Médecine Légale, Lyon, France

Laura Trentini
Department of Infectious Diseases, University of Turin,
Amedeo di Savoia Hospital, Turin, Italy

Shaida Varnous
Service de Chirurgie Cardio-vasculaire et Thoracique,
Institut de Cardiologie, Groupe Hospitalier Pitié-Salpêtrière,
Paris, France

Chapter 1

Natural History of HIV Infection and Evolution of Antiretroviral Therapy

G. Di Perri, S. Audagnotto, F. Gobbi, L. Trentini, A. Calcagno, S. Bonora

Introduction

The are probably few examples, if any, in the story of medicine like the one concerning the abrupt change that pharmacological research determined in the clinical evolution of HIV infection and AIDS. In few months since the introduction of the first triple drug association deserving the acronym HAART (Highly Active Antiretroviral Therapy), the life expectancy of persons infected with HIV switched from a few years to a still indefinable time that we can today estimate as several decades [1]. Those physicians who are sufficiently aged to have assisted HIV-infected patients both before and after the introduction of HAART, have probably experienced one of the most important events in their life. It is often difficult in these times to make young doctors (and young patients as well) aware of the magnitude of the change that took place in the overall life perspective of humans infected with HIV. While for the newcomers to antiretroviral therapy it is rather natural to see patients' immunity regain its competence under appropriate antiretroviral treatment, some of us still perceive something like a miracle in watching the reversal of such an otherwise deadly human disease. Most of our concerns today are related to side effects resulting from HAART rather than to its efficacy, and we are increasingly focusing on the long-term therapeutic balance (with issues like toxicity, tolerance and adherence) instead of life-threatening opportunistic infections. A short paragraph on the natural history of HIV infection is thus fully justified in the intention to remind others of how things were, and still are in many geographical regions, before the use of multi-drug therapy transformed HIV infection from a lethal disease to a condition often compatible with a reasonably normal life.

The Natural History of HIV Infection

In the years following the time when specific diagnostic molecular assays became available (HIV serology by means of ELISA and Western-Blot techniques), we eventually recognized the rather atypical clinical evolution of HIV infection. With infectious diseases resulting in physicians being more accustomed (with notable exceptions) to deal with acute disease forms, the multiphasic progression of HIV infection, with long-lasting asymptomatic periods, brought to our attention a totally new infectious disease model.

Well before HIV was identified as the causative agent of AIDS, a clear-cut correlation was established between the downgrading tendency of immune surveillance and the increasingly severe clinical manifestations leading eventually to death [2]. It is worth noting that 26 years after the first five AIDS patients were described as individuals developing unusual opportunistic infections and neoplasms in association to extremely low numbers of circulating CD4+ T-lymphocytes, no immunological markers better than CD4+ cells have been identified as indicator of immune status in patients with HIV infection [3]. Although exceptions are not so uncommon, the relationship between the CD4+ cell count and the likelihood of developing specific opportunistic diseases is still the best clinical rule for clinicians to rely upon in the diagnostic workup of patients with HIV infection. There are no other human diseases in which the relationship between an immunological marker and a given clinical condition is so coherent. Although the distinction between HIV infection (defined by a positive HIV serology) and AIDS (defined by a positive serology in association with some major associated disorders) is still made on a clinical ground, reliance on the number of circulating CD4+ cells is pivotal in the process of choosing diagnostic procedures and taking therapeutic decisions [4].

Based on these two markers (serology and CD4+ count), a more than approximate description of the natural history of HIV infection can be easily plotted on a graph, with the time elapsing since infection on the x axis and the absolute number of CD4+ T-lymphocytes/μl on the y axis (Fig. 1). In the 2nd half of the 90s, a molecular marker representing the plasma concentration of HIV-specific nucleic acids became available (HIV-RNA), which made it possible to quantify the presence of HIV in the blood and to successfully relate it to clinical and immune disease progression [5].

In clinical terms, the manifestations of HIV infection can be classified in four sequential phases. In the days following infection, an acute inflammatory syndrome may take place with a rather wide variety of signs and symptoms [6]. In more than 50% of symptomatic cases, fever, pharyngitis ("mononucleosis-like syndrome"), systemic adenopathy, cutaneous rash and diffuse musculoskeletal pain are usually present, but less common disease forms are also described, with involvement of the central nervous system [7]. Acute retroviral syndrome tends to subside in a few days to several weeks; and, depending on a variety of circumstantial factors (clinical presentation, physician's experience), it may actually be recognized or simply interpreted as a common flu-like disease. Today it is common

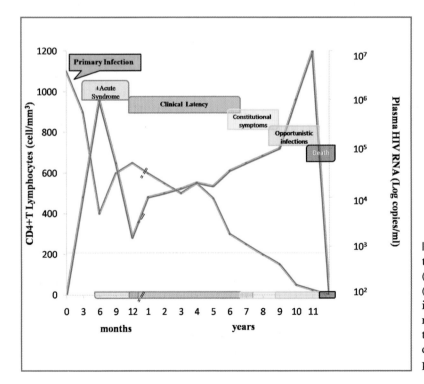

Fig. 1. The chronological relationship among immunological (CD4+T-cells) and virological (HIV-RNA) markers and the clinical evolution of HIV infection is represented. The *red line* refers to circulating CD4+T-lymphocytes and the *green line* refers to plasma HIV-RNA

practice to rely upon plasma HIV-RNA assays when serology is still negative and the clinical picture suggests the possibility of acute retroviral syndrome. While anti-HIV antibodies may take up to several months to become detectable, the molecular evidence of HIV infection in the plasma well anticipates seroconversion, thus allowing the diagnosis of newly acquired HIV infection in the absence of detectable anti-HIV antibodies [8]. It must be recognized, however, that it is not easy to estimate the rate of newly acquired HIV infection cases producing acute symptomatic disease, and the proportion of newly diagnosed infections presenting with an acute inflammatory disease form is rather low.

After primary infection (which may thus pass unnoticed in a substantial proportion of cases) a prolonged asymptomatic phase follows, which usually lasts several years [9]. With progression of immune decline, an early symptomatic phase may be recognized, with some minor clinical manifestations like pharyngeal candidiasis, systemic lymphadenopathy, seborrhoeic dermatitis [10]. When immune deterioration gets below the threshold of 200 CD4+ T-lymphocytes/μl, the patient enters in the phase of highest vulnerability to opportunistic disorders, as the risk of developing overtly symptomatic opportunistic disorders increases in inverse relationship with decreasing CD4+ T-lymphocytes [11]. The clinical phase corresponding to a CD4+ cell count <200/μl is thus the most symptomatic one and in the vast majority of patients, the clinical diagnosis of AIDS is made with a number of circulating CD4+ T-lymphocytes below such a value. In a minority of patients, however, AIDS-defining clinical manifestations may occur when their CD4+ cell count is still above this threshold, as may be the case with less strict opportunistic disorders like Kaposi's sarcoma, esophageal candidiasis, extrapulmonary tuberculosis or recurrent bacterial pneumonia [12, 13].

Among the major opportunistic infections occurring in patients with less than 200 CD4+ cells/μl, some difference is worth noting. While infections like *Pneumocystis jirovecii* pneumonia (formerly known as *P. carinii* pneumonia or PCP) and Toxoplasmosis may take place with any CD4+ cell count below 200/μl (with increasing frequency at lower values, however), some specific opportunistic infections like cryptococcosis, multi-organ disease by *Cytomegalovirus*, atypical mycobacteriosis or less frequent infections like that from *Rhodococcus equi* tend to develop in the very latest phase of the downgrading course of HIV-related immune deterioration, such as when the CD4+ cell count has dropped below the value of 50/μl [14]. In clinical practice, the diagnosis of one among these extremely opportunistic disorders corresponds, therefore, to a residual immune competence approaching exhaustion. From this viewpoint, it is worth noting that some increase in the incidence of these end-stage opportunistic infections was seen in the 90s such as when the life expectancy of AIDS patients also increased as a result of a more appropriate and timely management of opportunistic infections (both therapeutic and prophylactic) [15]. In the western world, the improvement over time of the medical ability in the overall management of AIDS patients made it more likely, for a sizeable proportion of them, to survive until their immune competence eventually consisted of only few remaining CD4+ cells. In regions of the world where highly specialized care was not available, opportunistic disorders typical of this very last phase of the HIV clinical course were rarer, since death was more likely to occur in earlier phases.

Furthermore, regarding these specific opportunistic entities, and several other infections and neoplastic diseases also listed among the AIDS-associated conditions, the clinical picture usually also includes constitutional signs and symptoms like significant weight loss (>10% of normal body weight), chronic fatigue and fever [16–18].

A particularly relevant position in the spectrum of the HIV-associated opportunistic infection is that of tuberculosis (TB). Active TB may develop in any human being regardless of the presence of specific immunosuppressant conditions, but as is the case with other predisposing factors, in the case of HIV infection, the risk increases several fold as compared to the general population [19]. In patients with HIV infection, the risk of developing active TB increases when the individual immune surveillance declines and such increased individual vulnerability has been demonstrated both in the case of reactivation of a pre-existing (latent) infection as well as in case of *de novo* exposure [20, 21]. Further to play the role of the most powerful factor predisposing to active TB, HIV infection was also found to alter the clinical presentation of the disease [22]. In a sizeable proportion of patients with low values of circulating CD4+ cells (<200/µl), the loss of the ability to mount an adequate cellular immune reaction often corresponds to unspecific pathologic pictures, with no or only poorly formed granulomas [23]. In terms of clinical presentation, the lesions appear less distinct from the surrounding parenchyma and the typical cavitations are often absent. This loss of immune control also translates into a higher frequency of extrapulmonary lesions as well as higher numbers of bacilli at the histopathologic level. Since the incidence of TB is closely related to the degree of disease endemicity, it is not surprising that TB represents the most frequent infectious disorder associated to HIV infection in the developing world [24].

The progressive multi-step clinical evolution of HIV infection might not be entirely observed in the individual patient, as is the case in the so-called "late presenters". This typically happens when subjects who are unaware of being HIV-infected develop a major, AIDS-defining, opportunistic disorder. In these increasingly encountered patients, the silent, asymptomatic loss of immune competence becomes recognizable only when the abrupt development of a totally unexpected opportunistic disorder discloses the diagnosis of AIDS.

In a small minority of patients, who are known as "long-term non-progressors", HIV infection does not seem to determine the same unfavourable immune deterioration which is described in most patients. Although it is not clear how the eventual outcome of HIV infection will be in these subjects, a number of reports have described a rather steady immunological condition up to 20 years since HIV was acquired [25, 26].

In the years preceding the release of effective antiretroviral regimens, the only therapeutic measures available to counteract the effects of the downgrading tendency of immune surveillance were drugs specifically active against opportunistic pathogens. Further to be used in the treatment of specific opportunistic infections, these drugs were also administered as prophylactic agents both for primary (e.g. for preventing *P. jirovecii* pneumonia in patients with less than 200 CD4+ T-lymphocytes/µl) or secondary prophylaxis (following the treatment of the first episode of opportunistic infection) of otherwise frequently occurring opportunistic infectious processes [27]. Although neither treatment or prophylaxis were able to reverse the tendency to lose immune competence over time, the life expectancy of HIV-infected patients who were carefully monitored on this basis was significantly increased in the years before HAART became available [15]. It is unclear to what extent the release of the first antiretroviral drugs contributed to this pre-HAART improvement in the life expectancy of AIDS patients. The use of azidothimidine (AZT) alone was found to delay the onset of AIDS, but no advantages were seen in terms of life duration [28].

The Effects of Highly Active Antiretroviral Therapy (HAART) in the Clinical Aspects of HIV Infection

It took a few months to realize how the use of existing nucleoside analogues inhibitors of the HIV reverse transcriptase (NRTIs) in combination with the newly released protease inhibitors (PIs) was associated to a spectacular reversal of the otherwise inescapable deterioration of immune competence [29, 30]. To better understand the changes that occurred with the introduction of HAART in those years, we must also consider the importance of the concomitant release of the test for measuring the amount of circulating HIV (plasma HIV-RNA by polymerase chain reaction–PCR) [31, 32].

Until that time we were dealing with a poorly active treatment (one or two NRTIs) whose efficacy was rather difficult to establish, since the rise in CD4+ cell count (of scarce extent, if any) took several weeks or months to became apparent and a short time to vanish. In the years preceding the use of HIV-RNA, the measurement of plasma p24 antigen levels, as a surrogate marker of the circulating viral burden, was employed to some extent but it never became part of the routinary analyses in HIV-infected patients, mostly for its limited clinical value [33]. In few months we acquired both much more potent therapeutic weapons and a pharmacodynamic marker more sensitive to treatment effects. Further to produce a quicker and more consistent effect on CD4+ cell count, HAART was also found to determine a rapid drop of logarithmic magnitude of the plasma HIV-RNA, which was demonstrable well before any rise in CD4+ cells [34]. The almost contemporary release of these two new instruments made it thus possible to both effectively treat HIV infection and to monitor treatment effects more timely and precisely than before. With the early evidence of HIV-RNA fall as indicator of therapeutic efficacy, with CD4+ cell increase ensuing thereafter, physicians administering HAART to their patients had thus increased confidence in this new treatment modality. From a more popular perspective, the now fully demonstrable and consistent association taking place between immunovirological and clinical benefit under HAART was the final and definitive answer to those persisting minor rumours against the role of HIV infection in the pathogenesis of AIDS [35]. The importance of relying upon plasma HIV-RNA as early efficacy marker is today emphasized by the common habit of designing short-lasting (10–14 days) phase I therapeutic trials aimed at assessing, as "proof of concept", the antiretroviral properties of new compounds before proceeding to conventional clinical studies [36].

In the years 1995–1997, with minor delays in some western regions, the introduction of combination therapy consisting of two NRTIs and one of the new PIs, determined a dramatic change in the natural course of HIV infection. In less than 2 years, according to the HIV Outpatient Study, mortality in patients with HIV infection dropped from 29.4 per 100-person-years to 8.8 [1]. In Italy the mortality of AIDS patients (determined as the number of yearly AIDS deaths per number of AIDS diagnoses in the same year) dropped from 67.3% in 1995 to 9.0% in 2005 [37]. A decline of similar magnitude was also seen in terms of lower incidence of opportunistic infections like *P. jirovecii* pneumonia, CMV retinitis and atypical mycobacteriosis, whose overall rate declined from 21.9 per 100-person-years to 3.7 in the period 1995–1997 [1]. The latter findings gave a working confirmation that immune recovery under HAART was not only numerical but also functional, thus leading to regained effective immune surveillance [38]. This was also testified by the spontaneous recovery from some opportunistic infections (without specific chemotherapy) in patients undergoing

HAART-associated immune reconstitution, which implies that the sole CD4+ cell increase may be sufficient to get rid of the ongoing active disorder by simply restoring a protective level of immune surveillance [39]. With few exceptions, which are likely to be attributable to some specific clonal deletion in immune reconstitution [40], the number of CD4+ to be restored in order to confer spontaneous protection against opportunistic pathogens was found to be the same as the one established before HAART was available. On this basis, once a patient has undergone a numerical recovery of CD4+ cells known to be sufficient to keep the patient out of a CD4+ defined risk of opportunistic infection, prophylaxis or maintenance therapy against specific opportunistic infections may be safely interrupted [41, 42].

A number of cohort studies have subsequently confirmed the unambiguous and sustained survival advantage provided by HAART. In the years following the astonishing debut of HAART in the HIV scenario, the exciting new wave of pharmaceutical research in antiretrovirals made it also possible to find the appropriate answers to a series of problems emerging from the ordinary antiretroviral practice such as resistance to existing drugs, insufficient antiretroviral potency, side effects and adherence, thus substantially keeping the initial promise of a really effective treatment. The effects of HAART in the clinical manifestations of HIV infection also translated into the emergence of new, HIV-unrelated, causes of death in patients with HIV infection [43]. This is to say that concomitant diseases like HCV chronic hepatitis, which were neglected in the pre-HAART era, became a priority in the management of patients with HIV infection. A number of pathophysiological factors well describe the complex pathogenetic interaction of diseases co-existing with HIV, but the single simple fact that HIV-infected patients receiving adequate antiretroviral therapy have many

more years to live, clearly implies that these conditions have a longer time to fully develop to clinically significant manifestations.

Today the management of HIV-infected patients has switched from mostly inpatient to mostly outpatient, since the most frequent service to be delivered is that of monitoring efficacy and toxicity of HAART in patients whose average quality of life has greatly improved and who do not require, in most circumstances, to be assisted in the hospital. A sizeable proportion of patients, however, still require intensive hospital-based treatment, as treatment failures occur for a variety of reasons: lack of patients' adherence to treatment, real treatment failures due to resistance to antiretrovirals, symptomatic chronic virus hepatitis, neoplastic diseases and other concurrent infectious and non-infectious conditions requiring close monitoring (e.g. active tuberculosis). In addition to these occurrences, we have also to face the increasingly important issue of the "late presenters" such as patients who present with a major opportunistic disorder without any prior clinical or serologic evidence of HIV infection. These are truly AIDS patients as we were accustomed to seeing in the pre-HAART era, and require the same therapeutic measures we had been applying in those years. Although HAART may be highly efficacious also in these cases, a measurable rate of early mortality is recorded in these patients, mainly due to the nature of the AIDS-defining disorder they present with. In Italy, the proportion of new cases of HIV infection meeting the case definition for AIDS increased from 18% in 1995 to nearly 50% in 2005 [37]. The reason why this has happened has probably some epidemiologic reasons, at least in countries like Italy, where the responsibility of sexual transmission as a risk factor for acquiring HIV infection increased from 27.5% in 1995 to 61.7% in 2005, while parenteral transmission among heroin addicts decreased from 66.7% in 1995 to 30.8% in 2005 [37]. Whereas, in the case of intravenous drug abusers, the outpatient facilities are able to detect HIV infection in earlier stages (as part of the ordinary serologic screening) in the majority of cases, the STD clinics can only screen that minority of the sexually active population who present with some disturbances. Although such a significant switch in HIV epidemiology might only be representative of regions like Italy, France and Spain, the phenomenon of "late presenters" is well present in most western countries. As a consequence, in order to curb this wave of AIDS presenters, efforts should clearly be made in the setting of the screening strategy, since the effectiveness of today's available HAART might prove to be useless in this not-so sizeable proportion of patients.

Antiretroviral Therapy Today

In late 2007, twenty antiretrovirals are available on the European market, with a further three drugs approaching official release in early 2008. In the last 10 years, by excluding some pharmaceutical remake and dual or triple drug co-formulations of existing drugs, the mean number of new antiretrovirals per year has been 1.5. Today, four drug classes are available (N/NtRTIs, NNRTIs, PIs, entry inhibitors), and a fifth (integrase inhibitors) is about to make its entry in the anti-HIV pharmacopea. Newer drugs classifiable in the existing classes and new classes are also in the pipeline (maturation inhibitors, monoclonal antibodies as entry inhibitors), thus testifying of the exciting liveliness of this pharmaceutical sector, probably the most active branch of pharmaceutical research in these times.

In the years following the first introduction of HAART, the therapeutic strategies underwent several changes on the basis of the new knowledge resulting from clinical evidence and according to the properties of the numerous new drugs that have been released over time. Therapeutic guidelines delivered by national and supranational health authorities (e.g. DHHS in USA and BHIVA in UK) are continuously updated in order to provide the best available indications for the overall management of HIV infection [44, 45].

The basic therapeutic potential of antiretroviral therapy today is that of providing significant inhibition of viral replication and then, as a result of the latter, recovery of CD4+ T-lymphocytes. This translates into clinical recovery in those who are symptomatic and in a condition of clinical stability for patients who begin their treatment while still in the asymptomatic stage. The response rate, which may vary according to numerous factors, may well be over 75% in patients starting HAART, and today numerous alternative options are available for those who do not respond to their first regimen. The most atypical and thorny aspect of HAART is that it must be administered for life. HIV infection is the only infectious disease requiring permanent therapy, as treatment interruption is followed by resumed viral replication, immunological impairment and progressive clinical deterioration, that is to say that HIV infection resumes its natural course. The only analogy may be that of chronic hepatitis B infection, for which, today, continuous suppressive treatment is also being advised [46].

The clinical demand has been changing over time as a consequence of different problems that arose in clinical practice. In the first years following the introduction of HAART, it soon became apparent that HIV was able to change its susceptibility to antiretrovirals and to become drug-resistant in a classic Darwinian way. By applying methods of molecular biology, it was possible to identify genotypic patterns of viral isolates that were correspondent to distinct phenomena of drug resistance. While In Vitro systems for testing viral sensitivity to antiretrovirals (phenotyping) were also developed, viral genotyping was found to be the most reliable and practical method for guiding antiretroviral selection in the case of resistant infections and today it remains the reference method [47].

A fundamental change in antiretroviral therapy took place when clinical pharmacology studies provided the means to overcome and prevent viral resistance. Among the first PIs released into the market, Ritonavir (RTV, which was subsequently abandoned as pure antiretroviral) was found to display remarkable properties in enhancing the pharmacokinetic (PK) exposure of other PI [48]. Through its interference with the isoenzyme CYP3A4 of the cytochrome P 450 system in the intestine and liver microsomes, RTV (at a daily dosage well lower than that recommended for its use as antiretroviral) was found to be able to increase PIs absorption and to decrease their metabolism, thus eventually leading to PK exposure of the co-administered PI which was up to 3 $logs_{10}$ higher than in the case of treatment without RTV. Such enhanced PK exposure led to the ability of RTV/PI-based treatments to overcome, to some significant extent, the pre-existing resistance selected by regimens containing a single PI, thus determining successful re-suppression of viral replication in patients who underwent virological failure with a single PI-based therapy. Furthermore, in the following years, it became apparent that the use of RTV/PI-based therapy was also able to almost totally avoid the selection of resistance when administered as first-line treatment in treatment-naïve patients [49]. The effect of this enhanced PK exposure on resistance prevention was found to also include the drugs co-administered with RTV/PI-based regimens, thus providing a benefit, in terms of long-term perspective, which goes far beyond the class of PIs and involves the entire pharmaceutical armamentarium we rely upon today for treating HIV infection. It must be stressed that the confidence we have today in the possibility to find a therapeutic solution for almost all individual patient conditions (e.g. resistance, intolerance, drug-drug interactions, pregnancy, organ failure, etc.) is largely based on the knowledge that RTV-boosted PI-based regimens will provide a concrete chance of therapeutic response in the vast majority of patients, unless very extensive resistance has been selected in the past. In this regard, it is worth noting that the process of multiple drug resistance selection resulting from the use of suboptimal regimens (which took place until the concept of boosting PI-based therapy with low-dose RTV was fully translated into large-scale use) has now come to its end, at least in the western world. This is to say that the use of RTV-boosted PI therapy does not generate the multiple resistance patterns selected by a single PI therapy any longer; and, thus, the size of the HIV-infected population carrying multiple drug resistance should not increase to any significant extent in the future [50].

Most of currently administered HAART regimens consist of two drugs belonging to the N/NtRTIs class (the so called "N/NtRTIs backbone") and a third drug to be selected among PIs or NNRTIs. When administered to patients in a treatment-naïve status, these regimens have repeatedly been proven to guarantee a long-term immunovirological and clinical benefit–provided they are taken regularly by the patients and no specific interferences are present. In the case of patients who are not eligible for these first-line recommended options because of prior resistance selection, a number of alternatives are available, both within the class of PIs (in the near future also in the class of NNRTIs) and in other newly developed drug classes [44, 45].

Although viral resistance is not the only problem in this therapeutic area, it is nevertheless the one that may definitively compromise the use of a drug class. While PIs are now recognized to be the drug class less vulnerable to resistance selection (in the RTV-boosted version), N/NtRTIs, NNRTIs and Enfuvirtide (the only entry inhibitor so far available) display various degrees of weakness in terms of genetic barrier. The term genetic barrier substantially indicates the number of mutations required to make HIV resistant to a drug or a drug class. The higher the number of mutations required to determine resistance, the stronger the genetic barrier. With the exception of PIs in association with RTV as a booster, for most of the other drugs, a single mutation (such as even a short exposure) may be sufficient to select for a drug-resistant infection. Considering that cross-resistance among members of the same class is rather common, attention is being increasingly paid to the best sequential strategy to be adopted in planning antiretroviral therapy. What has been learned after years of antiretroviral therapy is that the same principles applied almost 60 years ago in the multi-drug treatment of tuberculosis are also valid for antiretroviral therapy [51]. In other words, once resistance has developed and we have to face treatment failure, no single new active drug should be added to a failing regimen, since selection of resistant mutants will determine the emergence of virions which are also resistant to the newly introduced drug. In all clinical trials carried out to evaluate the effectiveness of new antiretrovirals, the best performances were seen when at least another component of the therapeutic regimen (further to the new experimental drug) was fully active against the virus. With only a single drug being active in any given regimen, the usual therapeutic result is that of a transient immunovirological response (often not complete) followed by a new therapeutic failure. As a consequence, in case of multi-drug failure, the best strategy is to select at least two active components to be included in the new regimen [52].

Side effects, both short and long-term, are another important issue in antiretroviral therapy. There are a number of drug-specific untoward effects to which patients are variably vulnerable [53]. Gastrointestinal reactions and hypertriglyceridaemia are more common with PIs, and among PIs there are effects like jaundice or nephrolithiasis which are attributable to specific drugs (respectively Atazanavir, ATV, and Indinavir, IDV). In this drug class, some differentiation is also worth making between ATV, Tipranavir (TPV) and the rest of the class in terms of disturbances of glucose homeostasis and decrease in insulin sensitivity; the former two, which do not interfere with the cellular receptor GLUT-4, are less prone to determine alterations in this setting. Cutaneous rash is more common with NNRTIs than with PIs, and neuropsychiatric disturbances (especially in the first weeks of treatment) are more common with Efavirenz (EFV) than with any other antiretroviral. Some degree of liver toxicity is attributed to NNRTIs, and their use should be cautious in case of co-existing viral hepatitis. On the side of the current most common "backbone" of HAART (N/NtRTIs), there are some specific reactions in the case of abacavir (ABV, genetically determined vulnerability for developing severe inflammatory reactions), tenofovir (TDF, reversible renal failure with concurrent factors), zidovudine (AZT, anaemia, lipoathrophy), Didanosine (peripheral neuropathy, pancreatitis) and stavudine (d4T, lipoathrophy), while the two citidine analogues lamivudine (3TC) and emtricitabine (FTC) are by far the best tolerated drugs in this class [54]. The outlook of side effects should also be analysed in longer terms such as in years of continuous treatment. In this perspective, complex pictures consisting of various degrees of metabolic and morphologic alterations are known to occur in recipients of antiretroviral therapy. From the metabolic side, disturbances in the glucose and lipid profiles are rather common and may form the basis for interpreting the higher incidence of cardiovascular events recorded in HAART intakers as compared to the age-matched population. While a small class-specific responsibility seems today to be attributable to PIs as compared to NNRTIs in the increased cardiovascular risk, many other concurrent factors should also be considered in this specific context, since traditional risk factors, like smoking, are also heavily represented in the HIV-infected population [55]. The other side of the coin, however, shows how a higher cardiovascular risk is also measurable in those with lower CD4+ cell counts, which means that in any case, the successful use of HAART is well favourable also in this specific regard [56].

The development of lipodystrophic syndromes (altered distribution of body fat), which have ambiguous links with the metabolic disturbances, is more likely to result from regimens containing d4T or, to a lesser extent, AZT, while the responsibility of other drugs is still sub judice. A recent ACTG trial (ACTG 5142) has actually capsized the belief that lipoathrophy was more common among PIs intakers as compared to NNRTIs; the results showed how the incidence of lipoathrophy was significantly higher in patients taking EFV as compared to those receiving lopinavir/RTV (LPV/r), regardless of the companion drugs also administered [57].

An additional point to consider in the long-term perspective is that of the incidence of non HIV-related diseases in the HIV-infected population. As said for the increased risk of cardiovascular events with lower CD4+ cell counts, the same applies for other conditions like renal failure, non-opportunistic infections and malignancies. This means that, in order to lower the risk of such occurrences over time as far as possible, our immunological target in antiretroviral therapy should be set at levels higher than 350 cells/µl. In the ongoing debate on the best therapeutic strategy for achieving the most convenient balance between treatment efficacy and side effects, this information certainly adds more weight on the side of the favourable effects of antiretroviral therapy [56].

From Now On

It is not easy today to depict which will be the real long-term perspective of HIV infection. There are several major points which deserve careful consideration. One is certainly epidemiology and the future trends of HIV diffusion in the different regions of the world. The major focus here is on developing countries, on the access to appropriate care in these regions and on the global impact that the ongoing preventive and therapeutic efforts will have on HIV epidemiology in the short-, mid- and long-term. Since a few years ago, a considerable amount of resources has been delivered to developing countries for the prevention and treatment of HIV infection, and an additional question relates to how long this will be affordable.

The epidemiologic tendency is also of great concern for western countries, where the extent to which preventive efforts are made is quite variable and there is much uncertainty about the future directions to be undertaken in this setting. The life expectancy of HIV-infected patients increased considerably following the introduction of HAART, a rather constant number of new infections are being diagnosed each year and, as a simple numerical consequence, the perspective is that of a growing proportion of our societies consisting of subjects with HIV infection, which corresponds to a growing number of subjects requiring antiretroviral treatment.

From a more technical viewpoint, that of chemotherapy, the question is whether the newly released antiretroviral drugs and those in the last portion of the pipeline will modify or not the current global treatment perspective. While viral eradication is still far beyond our current possibilities and continuous anti-HIV treatment remains substantially unavoidable, some recent results achieved in the use of new drug classes seem to indicate that our weapons against

HIV infection are about to grow remarkably. It is noteworthy that the virological threshold defining treatment success has now been established at 50 HIV-RNA copies/ml instead of the more permissive value of 400/ml, both in the case of fully susceptible treatment-naïve infections and of multi-experienced patients. Although the threshold of 400 copies/ml is still considered in the case of registration trials, the development of a new series of antiretrovirals in the last 3 years has also improved our current efficacy expectations in the case of prior multi-drug failure, thus making it possible to consider the value of 50 copies/ml as the target achievable in the vast majority of cases. New PIs (e.g. darunavir, DRV), new NNRTIs (etravirine, rilpivirine), new classes like integrase inhibitors and co-receptor (CCR5) inhibitors gave convincing evidence of their capacity to overcome existing viral resistance [58]. The rather abundant offer in terms of new drugs and new classes makes it now possible to use appropriate combinations to treat multiple-drug resistant infections by relying upon at least two new fully active compounds, which meets the basic principle of multi-drug therapy. The other side of the coin concerning these newly available antiretrovirals is their possible use in treatment-naïve patients. We have been successfully using N/NtRTIs in combination with PIs or NNRTIs as first-line treatment for years, but now additional options are about to be defined. This will make it easier to tailor antiretroviral treatment on the basis of individual characteristics. Individual issues like allergies, other forms of drug intolerance, family history of glucose intolerance or diabetes, pre-existing cardiovascular risk factors, concurrent use of other medications, or behavioural variables, will be more likely to find drug combinations adequate for long-term use. These new therapeutic resources are particularly welcome in the light of the changing perspectives of subjects living with HIV infection. Furthermore, regarding the risk of developing HIV-unrelated diseases requiring other forms of medical and/or surgical treatment (to be compatible with the ongoing antiretroviral treatment), persons living with HIV infection are also increasingly being considered eligible for extreme treatment modalities like organ transplantation. This clearly implies that the larger the choice of antiretrovirals, the wider the perspectives of successfully combining the continuous intake of antiretrovirals with the emerging therapeutic requirements of people whose life expectancy is well over the dramatic boundaries of the natural course of HIV infection.

References

1. Palella FJ, Delaney KM, Moorman AC et al (1998) Declining morbidity and mortality among patients with advanced human immunodeficiency virus infection. N Engl J Med 338:853–860
2. Gottlieb MS, Schroff R, Schanker HM et al (1981) Pneumocystis carinii pneumonia in homosexual men. N Engl J Med 305:1425–1431
3. CDC (1982) Kaposi's sarcoma and Pneumocystis carinii pneumonia in homosexual men: New York City and California. MMWR Morb Mortal Wkly Rep 30:305–330
4. Goeddert JJ, Biggar RJ, Melbye M et al (1987) Effect of T4 count and cofactors on the incidence of AIDS in homosexual men: an 11-year follow-up. JAMA 257:331–334
5. Wei X, Ghosh SK, Taylor ME et al (1995) Viral dynamics in human immunodeficiency virus type 1 infection. Nature 373:117–222
6. Cooper DA, Gold J, Maclean P et al (1985) Acute AIDS retrovirus infection: definition of a clinical illness associated with seroconversion. Lancet 1:537–540
7. Yanhems P, Routy JP, Hirschel B et al (2002) Clinical features of acute retroviral syndrome differ by route of infection but not by gender and age. J Acquir Immune Defic Syndr 31:318–321
8. Herard DR, Phillips J, Windsor I et al (1994) Detection of human immunodeficiency virus type 1 p24 antigen and plasma RNA: relevance to indeterminate serologic tests. Transfusion 34:376–380
9. Bacchetti P, Moss AR (1993) Incubation period of AIDS in San Francisco. Nature 338:251–253
10. Osmond D, Chaisson RE, Moss A et al (1987) Lym-

phadenopathy in asymptomatic patients seropositive for HIV. N Engl J Med 317:246

11. Masur H, Ognibene FP, Yarchoan R et al (1992) CD4 counts as predictors of opportunistic pneumonias in human immunodeficiency virus (HIV) infection. Ann Intern Med 111:223–231

12. Moore RD, Chaisson RD (1996) Natural history of opportunistic disease in an HIV-infected urban clinical cohort. Ann Intern Med 124:633–642

13. Janoff EN, Breiman RF, Daley CL et al (1992) Pneumococcal disease during HIV infection. Ann Intern Med 117:314–324

14. Petruckevich A, Del Amo J, Phillips AN et al (1998) Disease progression and survival following specific AIDS-defining conditions: a retrospective cohort study of 2048 HIV-infected persons in London. AIDS 12:107–113

15. Chaisson RE, Keruly J, Richman DD, Moore DD (1992) Pneumocystis prophylaxis and survival in patients with advanced human immunodeficiency virus infection treated with zidovudine. Arch Intern Med 152:2009–2013

16. Tang AM, Forrester J, Spiegelman D et al (2002) Weight loss and survival in HIV-positive patients in the era of highly active antiretroviral therapy. J Acquir Immune Defic Syndr 31:230–236

17. Sepkowitz KA, Telzak EE, Carrow M et al (1993) Fever among outpatients with advanced human immunodeficiency virus infection. Arch Intern Med 153:1909–1912

18. Serwadda D, Mugerwa RD, Sewankambo NK et al (1985) Slim disease: a new disease in Uganda and its association with HTLV-III infection. Lancet 2(8460):849–852

19. Theuer CP, Hopewell PC, Elias D et al (1990) Human immunodeficiency virus infection in tuberculosis patients. J Infect Dis 162:8–12

20. Selwyn PA, Hartel D, Lewis VA et al (1989) A prospective study of the risk of tuberculosis among intravenous drug abusers with human immunodeficiency virus infection. N Engl J Med 320:545–550

21. Di Perri G, Cruciani M, Danzi MC et al (1989) Nosocomial epidemic of active tuberculosis among HIV-infected patients. Lancet 2:1502–1504

22. Jones BE, Young SM, Antoniskis D et al (1993) Relationship of the manifestations of tuberculosis to CD4 cell count in patients with human immunodeficiency virus infection. Am Rev Respir Dis 148:1292–1297

23. Di Perri G, Cazzadori A, Vento S et al (1996) Comparative histopathology study of pulmonary tuberculosis in HIV-infected and non-infected patients. Tuberc Lung Dis 77:244–249

24. Corbett EL, Watt CJ, Walker N et al (2003) The growing burden of tuberculosis: global trends and interactions with the HIV epidemic. Arch Intern Med 163:1009–1021

25. Sheppard HW, Lang W, Ascher MS et al (1993) The characteristics of non-progressors: long-term HIV-1 infection with stable Cd4+ T-cell levels. AIDS 7:1159–1166

26. Cao Y, Quin L, Zhang L et al (1995) Virologic and immunologic characterization of long-term survivors of human immunodeficiency virus type 1 infection. N Engl J Med 332. 201–208

27. Gallant JE, Moore RD, Chaisson RE (1994) Prophylaxis for opportunistic infection in patients with HIV infection. Ann Intern Med 120:932–943

28. Graham NM, Zeger SL, Park LP et al (1991) Effects of zidovudine and Pneumocystis carinii pneumonia prophylaxis on progression of HIV-1 infection to AIDS. Lancet 338:265–269

29. Hogg RS, O'Shaughnessy MV, Gataric N et al (1997) Decline in deaths from AIDS due to new antiretrovirals. Lancet 349:1294

30. Mocroft A, Vella S, Benfield TL et al (1998) Changing patterns of mortality across Europe in patients infected with HIV-1. EuroSIDA Study Group. Lancet 352:1725–1730

31. Browne AE, Malone JD, Zhou SYJ et al (1997) Human immunodeficiency virus RNA levels in US adults: a comparison base on race and ethnicity. J Infect Dis 176:794–797

32. Yerly S, Perneger Tv, Hirshel B et al (1998) A critical assessment of the prognostic value of HIV-1 RNA levels and CD4+ cell counts in HIV-infected patients: The Swiss HIV cohort study. Arch Intern Med 158:247–252

33. Sterling TR, Hoover Dr, Astemborsky J et al (2002) Heat-denaturated human immunodeficiency virus type 1 protein p24 antigen: prognostic value in adults with early-stage disease. J Infect Dis 186:1181–1185

34. Wu H, Kuritzkes DR, McClerman Dr et al (1999) Characterization of viral dynamics in HIV type 1-infected patients treated with combination antiretroviral therapy: relationship to host factors, cellular restoration, and virologic end points. J Infect Dis 179:799–807

35. Balaram P (2003) The science and politics of AIDS. Curr Sci 85:117–118

36. Markovitz M, Morales-Ramirez JO, Nguyen BY et al (2006) Antiretroviral activity, pharmacokinetics and tolerability of MK-0518, a novel inhibitor of HIV-1 integrase, dosed as monotherapy for 10 days in treatment-naïve HIV-1-infected individuals. J Acquir Immune Defic Syndr 43:509–515

37. Suligoi B, Boros L, Camoni L et al (2005) Aggiornamento dei casi di AIDS notificati in Italia e delle nuove diagnosi di infezione da HIV. Commissione Nazionale per la Lotta contro l'AIDS. Ministero della Salute, Rome

38. Powderly WG, Landay A, Lederman MM (1998)

Recovery of the immune system with antiretroviral therapy: the end of opportunism? JAMA 280:72–77

39. Di Perri G, Bonora S, Vento S et al (1998) Highly active antiretroviral therapy. Lancet 351:1056–9

40. Pakker NG, Kroon ED, Roos MT et al (1999) Immune restoration does not invariably occur following long-term HIV-1 suppression during antiretroviral therapy. AIDS 13:203–212

41. Di Perri G, Vento S, Mazzi R et al (1999) Recovery of long-term natural protection against reactivation of CMV retinitis in AIDS patients responding to highly active antiretroviral therapy. J Infect 39:193–197

42. Schneider M, Borleffs JC, Stolk RP et al (1999) Discontinuation of prophylaxis for Pneumocystis carinii pneumonia in HIV-1 infected patients treated with highly active antiretroviral therapy. Lancet 353:201–3

43. Valdez H, Chowdhry TK, Assad R et al (2001) Changing spectrum of mortality due to human immunodeficiency virus: analysis of 260 deaths during 1995–1999: Clin Infect Dis 32:1487–1493

44. Department of Health and Human Services (2006) Guidelines for the use of antiretroviral agents in HIV-1 infected adults and adolescents. 10 Oct 2006. http://AIDSinfo.nih.gov

45. The British HIV Association (2005) BHIVA guidelines for the treatment of HIV-infected adults with antiretroviral therapy. HIV Med 6(S2):1–61

46. Dusheiko G, Antonakopoulos N. (2007) Treatment of hepatitis B. Gut. http://gut.bmj.com/cgi/content/abstract/gut.2005.077891v1

47. Hirsh MS, Brun-Vezinet F, Clotet B et al (2003) Antiretroviral drug resistance testing in adults infected with HIV type 1: 2003 recommendations of an international AIDS Society–USA panel. Clin Infect Dis 37:113–128

48. Kempf DJ, Marsh KC, Kumar G et al (1997) Pharmacokinetic enhancement of inhibitors of the HIV protease by coadministration with ritonavir. Antimicrob Ag Chemother 41:654–660

49. Walmsley S, Bernstein B, King M et al (2002) Lopinavir/ritonavir versus nelfinavir for the initial treatment of HIV infection. N Engl J Med 346:2039–2046

50. Di Giambenedetto S, Brocciale L, Colatigli M et al (2007) Declining prevalence of HIV-1 drug resistance in treatment-failing patients: a clinical cohort study. Antivir Ther 12:835–839

51. Canetti G, Grosset J (1961) Teneur des souches sauvages de Mycobacterium tuberculosis en variants resistants a l'isoniazide et en variants resistants a la streptomycine sur milieu de Lowenstein-Jensen. Ann Inst Pasteur 101:28–42

52. Lazzarin A, Clotet B, Cooper D et al (2003) Efficacy of enfuvirtide in patients infected with drug-resistant HIV-1 in Europe and Australia. N Engl J Med 348:2186–2195

53. Carr A, Cooper DA (2001) Adverse effects of antiretroviral therapy. Lancet 356:1423–1430

54. Calmy A, Hirschel B, Cooper DA, Carr A (2007) Clinical update: adverse effects of antiretroviral therapy. Lancet 370:12–14

55. DAD Study Group (2007) Class of antiretroviral drugs and the risk of myocardial infarction. N Engl J Med 356:1723–1735

56. SMART Study Group (2006) CD4+ count-guided interruption of antiretroviral treatment. N Engl J Med 355:2283–2296

57. Haubrich R, Riddler S, DiRienzo G et al (2007) Metabolic outcome of ACTG 5142; a prospective randomized phase III trial of NRTI-, PI- and NNRTI-sparing regimens for initial treatment of HIV-1 infection. Abstr. 38, 14th CROI, 25–28 Feb 2007, Los Angeles, CA

58. Edmunds-Ogbuokiri J (2007) Update: antiretroviral agents in expanded access. HIV Clin 19:4–5

Evolution and Pathogenesis of the Involvement of the Cardiovascular System in HIV Infection

G. Barbaro

Introduction

Cardiac illness related to human immunodeficiency virus (HIV) infection tends to occur late in the disease course and is therefore becoming more prevalent as therapy of the viral infection and longevity improve. Autopsy series and retrospective analyses performed before the introduction of highly active antiretroviral therapy (HAART) regimens suggest that cardiac lesions are present in 25–75% of patients with acquired immunodeficiency syndrome (AIDS) [1]. HAART regimens have significantly modified the course of HIV disease, with longer survival rates and improvement of life quality in HIV-infected subjects expected. However, early data raised concerns about HAART being associated with an increase in both peripheral and coronary arterial diseases. HAART is only available to a minority of HIV-infected individuals worldwide, and studies prior to HAART therapy remain globally applicable. As 36.1 million adults and children are estimated to be living with HIV/AIDS and 5.3 million adults and children are estimated to have been newly infected with HIV during the year 2000 [2], HIV-associated symptomatic heart failure may become one of the leading causes of heart failure worldwide. A variety of potential etiologies have been postulated for HIV-related heart disease, including myocardial infection with HIV itself, opportunistic infections, viral infections, autoimmune response to viral infection, drug-related cardiotoxicity, nutritional deficiencies, and prolonged immunosuppression (Table 1).

Congenital Cardiovascular Malformations in HIV-Infected Children

Most pediatric patients with HIV are infected in the perinatal period [22]. In a prospective longitudinal multicenter study, diagnostic echocardiograms were performed at 4- to 6-month intervals on two cohorts of children exposed to maternal HIV-1 infection: (1) a neonatal cohort of 90 HIV-infected, 449 HIV-uninfected, and 19 HIV-indeterminate children; and (2) an older HIV-infected cohort of 201 children with vertically transmitted HIV-1 infection recruited after 28 days of age [22]. In the neonatal cohort, 36 lesions were seen in 36 patients, yielding an overall congenital cardiovascular malformation prevalence of 6.5% (36/558), with 8.9% (8/90) prevalence in HIV-infected children and 5.6% (25/449) prevalence in HIV-uninfected children [22]. Two children (2/558, 0.4%) had cyanotic lesions. In the older HIV-infected cohort, there was a congenital cardiovascular malformation prevalence of 7.5% (15/201). The distribution of lesions did not differ significantly between the groups. There was no statistically significant difference in congenital cardiovascular malformation prevalence in the HIV-infected compared to the HIV-uninfected children born to HIV-infected women. With the use of early screening echocardiography, rates of congenital cardiovascular malformations in both the HIV-infected and HIV-uninfected children were five- to tenfold higher than rates reported in population-based epidemiologic

Table 1 Principal HIV-associated cardiovascular abnormalities. (From [3], with permission)

Type	Possible etiologies and associations	Incidence
Dilated cardiomyopathy	Infectious: HIV, *Toxoplasma gondii*, Coxsackievirus group B, Epstein-Barr virus, *Cytomegalovirus, Adenovirus* Autoimmune response to infection Drug-related Cocaine, possibly nucleoside analogs IL-2, doxorubicin, interferon Metabolic/endocrine Nutritional deficiency/wasting Selenium, B_{12}, carnitine Thyroid hormone, growth hormone Adrenal insufficiency, hyperinsulinemia Cytokines TNF-α, nitric oxide, TGF-β, endothelin-1 Hypothermia Hyperthermia Autonomic insufficiency Encephalopathy Acquired immunodeficiency HIV viral load, length of immunosuppression	15.9 patients/1,000 asymptomatic HIV- infected persons before the introduction of HAART [4]
Coronary heart disease	Protease-inhibitor-induced metabolic and coagulative disorders. Arteritis	Studies on the risk of coronary heart disease among HIV-infected individuals receiving protease inhibitor-including HAART have not shown a consistent association [5–13]
Systemic arterial hypertension	HIV-induced endothelial dysfunction. Vasculitis in small, medium, and large vessels in the form of leukocytoclastic vasculitis; atherosclerosis secondaryto HAART; aneurysms of the large vessels such as the carotid, femoral, and abdominal aorta with impairment of flow to the renal arteries; PI-induced insulin resistance with increased sympathetic activity and sodium retention	20%–25% of HIV-infected persons before the introduction of HAART [14] Up to 74% in HIV-infected persons with HAART-related metabolic syndrome [15, 18]
Pericardial effusion	Bacteria: *Staphylococcus, Streptococcus, Proteus, Nocardia, Pseudomonas, Klebsiella, Enterococcus, Listeria* Mycobacteria (*Mycobacterium tuberculosis, Mycobacterium avium intracellulare, Mycobacterium kansaii*) Viral pathogens HIV, herpes simplex virus, herpes simplex virus type 2, cytomegalovirus Other pathogens *Cryptococcus, Toxoplasma, Histoplasma* Malignancy Kaposi's sarcoma Malignant lymphoma Capillary leak/wasting/malnutrition Hypothyroidism Prolonged acquired immunodeficiency	11%/year in asymptomatic AIDS patients before the introduction of HAART [19]

cont. →

Table 1 *cont.*

Type	Possible etiologies and associations	Incidence
HIV-associated pulmonary hypertension	Recurrent bronchopulmonary infections, pulmonary arteritis, microvascular pulmonary emboli due to thrombus or drug injection. Plexogenic pulmonary arteriopathy. Mediator release from endothelium	1/200 of HIV-infected persons before the introduction of HAART [20]
AIDS-related tumors	Kaposi's sarcoma	12%–28% of AIDS patients before the introduction of HAART [20, 21]
	Non-Hodgkin's lymphomas	Mostly limited to case reports before the introduction of HAART

studies, but not higher than in normal populations similarly screened [22].

Dilated Cardiomyopathy

The estimated annual incidence of dilated cardiomyopathy with HIV infection before introduction of HAART was 15.9 in 1,000 cases [4]. Symptoms of heart failure may be masked in HIV-infected patients by concomitant illnesses such as diarrhea or malnutrition, or may be disguised by bronchopulmonary infections. The gross and microscopic findings for HIV-associated dilated cardiomyopathy are similar to those for idiopathic dilated cardiomyopathy in immunocompetent persons with four-chamber dilation and patchy myocardial fibrosis. Additional echocardiographic findings include diffuse left ventricular hypokinesis and decreased fractional shortening. The echocardiographic classification of HIV-associated cardiomyopathy with related clinical implications is reported in Fig. 1.

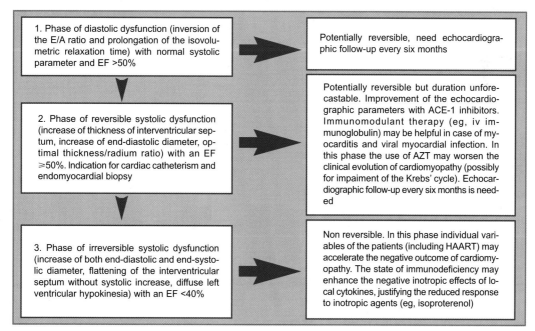

Fig. 1 Echocardiographic classification of HIV-associated cardiomyopathy with related clinical implications

Compared to patients with idiopathic dilated cardiomyopathy, those with HIV infection and dilated cardiomyopathy have markedly reduced survival rates (hazard ratio for death from congestive heart failure: 5.86) [23] (Fig. 2). The median survival to AIDS-related death is 101 days in patients with left ventricular dysfunction and 472 days in patients with a normal heart at a similar stage of HIV infection [3]. Although there is no evidence from prospective studies to suggest that HAART has a beneficial effect on HIV-associated cardiomyopathy and on HIV-associated pericardial effusion, some retrospective studies suggest that by preventing opportunistic infections and reducing the incidence of myocarditis, HAART might reduce the incidence of cardiomyopathy by about 33% (Fig. 3) and improve its course [24, 25]. However, the median incidence of HIV-associated cardiomyopathy is increasing in developing countries (about 32%), where the availability of HAART is limited and the pathogenetic impact of nutritional factors is greater [26].

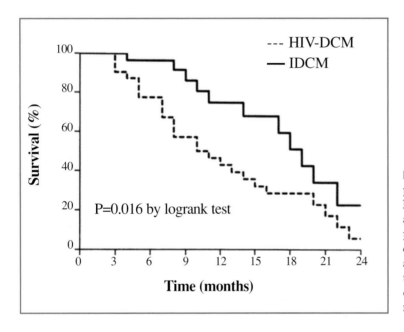

Fig. 2 Kaplan–Meier curves comparing the survival rate during follow-up between patients with HIV-associated cardiomyopathy and patients with idiopathic dilated cardiomyopathy. *HIV-DCM*, HIV-associated dilated cardiomyopathy; *IDCM*, idiopathic dilated cardiomyopathy. (From [23], with permission)

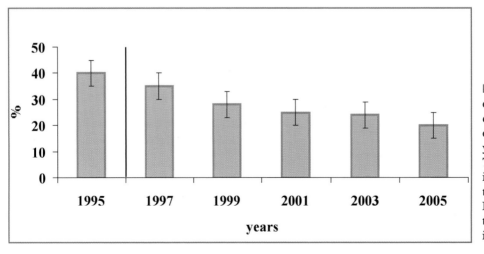

Fig. 3 Prevalence of HIV-associated dilated cardiomyopathy in the years 1995–2005. The *vertical line* indicates the introduction of HAART in the treatment of HIV infection

Animal Models

Simian immunodeficiency virus (SIV) infection in rhesus macaques is valuable for understanding the pathogenesis of cardiac injury associated with retroviral infection in a relevant nonhuman primate model of AIDS [27]. Chronic SIV infection resulted in depressed left ventricular systolic function and an extensive coronary arteriopathy suggestive of injury due to cell-mediated immune response [27]. Two-thirds of chronically infected macaques that died of SIV had related myocardial effects. Lymphocytic myocarditis was seen in 9 of 15 macaques and coronary arteriopathy in 9 of 15 (6 alone and 3 in combination with myocarditis) upon necropsy. In infected macaques, coronary arteriopathy was extensive, with evidence of vessel occlusion and recanalization and related regions of myocardial necrosis in four macaques. At necropsy, two animals had marantic endocarditis and one had a left ventricular mural thrombus. Macaques with cardiac pathology were emaciated to a greater extent than macaques with SIV and similar periods of infection who did not experience cardiac pathology [25, 27].

Myocarditis and Viral Myocardial Infection as Causes of Cardiomyopathy

Myocarditis and myocardial infection with HIV are the best-studied causes of dilated cardiomyopathy in HIV disease [28]. HIV-1 virions appear to infect myocardial cells in a patchy distribution with no direct association between the presence of the virus and myocyte dysfunction [28]. The myocardial fiber necrosis is usually minimal, with accompanying mild to moderate lymphocytic infiltrates. It is unclear how HIV-1 enters myocytes, which do not have CD4 receptors, although dendritic reservoir cells may play a role by activating multifunctional cytokines that contribute to progressive and late tissue damage such as tumor necrosis factor-alpha (TNF-α), interleukin-1 (IL-1), interleukin-6 (IL-6), and interleukin-10 (IL-10) [23]. Coinfection with other viruses (usually coxsackievirus B3 and cytomegalovirus) may also play an important pathogenetic role [21, 23].

Autoimmunity as a Contributor to Cardiomyopathy

Cardiac-specific autoantibodies (anti-alpha-myosin autoantibodies) are more common in HIV-infected patients with dilated cardiomyopathy than in HIV-infected patients with healthy hearts. Currie et al. reported that HIV-infected patients were more likely to have specific cardiac autoantibodies than were HIV-negative control subjects [29]. Those with echocardiographic evidence of left ventricular dysfunction were particularly likely to have cardiac autoantibodies, supporting the theory that cardiac autoimmunity plays a role in the pathogenesis of HIV-related heart disease and suggesting that cardiac autoantibodies could be used as markers of left ventricular dysfunction in HIV-positive patients with previously normal echocardiographic findings [29].

In addition, monthly intravenous administration of immunoglobulin in HIV-infected pediatric patients minimizes left ventricular dysfunction, increases left ventricular wall thickness, and reduces peak left ventricular wall stress, suggesting that both impaired myocardial growth and left ventricular dysfunction may be immunologically mediated [30]. These effects may be the result of immunoglobulins inhibiting cardiac autoantibodies by competing for Fc receptors, or they could be the result of immunoglobulins dampening the secretion or effects of cytokines and cellular growth factors [30]. These findings suggest that immunomodulatory therapy might be helpful in adults and children with declining left ventricular function, although further study of this possible therapy is needed.

Myocardial Cytokine Expression as a Factor in Cardiomyopathy

Cytokines play a role in the development of HIV-related cardiomyopathy [23]. Myo-carditis and dilated cardiomyopathy are associated with markedly elevated cytokine production, but the elevations may be highly localized within the myocardium, making peripheral cytokine levels uninformative [23].

When myocardial biopsy samples from patients with HIV-associated cardiomyopathy are compared to samples from patients with idiopathic dilated cardiomyopathy, the former stain more intensely for both TNF-α and inducible nitric oxide synthase (iNOS)

(Fig. 4). Staining is particularly intense in samples from patients with a myocardial viral infection and is correlated with CD4 count, independent of antiretroviral treatment [23] (Fig. 5). Staining is also more intense in samples from patients with HIV-associated cardiomyopathy coinfected with coxsackievirus B3, cytomegalovirus, or other viruses [23]. Moreover, staining for iNOS is more intense in samples from patients coinfected with HIV-1 and coxsackievirus B3 or cytomegalovirus than in samples from patients with idiopathic dilated cardiomyopathy and myocardial infection with coxsackievirus B3 or those who had adenovirus infection alone [23].

In patients with HIV-associated dilated cardiomyopathy and more intense iNOS staining, the survival rate was significantly lower: those whose samples stained more than 1 optical density unit had a hazard ratio of mortality of 2.57 (95% confidence interval: 1.11–5.43). Survival in HIV-infected patients with less intense staining was not significantly different from survival in

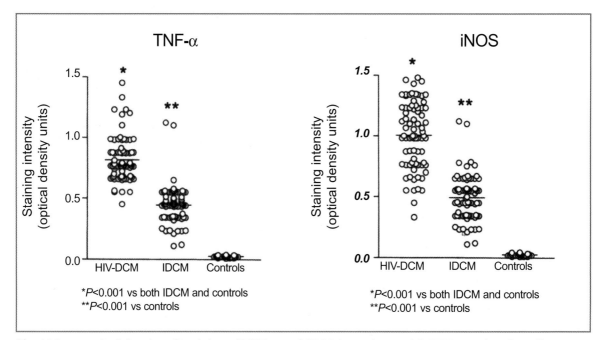

Fig. 4 Mean optical density of staining of TNF-α and iNOS in patients with HIV-associated cardiomyopathy (HIV-DCM), with idiopathic dilated cardiomyopathy (*IDCM*), and control subjects. *Horizontal bars* represent mean values. (From [23], with permission)

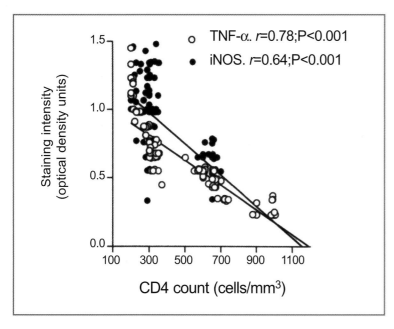

Fig. 5 Correlation between myocardial optical density units of TNF-α and iNOS and *CD4* count. (From [23], with permission)

patients with idiopathic dilated cardiomyopathy [23].

The inflammatory response may be enhanced by HIV-1 myocardial infection, by the interaction between HIV-1 and cardiotropic viruses, and by immunodeficiency. These factors may increase both the expression and the cytotoxic activity of specific cytokines such as TNF-α and iNOS and blunt the expected increase of anti-inflammatory cytokines such as IL-10 [31].

Relationship Between HIV-Associated Cardiomyopathy and Encephalopathy

HIV-infected patients with encephalopathy are more likely to die of congestive heart failure than are those without encephalopathy (hazard ratio: 3/4) [32, 33]. Cardiomyopathy and encephalopathy may both be traceable to the effects of HIV reservoir cells in the myocardium and the cerebral cortex. These cells may hold HIV-1 on their surfaces for extended time periods even after antiretroviral treatment, and they may

chronically release cytotoxic cytokines (TNF-α, IL-6, and endothelin-1), which contribute to progressive and late tissue damage in both systems (Fig. 6). Because the reservoir cells are not affected by treatment, the effect is independent of whether the patient receives HAART.

Nutritional Deficiencies as a Factor in Left Ventricular Dysfunction

Nutritional deficiencies are common in HIV infection and may contribute to ventricular dysfunction independently of HAART. Malabsorption and diarrhea can both lead to trace-element deficiencies which have been directly or indirectly associated with cardiomyopathy [34–36]. Selenium replacement may reverse cardiomyopathy and restore left ventricular function in selenium-deficient patients [34–36]. HIV infection may also be associated with altered levels of vitamin B12, carnitine, growth hormone, and thyroid hormone, all of which have been associated with left ventricular dysfunction [36].

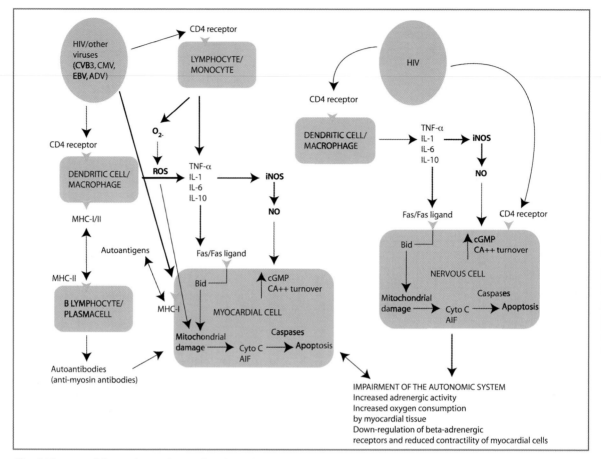

Fig. 6 The possible pathogenic mechanisms involved in the development of HIV-associated cardiomyopathy and encephalopathy and their relationship. The infection of dendritic cells, of CD4 lymphocytes, and of myocardial or neuronal cells by HIV-1 or by other viruses may be responsible for the release of specific cytokines (TNF-α, IL-1, IL-6, IL-10) that activate the inducible form of nitric oxide synthase (iNOS). The interaction between cytotoxic T lymphocytes and the receptoral complex Fas/Fas ligand located on the surface of the target cell may cause mitochondrial damage with release of mitochondrial pro-apoptosis factors–cytochrome c, apoptosis inducing factor (AIF). Similar mitochondrial damage may be caused by reactive oxygen species (ROS) released by activated lymphomonocytes. The interaction between autoantigens and major histocompatibility complex (MHC) molecules on the surface of dendritic cells/macrophages, of myocardial cells (MHC-I), and of B lymphocytes (MHC-II) determines the production of autoantibodies (e.g., alpha-antimyosin) that are responsible for direct cellular damage. The neuronal damage, specifically the impairment of the autonomic system, may enhance the functional damage to myocardial cells because of increased adrenergic activity and down-regulation of beta-adrenergic receptors. *CVB3*, coxsackievirus B3; *CMV*, cytomegalovirus; *EBV*, Epstein-Barr virus; *ADV*, adenovirus; *Ca++*, calcium; *cGMP*, cyclic guanine monophosphate; Bid, a protein of the bcl 2 family involved in apoptosis. (From the Lancet [20], with permission from Elsevier)

Left Ventricular Dysfunction Caused by Drug Cardiotoxicity

Studies of transgenic mice suggest that zidovudine is associated with diffuse destruction of cardiac mitochondrial ultrastructure and inhibition of mitochondrial DNA replication [37, 38]. This mitochondrial dysfunction may result in lactic acidosis, which could also contribute to myocardial cell dysfunction. However, in a study of infants born to HIV-positive mothers followed up from birth to age 5, perinatal exposure to zidovudine was not found to be associated with acute or chronic abnormalities in left ventricular structure or function [39]. Other nucleoside reverse transcriptase inhibitors, such as didanosine and zalcitabine, do not seem to either promote or prevent dilated cardiomyopathy.

Pericardial Effusion

Before the introduction of HAART, the prevalence of pericardial effusion in asymptomatic AIDS patients was estimated at 11% per year [19]. Although prospective data are lacking, retrospective data suggest that HAART has reduced the overall incidence of pericardial effusion in HIV disease by about 30% [24] (Fig. 7). AIDS patients with pericardial effusion survive a median of 6 months, significantly shorter than do AIDS patients without effusion. Survival is independent of CD4 count and albumin levels [19].

A 5-year prospective evaluation of cardiac involvement in AIDS found 16 of 231 patients had or developed pericardial effusions [19]. Three subjects had an effusion on enrollment, and 13 developed effusions during follow-up (12/13 with AIDS at enrollment). Pericardial effusions were generally small (80%) and asymptomatic (87%). The calculated incidence of pericardial effusion among those with AIDS was 11% per year. The prevalence of effusion in AIDS patients may rise over time, reaching an estimated mean of 22% after 25 months of follow-up in asymptomatic patients [19].

Among subjects with AIDS and pericardial effusion, 36% were alive after 6 months of follow-up, whereas 93% of those without effusion were alive at 6 months [19]. Two patients developed pericardial tamponade as assessed by clinical and echocardiographic criteria [19]. Several studies have suggested spontaneous resolution of pericardial effusion over time in 13–42% of affected patients [19]. However, mortality remains markedly increased in patients who had developed an effusion, whether or not the effusion resolved [19].

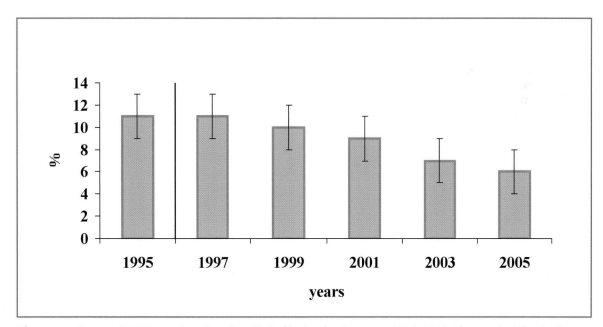

Fig. 7 Prevalence of HIV-associated pericardial effusion in the years 1995–2005. The *vertical line* indicates the introduction of HAART in the treatment of HIV infection

Endocardial Involvement

The prevalence of infective endocarditis in HIV-infected patients is similar to that of patients in other risk groups, such as intravenous drug users [40]. Estimates of endocarditis prevalence vary from 6.3 to 34% of HIV-infected patients who use intravenous drugs independently of HAART regimens [21]. Right-sided valves are predominantly affect-ed and the most frequent agents are *Staphylococcus aureus* (>75% of cases), *Streptococcus pneumoniae* (15–20% of cases), *Haemophilus influenzae* (10% of cases), *Candida albicans*, and *Aspergillus fumigatus* [21, 41]. Patients with HIV generally have similar presentations and survival (85 vs 93%) from infective endocarditis as those without HIV [41] (Figs. 8–11). However, in relation to the state of immunodeficiency, patients with late-stage HIV disease have a mortality rate

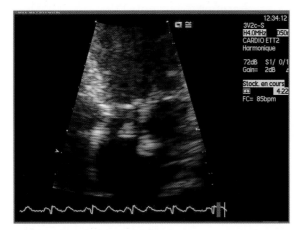

Fig. 8 Voluminous mobile vegetation on the anterior and posterior mitral leaflet in an HIV-infected patient, detected by transthoracic echocardiography (apical four-chamber view)

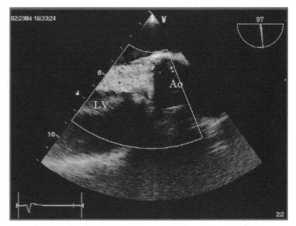

Fig. 10 Significant aortic regurgitation (grade IV) in an HIV-infected patient, detected by color Doppler transesophageal echocardiography. *Ao,* aorta; *LV,* left ventricle

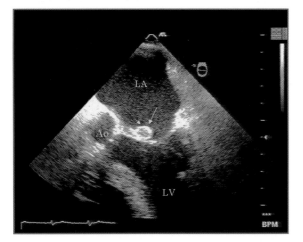

Fig. 9 Large anterior mitral vegetation in an HIV-infected patient, detected by transesophageal echocardiography. *Ao,* aorta; *LA,* left atrium; *LV,* left ventricle

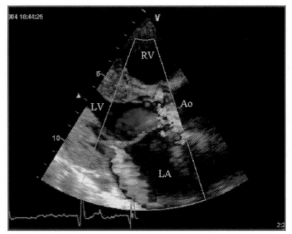

Fig. 11 Significant mitral regurgitation in HIV-infected patients with endocarditis, detected by color Doppler trans-thoracic echocardiography (parasternal long-axis view). *RV,* right ventricle; *LV,* left ventricle; *Ao,* aorta; *LA,* left atrium

from infective endocarditis of about 30% higher than do asymptomatic HIV-infected patients [41]. Nonbacterial thrombotic endocarditis–which was described with a prevalence of 3–5% in AIDS patients before the introduction of HAART, and mostly in patients with HIV wasting syndrome–is now more frequently observed in developing countries with a high incidence (about 10–15%) and mortality rate for systemic embolization [26]. Death from marantic endocarditis is rare in HIV-infected patients receiving HAART.

HIV Infection, Opportunistic Infections, and Vascular Disease

A wide range of inflammatory vascular diseases, including polyarteritis nodosa, Henoch-Schönlein purpura, and drug-induced hypersensitivity vasculitis may develop in HIV-infected individuals. Kawasaki-like syndrome [42] and Takayasu's arteritis [43] have also been described. The course of vascular disease may be accelerated in HIV-infected patients because of atherogenesis stimulated by HIV-infected monocyte-macrophages, possibly via altered leukocyte adhesion or arteritis [44].

Some patients with AIDS have a clinical presentation resembling systemic lupus erythematosus (SLE), including vasculitis, arthralgias, myalgias, and autoimmune phenomena with a low-titer positive antinuclear antibody, coagulopathy with lupus anticoagulant, hemolytic anemia, and thrombocytopenic purpura. Hypergammaglobulinemia from polyclonal B-cell activation may be present, but often diminishes in the late stages of AIDS. Specific autoantibodies to double-stranded DNA, Sm antigen, RNP antigen, SSA, SSB and other histones may be found in a majority of HIV-infected persons, but their significance is unclear [44].

Endothelial Dysfunction

Endothelial dysfunction and injury have been described in HIV infection [45]. Circulating markers of endothelial activation such as soluble adhesion molecules and procoagulant proteins are elaborated in HIV infection. HIV may enter the endothelium via CD4 or galactosylceramide receptors [45]. Other possible mechanisms of entry include chemokine receptors [46]. Endothelium isolated from the brain of HIV-infected subjects strongly expresses both CCR3 and CXCR4 HIV-1 coreceptors, whereas coronary endothelium strongly expresses CXCR4 and CCCR2A coreceptors [46]. CCR5 is expressed at a lower level in both types of endothelium. The fact that CCR3 is more common in brain endothelium than in coronary endothelium could be significant in light of the different susceptibilities of the heart and brain to HIV-1 invasion. Endothelial activation in HIV infection may also be caused by cytokines (e.g., TNF-α) secreted in response to mononuclear or adventitial cell activation by the virus, or it may be a direct effect of the secreted HIV-associated proteins gp 120 (envelope glycoprotein) and tat (transactivator of viral replication) on endothelium with the possible induction of an apoptosis process [47]. Opportunistic agents such as cytomegalovirus, frequently coinfect HIV-infected patients and may contribute to the development of endothelial damage. It has also been hypothesized that human herpes virus-8 (a virus that is found in all forms of Kaposi's sarcoma) may trigger or accelerate the development of atheroma in the presence of HAART-related hyperlipidemia [48]. In spite of all these observations, the clinical consequences of HIV-1 and opportunistic agents on endothelial function have not been elucidated yet.

HIV Infection and Coronary Arteries

The association between viral infection (cytomegalovirus or HIV-1 itself) and coronary artery lesions is not clear. HIV-1 sequences have been detected by in situ hybridization in the coronary vessels of an HIV-infected patient who died of acute myocardial infarction [49]. Potential mechanisms through which HIV-1 may damage coronary arteries include activation of cytokines and cell-adhesion molecules and alteration of major histocompatibility complex class I molecules on the surface of smooth muscle cells [49]. It is also possible that HIV-1-associated protein gp 120 may induce smooth muscle cell apoptosis through a mitochondrion-controlled pathway by activation of inflammatory cytokines (e.g., TNF-α) [47].

Opportunistic Infections

Toxoplasma gondii can produce a gross pattern of patchy irregular white infiltrates in the myocardium, similar to non-Hodgkin's lymphoma. Microscopically, the myocardium shows scattered mixed inflammatory cell infiltrates with polymorphonuclear leukocytes, macrophages, and lymphocytes. True *Toxoplasma gondii* cysts or pseudocysts containing bradyzoites are often hard to find, even if inflammation is extensive. Immunohistochemical staining may reveal free tachyzoites, otherwise difficult to distinguish, within the areas of inflammation. *Toxoplasma gondii* myocarditis can produce focal myocardial fiber necrosis and heart failure can ensue [40].

Other opportunistic infections of the heart are infrequent. They are often incidental findings at autopsy, and cardiac involvement is probably the result of widespread dissemination, as exemplified by

Candida and by the dimorphic fungi *Cryptococcus neoformans*, *Coccidioides immitis*, and *Histoplasma capsulatum*. Patients living in endemic areas for *Trypanosoma cruzi* may rarely develop a pronounced myocarditis and dilated cardiomyopathy [40].

Common HIV Therapies and the Heart

In AIDS patients with Kaposi's sarcoma, reversible cardiac dysfunction was associated with prolonged, high-dose therapy with interferon alpha [20]. Doxorubicin (Adriamycin) used to treat AIDS-related Kaposi's sarcoma and non-Hodgkin's lymphoma has a dose-related effect on dilated cardiomyopathy, as does foscarnet sodium used to treat cytomegalovirus esophagitis [20]. Cardiac arrhythmias have been described with the administration of amphotericin B [50], ganciclovir [51], trimethoprim-sulfamethoxazole [52], and pentamidine [14]. The principal cardiovascular actions/interactions of common HIV therapies are reported in Table 2.

Cardiovascular Malignancy

Cardiac Kaposi's sarcoma in AIDS may cause visceral and parietal pericardial lesions and, less frequently, myocardial lesions. The prevalence has ranged from 12 to 28% in retrospective autopsy studies performed before the introduction of HAART [21]. Cardiac Kaposi's sarcoma is not usually obstructive or associated with clinical cardiac dysfunction, morbidity, or mortality [40].

Malignant lymphoma involving the heart is infrequent in AIDS [21]. Lymphomatous infiltration may be diffuse or may result in discrete isolated lesions, which are usually derived from the Burkitt or immunoblastic type B cells [40]. The lesions are usually

Table 2 Cardiovascular actions/interactions of common HIV therapies. Modified from [3], with permission

Class	Drugs	Cardiac drug interactions	Cardiac side effects
Antiretroviral 1. Nucleoside reverse transcriptase inhibitors (RTI)	Abacavir (Ziagen), zidovudine (AZT, Retrovir)	Dipyridamole	Lactic acidosis (rare), hypotension, skeletal muscle myopathy (mitochondrial dysfunction hypothesized, but not seen clinically)
2. Nucleotide RTI	Tenofovirs (Viread)		
3. Non-nucleoside RTI	Delavirdine (Rescriptor), efavirenz (Sustiva), nevirapine (Viramune)	Warfarin (class interaction), calcium channel blockers, beta blockers, quinidine, steroids, theophylline	Delavirdine can cause serious toxic effects if given with anti-arrythmic drugs and myocardial ischemia if given with vasoconstrictors
4. Protease inhibitors	Amprenavir (Agenerase), indinavir (Crixivan), nelfinavir (Viracept), ritonavir (Norvir), saquinavir (Invirase, Fortovase), atazanavir (Reyataz)	All are metabolized by cytochrome p-450 and interact with: sildenafil, amiodarone, lidocaine, quinadine, warfarin, statins Calcium channel blockers, beta-blockers (1.5–3 x increase), prednisone, quinine, theophylline (decrease concentrations)	Implicated in premature atherosclerosis, dyslipidemia, insulin resistance, and lipodystrophy/lipoatrophy
Anti-infective 1. Antibiotics	Erythromycin, clarithromycin	Cytochrome p-450 metabolism and drug interactions	Orthostatic hypotension, ventricular tachycardia, bradycardia, QT prolongation
	Rifampicin	Reduces therapeutic effect of digoxin by induction of intestinal P-glycoprotein	
	Trimethoprim/sulfamethoxazole (Bactrim)	Increases warfarin effects	Orthostatic hypotension, QT prolongation
2. Antifungal agents	Amphotericin B	Digoxin toxicity	Hypertension, renal failure, hypokalemia, thrombophlebitis
	Ketoconazole, itraconazole	Cytochrome p-450 metabolism and drug interactions-increases levels of sildenafil, warfarin, "statins", nifedipine, digoxin	Angioedema, dilated cardiomyopathy, arrhythmias
3. Antiviral agents	Foscarnet, ganciclovir	Zidovudine	Reversible cardiac failure (dose-related effect), electrolyte abnormalities, ventricular tachycardia (QT prolongation), hypotension
4. Antiparasitic	Pentamidine (intravenous)		Hypotension, arrhythmias (torsade de pointes, ventricular tachycardia), hyperglycemia, hypoglycemia, sudden death

Note: Contraindicated if base-line QTc >0.48

nodular or polypoid masses, and they predominantly involve the pericardium, with variable myocardial infiltration. The prognosis of patients with HIV-associated cardiac lymphoma is generally poor, although clinical remission has been observed with combination chemotherapy. The introduction of HAART led to an approximately 50% reduction in the overall incidence of cardiac involvement by Kaposi's sarcoma and non-Hodgkin's lymphomas (Fig. 12). The fall may be attributable to the improved immunologic state of the patients and the prevention of opportunistic infections (human herpes virus-8 and Epstein-Barr virus) known to play an etiologic role in these neoplasms [53].

Antiretroviral Therapy and Metabolic Disorders

The introduction of HAART in recent years has significantly modified the course of HIV disease, prolonging survival and improving patients' quality of life. However, early data have raised concern that HAART regimens, especially those including protease inhibitors (PIs), except atazanavir, are associated with an increased incidence of metabolic (hyperlipidemia, insulin resistance) and somatic (lipodystrophy/lipoatrophy) changes that in the general population are associated with an increased risk for cardiovascular disease (coronary and peripheral artery disease and stroke), producing an intriguing clinical scenario [54].

HIV-associated lipodystrophy/lipoatrophy, first described in 1998 [55], is characterized by prominence of the dorsocervical fat pad ("buffalo hump"), increased abdominal girth and breast size, lipoatrophy of subcutaneous fat of the face, buttocks, and limbs, and prominence of the veins on the limbs [55]. The overall prevalence of at least one physical abnormality is about 50% in otherwise healthy outpatients. The differences between these prevalence rates (which ranged from 18 to 83%) may also have been confounded by patient sex and age, the type and duration of antiretroviral therapy, and the lack of an objective and validated case definition. Metabolic features significantly associated with lipodystrophy include dyslipidemia (about 70% of patients), insulin resistance (elevated C-peptide and insulin), type 2 diabetes mellitus (8–10% of the patients), lactic acidemia, and elevated hepatic transaminases (non-alcoholic steatohepatitis) [56]. These metabolic abnormalities are more profound in those with more severe physician-assessed

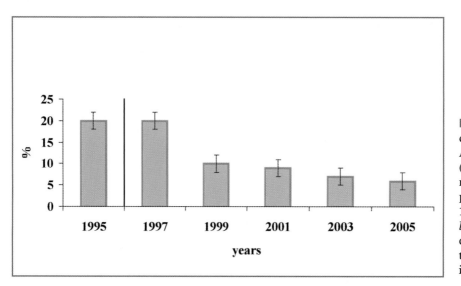

Fig. 12 Prevalence of cardiac involvement of AIDS-associated tumors (Kaposi's sarcoma and non-Hodgkin's lymphoma) in the years 1995– 2005. The *vertical line* indicates the introduction of HAART in the treatment of HIV infection

lipodystrophy and are associated with an increased risk in cardiovascular events (about 1.4 cardiac events per 1,000 years of therapy according to the Framingham score) [56].

A detailed description of HAART-associated metabolic syndrome and coagulation disorders, and of HAART-associated coronary and peripheral artery disease and stroke is provided by J. Capeau, L. Drouet, F. Boccara, P. Mercié, and A. Moulignier in separate chapters in this volume.

References

1. Barbaro G, Di Lorenzo G, Grisorio B, Barbarini G and the Gruppo Italiano per lo Studio Cardiologico dei pazienti affetti da AIDS Investigators (1998) Cardiac involvement in the acquired immunodeficiency syndrome: a multicenter clinical-pathological study. AIDS Res Hum Retroviruses 14:1071–1077

2. Temesgen Z (1999) Overview of HIV infection. Ann Allergy Asthma Immunol 83:1–5

3. Barbaro G (2002) Cardiovascular manifestations of HIV infection. Circulation 106:1420–1425

4. Barbarini G, Barbaro G (2003) Incidence of the involvement of the cardiovascular system in HIV infection. AIDS 17:S46–S50

5. Holmberg SD, Moorman AC, Williamson JM et al (2002) Protease inhibitors and cardiovascular outcomes in patients with HIV-1. Lancet 360:1747–1748

6. Bozzette SA, Ake CF, Tam HK et al (2003) Cardiovascular and cerebrovascular events in patients treated for human immunodeficiency virus infection. N Engl J Med 348:702–710

7. Friis-Moller N, Weber R, Reiss P et al (2003) Cardiovascular risk factors in HIV patients: association with antiretroviral therapy: results from DAD study. AIDS 17:1179–1193

8. Klein D, Hurley LB, Quesenberry Jr CP, Sidney S (2002) Do protease inhibitors increase the risk for coronary heart disease in patients with HIV-1 infection? J AIDS 30:471–477

9. Coplan PM, Nikas A, Japour A et al (2003) Incidence of myocardial infarction in randomized trials of protease inhibitor-based antiretroviral therapy: an analysis of four different protease inhibitors. AIDS Res Hum Retroviruses 19:449–455

10. Mary-Krause M, Cotte L, Simon A et al and the Clinical Epidemiology Group from the French Hospital Database (2003) Increased risk of myocardial infarction with duration of protease inhibitor therapy in HIV-infected men. AIDS 17:2479–2486

11. Barbaro G, Di Lorenzo G, Cirelli A et al (2003) An open-label, prospective, observational study of the incidence of coronary artery disease in patients with HIV receiving highly active antiretroviral therapy. Clin Ther 25:2405–2418

12. The Data Collection on Adverse Events of Anti-HIV Drugs (DAD) Study Group (2003) Combination antiretroviral therapy and the risk of myocardial infarction. N Engl J Med 349:1993–2003

13. The Data Collection on Adverse Events of Anti-HIV Drugs (DAD) Study Group (2007). Class of antiretroviral drugs and the risk of myocardial infarction. N Engl J Med 356:1723–1735

14. Stein KM, Haronian H, Mensah GA et al (1990) Ventricular tachycardia and Torsades de pointes complicating pentamidine therapy of Pneumocystis carinii pneumonia in the acquired immunodeficiency syndrome. Am J Cardiol 66:888–889

15. Aoun S, Ramos E (2000) Hypertension in the HIV-infected patient. Curr Hypertens Rep 2:478–481

16. Sattler FR, Qian D, Louie S et al (2001) Elevated blood pressure in subjects with lipodystrophy. AIDS 15:2001–2010

17. Gazzaruso C, Bruno R, Garzaniti A et al (2003). Hypertension among HIV patients: prevalence and relationship to insulin resistance and metabolic syndrome. J Hypertens 21:1377–1382

18. Crane H, Van Rompaey S, Kitahata M (2006) Antiretroviral medications associated with elevated blood pressure among patients receiving highly active antiretroviral therapy. AIDS 20:1019–1026

19. Heidenreich PA, Eisenberg MJ, Kee LL et al (1995) Pericardial effusion in AIDS: incidence and survival. Circulation 92:3229–3234

20. Barbaro G, Fisher SD, Lipshultz SE (2001) Pathogenesis of HIV-associated cardiovascular complications. Lancet Infect Dis 1:115–124

21. Barbaro G, Di Lorenzo G, Grisorio B, Barbarini G and the Gruppo Italiano per lo Studio Cardiologico dei pazienti affetti da AIDS investigators (1998) Cardiac involvement in the acquired immunodeficiency syndrome: a multicenter clinical-pathological study. AIDS Res Hum Retroviruses 14:1071–1077

22. Lai WW, Lipshultz SE, Easley KA et al (1998) Prevalence of congenital cardiovascular malformations in children of human immunodeficiency virus-infected women: the prospective P2C2 HIV Multicenter Study. P2C2 HIV Study Group, National Heart, Lung, and Blood Institute, Bethesda, Maryland. J Am Coll Cardiol 32:1749–1755

23. Barbaro G, Di Lorenzo G, Soldini M et al (1999) Intensity of myocardial expression of inducible ni-

tric oxide synthase influences the clinical course of human immunodeficiency virus-associated cardiomyopathy. Circulation 100:933–939

24. Pugliese A, Isnardi D, Saini A et al (2000) Impact of highly active antiretroviral therapy in HIV-positive patients with cardiac involvement. J Infect 40:282–284

25. Bijl M, Dieleman JP, Simoons M, Van Der Ende ME (2001) Low prevalence of cardiac abnormalities in an HIV-seropositive population on antiretroviral combination therapy. J AIDS 27:318–320

26. Nzuobontane D, Blackett KN, Kuaban C (2002) Cardiac involvement in HIV-infected people in Yaounde, Cameroon. Postgrad Med J 78:678–681

27. Shannon RP, Simon MA, Mathier MA et al (2000) Dilated cardiomyopathy associated with simian AIDS in nonhuman primates. Circulation 101:185–193

28. Barbaro G (2003) Pathogenesis of HIV-associated heart disease. AIDS 17:S12–S20

29. Currie PF, Goldman JH, Caforio AL et al (1998) Cardiac autoimmunity in HIV-related heart muscle disease. Heart 79:599–604

30. Lipshultz SE, Easley KA, Orav EJ et al (2000) Cardiac dysfunction and mortality in HIV-infected children: the Prospective P2C2 HIV Multicenter study. Circulation 102:1542–1548

31. Freeman GL, Colston JT, Zabalgoitia M, Chandrasekar B (1998) Contractile depression and expression of proinflammatory cytokines and iNOS in viral myocarditis. Am J Physiol 274:249–258

32. Lipshultz SE, Easley KA, Orav EJ et al (1998) Left ventricular structure and function in children infected with human immunodeficiency virus: the prospective P2C2 HIV multicenter study. Circulation 97:1246–1256

33. Cooper ER, Hanson C, Diaz C et al (1998) Encephalopathy and progression of human immunodeficiency virus disease in a cohort of children with perinatally acquired human immunodeficiency virus infection. J Pediatr 132:808–812

34. Miller TL, Orav EJ, Colan SD, Lipshultz SE (1997) Nutritional status and cardiac mass and function in children infected with the human immunodeficiency virus. Am J Clin Nutr 66:660–664

35. Miller TL (1998) Cardiac complications of nutritional disorders. In: Lipshultz SE (ed) Cardiology in AIDS. Chapman and Hall, New York, pp 307–316

36. Hoffman M, Lipshultz SE, Miller TL (1999) Malnutrition and cardiac abnormalities in the HIV-infected patients. In: Miller TL, Gorbach S (eds) Nutritional aspects of HIV infection. Arnold, London, pp 33–39

37. Lewis W, Simpson JF, Meyer RR (1994) Cardiac mitochondrial DNA polymerase gamma is inhibited competitively and noncompetitively by phosphorylated zidovudine. Circ Res 74:344–348

38. Lewis W, Grupp IL, Grupp G et al (2000) Cardiac dysfunction in the HIV-1 transgenic mouse treated with zidovudine. Lab Invest 80:187–197

39. Lipshultz SE, Easley KA, Orav EJ et al (2000) Absence of cardiac toxicity of zidovudine in infants. N Engl J Med 343:759–766

40. Barbaro G, Klatt EC (2002) HIV infection and the cardiovascular system. AIDS Rev 4:93–103

41. Nahass RG, Weinstein MP, Bartels J, Gocke DJ (1990) Infective endocarditis in intravenous drug users: a comparison of human immunodeficiency virus type 1-negative and -positive patients. J Infect Dis 162:967–970

42. Johnson RM, Little JR, Storch GA (2001) Kawasaki-like syndromes associated with human immonodeficiency virus infection. Clin Infect Dis 32:1628–1634

43. Shingadia D, Das L, Klein-Gitelman M, Chadwick E (1999) Takayasu's arteritis in a human immunodeficiency virus-infected adolescent. Clin Infect Dis 29:458–459

44. Gisselbrecht M (1999) Vasculitis during human acquired immunodeficiency virus infection. Pathol Biol (Paris) 47:245–247

45. Chi D, Henry J, Kelley J et al (2000) The effects of HIV infection on endothelial function. Endothelium 7:223–242

46. Berger O, Gan X, Gujuluva C et al (1999) CXC and CC chemokine receptors on coronary and brain endothelia. Mol Med 5:795–805

47. Twu C, Liu QN, Popik W et al (2002) Cardiomyocytes undergo apoptosis in human immunodeficiency virus cardiomyopathy through mitochondrion and death receptor-controlled pathways. Proc Natl Acad Sci USA 99:14386–14391

48. Grahame-Clarke C, Alber DG, Lucas SB et al (2001) Association between Kaposi's sarcoma and atherosclerosis: implications for gammaherpesviruses and vascular disease. AIDS 15:1902–1905

49. Barbaro G, Barbarini G, Pellicelli AM (2001) HIV-associated coronary arteritis in a patient with fatal myocardial infarction. N Engl J Med 344:1799–1800

50. Arsura EL, Ismail Y, Freeman S, Karunakav AR (1994) Amphotericin B-induced dilated cardiomyopathy. Am J Med 97:560–562

51. Cohen AJ, Weiser B, Afzal Q, Fuhrer J (1990) Ventricular tachycardia in two patients with AIDS receiving ganciclovir (DHPG). AIDS 4:807–809

52. Lopez JA, Harold JG, Rosenthal MC et al (1987) QT prolongation and Torsades de pointes after administration of trimethoprim-sulfamethoxazole. Am J Cardiol 59:376–377

53. Dal Maso L, Serraino D, Franceschi S (2001) Epidemiology of HIV-associated malignancies. Cancer Treat Res 104:1–18

54. Barbaro G, Klatt EC (2003) Highly active antiretroviral therapy and cardiovascular complications in HIV-infected patients. Curr Pharm Des 9:1475–1481

55. Carr A, Samaras K, Burton S et al (1998) A syndrome of peripheral lipodystrophy, hyperlipidaemia and insulin resistance in patients receiving HIV protease inhibitors. AIDS 12:F51–F58

56. Carr A (2003) HIV lipodystrophy: risk factors, pathogenesis, diagnosis and management. AIDS 17:S141–S148

Chapter 3

Pathogenesis of Antiretroviral Treatment-Associated Metabolic Syndrome

J. Capeau, M. Caron, F. Boccara

Highly active antiretroviral therapy (ART) with protease inhibitors (PIs) and nucleoside analogue inhibitors of viral reverse transcriptase (NRTI) allowed a major reduction in the severity and morbidity of HIV infection; however, these drugs were associated with the occurrence of secondary effects collectively termed "ART-related lipodystrophy or metabolic syndrome." This syndrome is defined by alterations in body-fat repartition with peripheral fat loss and/or central fat accumulation together with metabolic disorders such as hypertriglyceridemia (hyper-TG), hypercholesterolemia, and insulin resistance sometimes with altered glucose tolerance. This set of abnormalities shows some similarities with those present in the very common metabolic or insulin-resistance syndrome and some of the pathophysiological mechanisms are probably the same. In addition, the ART-related metabolic syndrome probably results from alterations directly related to the treatment and also probably to the ongoing infection in the context of altered immunity and modified cytokine profile, which most likely enhances its severity and could be responsible for its specific features.

Definition of the Metabolic Syndrome in Non-HIV-Infected Patients

Metabolic syndrome (MetS)–also previously called syndrome X, insulin resistance syndrome, or dysmetabolic syndrome–was defined, according to the WHO [1], by the presence of:

1. Impaired glucose regulation (either impaired fasting glucose or glucose intolerance or diabetes) or insulin resistance (the HOMA values being in the top quartile)
2. With at least two of the following criteria: triglycerides (TG) >1.7 mmol/L (1.5 g/L), high-density lipoprotein cholesterol (HDL) <0.9 mmol/L (0.35 g/L) for men or <1.0 mmol/L (0.39 g/L) for women, SBP/DBP >140/90 mmHg, body-mass index (BMI) >30 kg/m2 or waist-to-hip ratio (WHR) >0.9 for men and 0.85 for women, albuminuria/creatinine ratio ≥30 mg/g

A simplified definition was proposed by the NCEP ATP-III guidelines in 2001 modified in 2005 for the level of fasting glycemia [1]. Moreover, a new definition has been proposed by the IDF (International Diabetes Federation) [2] with a limit for the waist circumference lower than that used in the NCEP III definition, which is a necessary factor for the diagnosis (Table 1).

In France, the prevalence of the metabolic syndrome in the general population is about 10 and 7% of adult men and women, respectively, while in the USA it varies from 20 to more than 50% according to the ethnic origin of the subjects.

The main biological components clustered in the metabolic syndrome are linked to the presence of a state of insulin resistance due to an accumulation of visceral fat resulting in visceral obesity, altered glucose tolerance or diabetes, dyslipidemia with decreased HDL, increased small and dense LDL particles, increased TG and increased blood pressure.

Table 1 Different definitions of the metabolic syndrome

	Definitions
OMS (1999)	Glucose intolerance associated with at least 2 of the following abnormalities: - Hyerpertension ≥ 140/90 mmHg - Elevated triglycerides ≥ 1.7 mmol/L and/or decreased of HDL cholestérol < 0.9 mmol/L in men or < 1.0 mmol/L in women - Central obesity waist to hip ratio > 0.90 in men and > 0.85 in women or body mass index > 30 kg/m^2 - Micro-albuminuria ≥ 20 μg/min
NCEP ATPIII (2005)	At least three criteria of the following: - Abdominal perimeter ≥ 102 cm in men and ≥ 88 cm in women - Triglycerides ≥ 1.7 mmol/L (1.5 g/L) - HDL cholesterol < 1.03 mmol/L (0.4 g/L) in men and < 1.29 mmol/L (0.5 g/L) in women - Systolic arterial pressure ≥ 130 and/or diastolic arterial pressure ≥ 85 mmHg - Fasting glycemia ≥ 5.6 mmol/L (1 g/L)
IDF (2005)	Central obesity defined by an abdominal perimeter ≥ 94 cm for men and ≥ 80 cm for European women associated with at least 2 of the following criteria: - Triglycerides ≥ 1.7 mmol/L, (1.5 g/L) or specific treatment - HDL cholesterol < 1.03 mmol/L (0.4 g/L) in men and < 1.29 mmol/L (0.5 g/L) in women or treatment - Systolic arterial pressure ≥ 130 and/or diastolic arterial pressure ≥ 85 mmHg or treatment - Fasting glycemia ≥ 5.6 mmol/L (1 g/L)

Moreover, a number or other components can be present such as increased uric acid and plasminogen activator inhibitor (PAI)-1 levels, steatosis, presence of a syndrome of polycystic ovaries and of sleep apneas. The risks associated with the metabolic syndrome are predominantly of cardiovascular disease (two or three-fold higher) and diabetes mellitus (six to sevenfold). Other risks are at the liver level, with the occurrence of NASH (non-alcoholic steatohepatitis) and the possible evolution towards cirrhosis.

Prevalence of the Metabolic Syndrome in the HIV-infected Population

Different studies evaluated the prevalence of the MetS in HIV-infected patients according to the two most used definitions in the general population.

Prevalence According to ATPIII-NCEP Definition

North American populations with elevated body mass index:

Mondy et al. [3] found a prevalence of 25.5 and 26.5% in HIV and non-HIV-infected subjects, respectively. Jacobson et al. [4] found a prevalence of 24% in HIV-infected subjects and 34% in the general population (NHAHES cohort) with a higher body mass index (BMI). When adjusted on BMI, this difference disappeared.

European Populations:

Bonfanti et al. [5] in the Italian population found a prevalence of 22% compared to 15.8% in the general population (PAMELA cohort). In the Spanish population, Estrada et al. [6] reported a prevalence of 15.8% in HIV-infected subjects compared to 3.2% in the general population with the same BMI

(23 kg/m²). In the APROCO-COPILOTE French cohort, we found a prevalence of 15–20% according to the period of the study, which is much more than that of the general population, inasmuch as the mean BMI was low around 22–23 kg/m². We can conclude that for European studies, the prevalence of MetS is increased in HIV-infected patients compared to the general population.

Prevalence According to IDF definition

Generally, the prevalence is lower when using this definition because of the necessary criteria of the abdominal perimeter. This element is uncommon in HIV-infected patients with a lipodystrophic syndrome. Samaras et al. [7], in an international cohort, reported a near similarly prevalence of 18% (ATP III-NCEP) and 14% (IDF) according to the two definitions. However, in the APROCO-COPILOTE cohort, the prevalence was 5–7% according to the period of the study, much lower that the prevalence identified by the ATP definition.

In HIV-infected patients, the most frequent criteria of the metabolic syndrome are elevated triglycerides and low HDL. Increased abdominal girth is rarely found, whereas in the general population, this criterion is predominant.

Physiology of Insulin Signaling and Adipose Tissue

Insulin acts on glucose and lipid metabolism, favoring the storage of energy after meals. At the clinical level, insulin resistance is defined as the inability or decreased ability of insulin to control glycemia, which means that a high level of insulin is required to maintain normoglycemia or that, when glycemia is increased, the levels of insulinemia are disproportionately elevated. To evaluate insulin resistance, the most used index is HOMA (homeostasis model assessment), which is calculated from fasting glycemia levels (mmol/L) multiplied by fasting insulin levels (mU/ml) divided by 22.5. This index, or its derivatives (FIRI, QUICKI), is correlated with the evaluation of insulin sensitivity given by the gold standard test, i.e., the euglycemic hyperinsulinemic clamp but, at the individual level, this correlation is rather low [8]. The measurement of fasting glycemia and insulinemia mainly relies on the effect of insulin on the liver, where insulin inhibits hepatic glucose production by inhibiting glycogenolysis and gluconeogenesis. During the clamp test, or when a post-prandial measurement is performed, the presence of elevated levels of glycemia and insulin is mainly due to the defective entry and utilization of glucose at the muscle level.

At the cellular level, the mechanisms whereby insulin transduces its signal have been studied for a long time, as have the mechanisms responsible for insulin resistance. In addition to the liver and muscles, adipose tissue is an important target tissue of insulin (Fig. 1). Insulin signals inside the cell by activating its receptor, which possesses a tyrosine kinase activity, and afterwards, insulin binding phosphorylates its intracellular domain, therefore allowing cytosol substrate proteins to associate with the receptor. The insulin receptor substrate (IRS) class of proteins transduces the signal towards different intracellular pathways: briefly, the metabolic signals are mainly transduced through the phosphatidylinositol 3 kinase (PI3K) pathway, while the mitogenic signals are mainly transmitted through the mitogen-activated protein (MAP) kinase pathway, which can use the IRS and SHC classes of proteins as receptor substrates. At the level of the liver, insulin acts on glycogen synthesis and increases lipogenesis, in particular from glucose. It inhibits hepatic glucose production by impairing glycogenolysis and gluconeogenesis. In muscle cells, insulin recruits the glucose

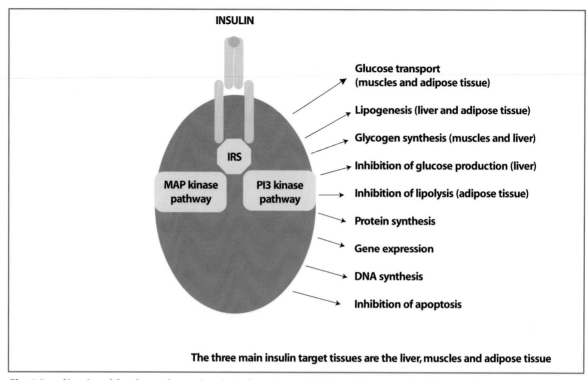

Fig. 1 Insulin signal leads to the activation of major anabolic pathways. *MAP kinase*, mitogen activated kinase; *PI3 kinase*, phosphatidylinositol 3 kinase

transporters GLUT4 to the plasma membrane and activates glucose entry together with its storage as glycogen and its oxidation. In adipocytes, insulin plays a strong metabolic role by increasing TG storage through the activation of lipoprotein lipase and glucose entry and by decreasing TG hydrolysis through the inhibition of the hormone-sensitive lipase involved in lipolysis [9], a pathway stimulated by catecholamines in humans.

In 1963, Randle [10] described the glucose–fatty acid cycle and its role in physiology and pathology. He showed that free fatty acids (FFA) are used in preference to glucose by the heart and diaphragm muscles, leading to decreased glucose utilization. This concept has been revisited by Perseghin et al. [11]. By performing both human and animal studies in vivo, they revealed that FFA entering the muscle cell are transformed into acyl-CoA derivatives and they activate the PKCθ isoform and IKKβ, which in turn activate IRS phosphorylation on ser-

ine residues. This serine phosphorylation has been shown by numerous groups to stop insulin signaling and to impede the activation of the downstream steps, including the recruitment of GLUT4 transporters from their intracellular location to the plasma membrane. In that situation, muscle and liver cells use FFA to produce the energy required for their metabolism.

In addition to its metabolic function, adipose tissue now appears to play an important endocrine role: it can release a number of hormones, proteins, and cytokines acting through endocrine or autocrine/paracrine mechanisms and collectively called adipokines (Fig. 2) [12–14].

Leptin

Leptin is a 16-kDa protein mainly produced by subcutaneous adipose tissue, and it acts as an endocrine factor at the hypothalamic

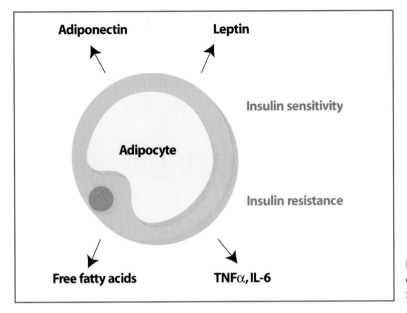

Fig. 2 Adipocytes secrete a range of adipocytokines which control insulin sensitivity

level to reduce food intake and to regulate energy production and utilization. In addition, leptin exerts pleiotropic actions and plays a role in peripheral energy and bone metabolism, reproduction, and immunity. Leptin receptors located on muscle cells have been shown to activate AMP kinase (AMPK) and thereby to favor FFA oxidation (see the following section).

Adiponectin

Adiponectin or adipoQ or ACRP30 is secreted at high levels by adipose tissue, and circulating levels are between 5 and 10 µg/ml in human plasma. They are negatively correlated with BMI and with the content in visceral fat [15] and are decreased in diabetic and obese patients. It has been reported in numerous studies that the level of circulating adiponectin is inversely related to insulin resistance. Adiponectin is also decreased in patients with ischemic heart disease.

The mechanisms whereby adiponectin acts are now starting to be understood. Two receptors have been cloned, but the transduction pathway is still poorly understood.

The activation of the two adiponectin receptors leads to the activation of the transcription factor PPARα and AMPK in the liver and muscles [16]. There has been a major interest in the role of this enzyme in cell metabolism. AMPK is activated by AMP, the level of which is increased when ATP has been hydrolyzed. AMPK now appears as an energy level-detecting enzyme, which plays a key role in redirecting the energy-synthesizing pathways of glucose and lipid metabolism. First, activated AMPK is able to indirectly activate the entry of acyl-CoA into the mitochondria to be degraded by the β-oxidation pathway in the liver and muscles and to be converted into energy. In liver cells, AMPK is also able to inhibit the expression of the gluconeogenic enzymes required for hepatic glucose production. In muscle cells, AMPK can recruit glucose transporters GLUT4 to the membrane, even in the absence of insulin, allowing glucose entry and utilization [12]. In addition to its insulin-sensitizing effect, adiponectin can act at the level of the arterial wall. Atherosclerotic cellular changes include monocyte adhesion to endothelial cells due to the expression of adhesion molecules, uptake of oxidized LDL by macrophages through scavenger receptors, and proliferation of vascular smooth muscle cells in response to PDGF. Adiponectin has been found to inhibit tumor necrosis factor TNF-α production and TNF-α-induced adverse effects on the vascular wall, therefore inhibiting all these atherogenic processes [15, 17]. Thus, it probably has a potent anti-atherogenic role and could protect injured vessels against the development of atherogenic lesions. The expression of adiponectin has been found to be inhibited in vitro by TNF-α and interleukin (IL)-6.

Tumor Necrosis Factor-α

TNF-α is synthesized as a 26-kDa plasma membrane-bound monomer. A secreted trimer is formed by proteolysis of the precursor, giving rise to a 17-kDa cytokine, which binds to two receptors, type I and II, and activates the classic inflammatory NFκB pathway [18]. In physiological conditions, adipose tissue production is very low.

However, its production has been found to be increased in pathological conditions, even if the reason for this increased production remains unclear. Animal studies have revealed that in cases of obesity and insulin resistance, the secretion of TNF-α was increased and could be involved in insulin resistance. In particular, TNF-α has been found to act at the local level on adipocytes and to inhibit insulin signal transduction through the inhibitory phosphorylation of the IRS1 protein together with a decreased expression of GLUT4 [12]. In human studies, the deleterious role of TNF-α has been questioned. Several studies reported that the circulating levels of TNF-α were related with obesity and insulin resistance. However, systemic inhibition of TNF-α in type 2 diabetic patients was not able to decrease insulin resistance. It could be proposed that TNF-α acts mainly at the local and not the systemic level and that it induces adipose tissue resistance, which results in increased lipolysis and FFA fluxes (Fig. 3). In addi-

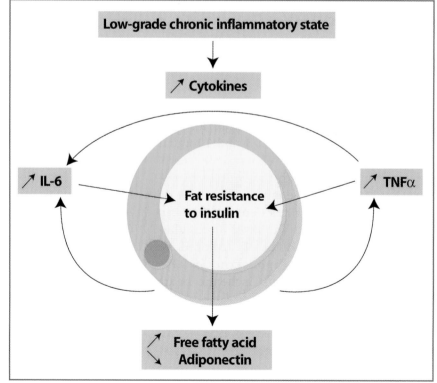

Fig. 3 Proinflammatory cytokines induce insulin resistance

tion, TNF-α acts on adipocytes by decreasing adiponectin and increasing IL-6 expression. These latter cytokines, which act at a distance from adipose tissue, probably play a major role in insulin sensitivity and indirectly trigger the insulin-resistant effect of TNF-α.

In addition, in patients with HIV-related metabolic syndrome, several studies consistently revealed increased levels of TNF-α, pointing to a major role for this cytokine in this condition (see the following section).

Interleukin-6

Interleukin-6 is a pro-inflammatory cytokine produced by several tissues and cells and, in particular, by adipose tissue: 10–30% of circulating Interleukin-6 could be produced by adipose tissue. Interleukin-6 may exert its effects at the central level on the hypothalamus. At the liver level, Interleukin-6 induces the production of acute-phase proteins and in particular of C-reactive protein (CRP). The levels of circulating Interleukin-6 were shown to be increased in obesity and were related to insulin resistance. Interleukin-6 also acts by paracrine/autocrine mechanisms on adipocytes and induces insulin resistance and altered differentiation in particular by inducing the expression of SOCS3 [19].

Plasminogen Activator Inhibitor-1

Plasminogen activator inhibitor-1 (PAI-1) is a protein involved in thrombosis, which compromises the clearance of fibrin. Its level is increased in obesity, type-2 diabetes, and metabolic syndrome. In addition, it is strongly associated with vascular disease including myocardial infarction and venous thrombosis [13].

Regional Differences in Fat Distribution and Physiology

The visceral fat depot is contained within the body cavity surrounding the internal organs and is composed of mesenteric and omental depots. Visceral fat represents about 20 and 6% of total body fat in men and women, respectively. The subcutaneous fat depot is located under the skin, particularly in the abdominal region. In the lower body, all adipose depots are subcutaneous and the largest sites of storage are the gluteal and femoral regions [20]. Visceral and subcutaneous fat express and secrete various amounts of different cytokines. Leptin is mainly secreted by peripheral fat, while adiponectin and Interleukin-6 are secreted in higher quantities by visceral fat. For TNF–α, the results are less clear. In addition, visceral fat is more sensitive to catecholamines, and therefore to lipolysis, and more resistant to insulin than subcutaneous fat [21].

It has long been known that glucocorticoids act on adipose tissue and can inhibit proliferation but enhance lipid storage leading to fat hypertrophy. Visceral adipocytes, which contain higher levels of glucocorticoid receptors, are more sensitive to the effect of this hormone. Accordingly, in Cushing's syndrome with hypercorticism, visceral fat is particularly increased. More recently, profound differences have been demonstrated in the level of the enzyme that can convert inactive cortisone to active cortisol, 11β-hydroxysteroid dehydrogenase type 1 (11β-HSD1), with very high activity in visceral fat and barely detectable activity in subcutaneous fat [20, 22]. Therefore, visceral fat is able to produce cortisol locally, which could act inside adipocytes and increase lipid accumulation. Interestingly, this enzyme is activated by TNF-α (Fig. 4).

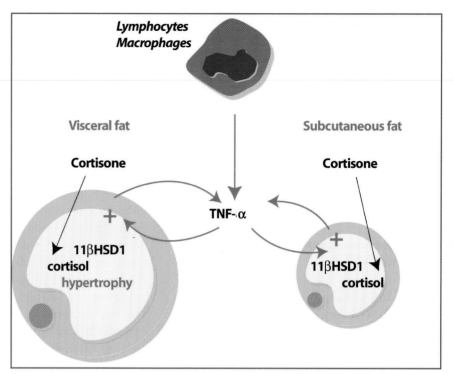

Fig. 4 Pathophysiology of visceral fat hypertrophy: hypothetical mechanisms

Pathology of Insulin Signaling and Adipose Tissue

When adipose tissue is hypertrophic and resistant to insulin, as seen for visceral fat in metabolic syndrome, lipolysis is increased, resulting in increased levels of circulating free fatty acids (FFA). An increased level of FFA plays a detrimental role on glucose utilization in the liver and muscles and leads to insulin resistance. The mechanisms responsible for this resistance to insulin can be hypothesized from the studies performed by Perseghin et al. [11] and are related to the inhibition of the insulin signaling pathway induced by acyl-CoA derivatives as indicated above. In addition, this excess of acyl-CoA inside the cytosol, exceeding the capacities of degradation in the mitochondria and peroxysomes, leads to accumulation of TG in hepatocytes and muscle cells. Such an accumulation has been reported in numerous studies of patients with insulin resistance,

metabolic syndrome, obesity, and diabetes. Moreover, it has been consistently reported that the extent of fat accumulation in the liver is related to the amount of visceral fat and also to insulin resistance evaluated by HOMA or clamp tests [23]. Similarly, the amount of intramyocellular fat has been related to insulin resistance in obese and diabetic patients [24]. This set of alterations has been named lipotoxicity [25]. The location of adipose tissue is probably important; visceral fat, which is highly sensitive to catecholamines and resistant to insulin, is prone to release large amounts of FFA in the portal system which will be driven mainly to the liver. Subcutaneous fat, which is more resistant to lipolysis, would release lower levels of FFA, particularly towards peripheral tissues such as muscles.

Metabolic syndrome, type 2 diabetes, and obesity are now considered as low-grade chronic inflammatory states, like atherosclerosis, leading to coronary heart disease. Hyperinsulinemia and insulin resistance are considered as common preceding factors of hypertension, decreased HDL concentrations, hyper-TG, and altered glucose tolerance (Fig. 5). Part of the features of insulin resistance syndrome can be explained by the altered secretion of products from adipose tissue (and in particular from expanded visceral fat) with increased levels of proinflammatory cytokines, TNF-α and IL-6, responsible for this inflammatory profile. Interestingly, it has been shown in animal models of obesity and in human subcutaneous and visceral fat, that white adipose tissue presents macrophage accumulation, which is responsible for increased TNF-α expression [26–29]; increased endogenous production of cortisol increases insulin resistance participating in a vicious cycle (Fig. 6). Even if visceral fat is more difficult to study than subcutaneous fat in patients, it is highly probable that visceral fat is prone to release higher amounts of FFA and IL-6 and decreased amounts of adiponectin. They are released in the portal

system and reach the liver first. This will result in increased production of acute inflammation proteins, such as CRP, and in increased glucose production and very-low-density lipoprotein (VLDL) synthesis resulting in hyper-TG [20].

Subcutaneous abdominal fat, if insulin-resistant, will produce increased FFA used by muscles, resulting in reduced glucose utilization at that level. The causes for this altered adipocyte function remain speculative: insulin can alter TNF–α and IL-6 secretion and, therefore, in the case of insulin resistance, these cytokines could be increased. Otherwise, insulin resistance could be a consequence of TNF-α and IL-6 oversecretion (Fig. 6). Increased levels of these cytokines at the level of the arterial wall lead to inflammatory lesions of atherosclerosis. Factors such as aging, smoking, and obesity can be responsible for increased proinflammatory cytokines [30]. This set of alterations will create a vicious

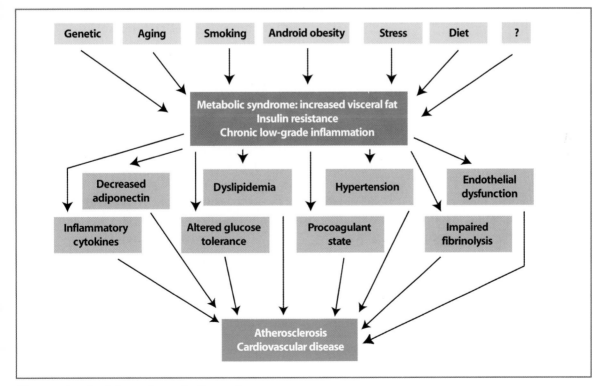

Fig. 5 Pathophysiology of metabolic syndrome

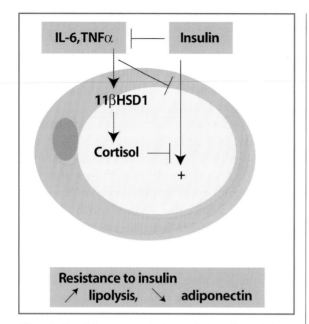

Fig. 6 Cytokines, cortisol, and insulin vicious cycle resulting in insulin resistance

cycle resulting in metabolic and vascular changes, ultimately leading to atherosclerosis and cardiovascular disease.

Description and Pathophysiology of the ART-Related Metabolic Alterations

Dyslipidemia

Increased levels of TG and cholesterol, together with decreased HDL and increased LDL cholesterol, have been described in HIV patients undergoing ART [31]. These alterations probably have multiple origins. The HIV infection itself has been shown to be associated with increased levels of TG, decreased levels of HDL and, in patients with AIDS, of LDL cholesterol. These alterations could result from the high level of proinflammatory cytokines (TNF-α, IL-6, IL-1) observed in these patients with an active infection, due to their increased secretion by activated monocytes and macrophages.

TNF-α and IL-6 can decrease the expression and activity of lipoprotein lipase, which is involved in TG clearance from circulation lipoproteins. Moreover, acute-phase proteins can bind to HDL particles, promoting their uptake by macrophages and therefore increasing their clearance rate. These phenomena are seen in infection with severe inflammation whatever its origin [32].

After the introduction of HAART, increased levels of lipids were constantly reported [31, 33]. Regarding the NRTIs, stavudine was associated with increased levels of TG [34]. However, the major contributor to dyslipidemia was the class of PIs. Studies performed in non-HIV-infected control subjects revealed that RTV was able, after a few days, to alter lipid parameters with hyper-TG and increased cholesterol levels. Similarly, boosting concentrations of RTV in association with LPV increased TG levels. By contrast, atazanavir was associated with a safe metabolic profile [35]. NNRTIs are also able to modify lipid parameters: NVP increases total and HDL cholesterol levels but not TG [36]. EFV has a similar effect but increases cholesterol and TG. Various phenotypes of dyslipidemia were reported in patients undergoing ART with PIs, but the major alterations are increased levels of TG, decreased levels of HDL, and increased content in small dense LDLs, a profile very similar to that seen in the classic metabolic syndrome. An important prevalence of lipid alterations was observed in PI-treated patients when first generation PI were introduced; in an Australian cohort, 14 months after initiating treatment with PIs, 50% of the patients had TG levels above 2 mmol/L and 60% had cholesterol levels above 5.5 mmol/L, whereas these values were 22% and 11%, respectively, in patients under NRTI treatment without PIs [37]. In the French cohort APROCO-TM, after 1 and 3 years of PI treatment, respectively, the prevalence of hyper-TG increased from 26 to 36% in men and from 20 to 25% in women. The prevalence of hypercholesterolemia was elevated between 55 and 60% in both groups [34]. At present, the use of PI with a more friendly metabolic effect such as atazanavir and the more generalized dietary and lipid-lowering drugs prescriptions allowed a reduction of the lipid values in this population [31].

The PI-induced alterations could result from a direct effect of the drugs, particularly at the liver level, resulting in modified lipid metabolism (Fig. 7). The synthesis and secretion of apoB, the major VLDL-linked apoprotein, are partly regulated by the balance between the association to lipids and the degradation in the proteasome system involved in overall cellular protein degradation. Thus, it has been shown, in in vitro models of hepatic cells, that RTV and SQV could inhibit the degradation of apoB by inhibiting the proteasome, which results in increased VLDL secretion [38]. When animals were fed a high-fat diet, an increased synthesis of TG on VLDL was observed [39]. Moreover, RTV is able to increase VLDL secretion in mice through the activation of the lipogenic transcription factor SREBP-1 in the liver [40]. Regarding VLDL catabolism, Bonnet et al. presented interesting data [41] indicating that, in PI-treated patients, there was an accumulation of lipoparticles containing apoC-III and apo-E in association with apoB. These complex particles would represent persistent potentially atherogenic cholesterol-rich remnant particles derived from TG-rich lipoproteins. The observed excess in apoC-III on lipoproteins might be a major determinant of a slower catabolism of TG-rich lipoproteins, since apoC-III is an inhibitor of lipoprotein lipase activity and it also impairs the interaction of apoB and apoE with the LDL-receptor and LRP. This will result in an increased level of remnant lipoprotein returning to the liver.

In addition to a direct effect of some PIs on lipid metabolism, the altered repartition of body fat is probably also involved in lipid alterations. As explained above, for the

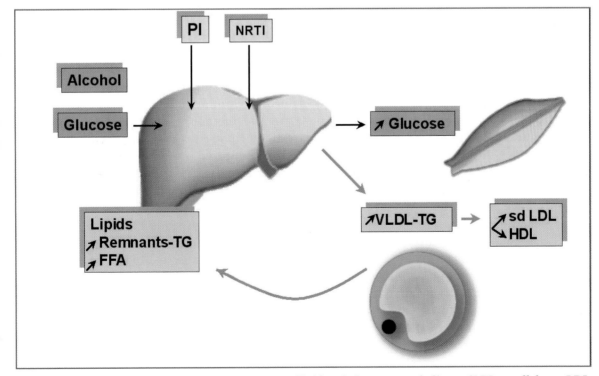

Fig. 7 Adverse effects of antiretroviral treatment on lipid and glucose metabolism. *sdLDL*, small dense LDL

metabolic syndrome, increased content in visceral fat as well as decreased peripheral adipose tissue are associated with an increased level of lipolysis and of FFA fluxes together with altered adipocytokine production: increased levels of TNF-α, IL-1, and IL-6 and decreased levels of adiponectin [42, 43]. Thus, even after the introduction of HAART, the severity of the inflammatory syndrome is markedly decreased as compared to the state of active infection. Patients with ART-related metabolic syndrome still present a state of low-grade inflammation with increased cytokines and acute-phase proteins such as CRP, which could contribute to the dyslipidemia observed in these patients.

Altered Glucose Tolerance, Diabetes and Insulin Resistance

The presence of altered glucose tolerance is observed in a minority of PI-treated patients, but its prevalence was high with the first generation PI and in particular with the wide use of indinavir. In the APRO-CO-TM French cohort, increased glycemia (either fasting hyperglycemia or glucose intolerance) increased from 17 to 27% in men after 1 and 3 years of treatment with PI, respectively, while diabetes increased from 4 to 9%. In women, alterations in glucose tolerance remained stable at 25% but the prevalence of diabetes increased from 2 to 11%. More recent data, 6 years after the introduction of PI in the treatment of these patients, reveal that the incidence of diabetes is increased [44]. In a recent study on the Swiss cohort [45], an increased incidence of diabetes was noted in particular in the oldest patients as compared to the general population and the occurrence of diabetes was estimated at 4.4 cases per 1,000 person-years of follow-up (PYFU) and was strongly associated with the treatment with PI (except atazanavir), stavudine and didanosine. This incidence is much higher in the US population, with a higher BMI since it has been reported to be of 47 cases per 1,000 PYFU [46]. These data suggest that the prevalence and the severity of glucose alterations tend to increase with the duration of the treatment. Insulin resistance, which can be evaluated by the simple HOMA test, was highly prevalent in these patients when indinavir was used and is less frequent at present [31, 47].

Studies performed with non-HIV-infected control subjects revealed that IDV was able to induce insulin resistance and to modify glycemia after a few days [48]. After a single dose, IDV was able to decrease glucose uptake during a clamp test, indicating insulin resistance, which was rapid and reversible [49]. It is hypothesized that this effect could be due to inhibition of the insulin-sensitive glucose transporter GLUT4 that has been evidenced in in vitro studies. Similarly, LPV boosted by RTV induced an increased glycemia and insulinemia after 4 weeks in normal volunteers [35].

The prevalence of glucose alterations and insulin resistance has been consistently found to be higher in patients with lipodystrophy than in patients without lipodystrophy. A role for adipose tissue in insulin resistance resulting from altered cytokine production and increased lipolysis can be easily hypothesized, which would accentuate the metabolic disorders. As explained below, lipodystrophic adipose tissue presents an altered profile of secreted cytokines with increased TNF-α and IL-6. These cytokines are responsible for insulin resistance at the adipocyte level resulting in increased lipolysis and FFA fluxes, which in turn induce insulin resistance at the level of the liver and muscles. In addition, lipodystrophic adipose tissue has a decreased secretion of adiponectin, which could result in decreased lipid oxidation and glucose intake in the muscles, and in decreased lipid oxidation and increased glucose production in the liver as explained above. Therefore, the drug-induced alterations in glucose metabolism and in insulin sensitivity are aggravated by the altered adipose tissue function due to lipodystrophy.

Description and Pathophysiology of the ART-Related Abnormal Fat Distribution

Description

Different forms of abnormal fat distribution or lipodystrophies are seen in HIV-infected patients undergoing HAART. Lipoatrophy mainly affects peripheral fat at the level of the limbs, buttocks, face, and abdomen and could be clinically evaluated by the reduced skin-fold due to the decrease in subcutaneous fat. Results from the US FRAM study revealed that, in this population with high BMI in the control group, both peripheral and central lipoatrophy was associated with HIV infection [50]. Central lipoatrophy, inside the abdomen, can be diagnosed by imaging technologies such as MRI or CT scans. In addition, fat is increased in some regions located primarily in the visceral area but also in the chest and neck, giving an aspect of a buffalo hump. When lipoatrophy and lipohypertrophy are associated, a phenotype of mixed lipodystrophy is present. This syndrome resembles the typical metabolic syndrome but is more striking since both the loss of the peripheral fat and the increase in visceral fat can be very marked in the same patient.

A number of studies have now clearly shown that peripheral lipoatrophy is related to the duration of the treatment with stavudine or to a lesser extent with zidovudine and that switch strategies towards other NRTI have allowed a slow recovery [51]. While the prevalence of lipodystrophies was important when these NRTI and first generation PIs were widely used, their occurrence seems to be low with the new-generation ART. Atazanavir, appears to exert few adverse effects on the fat tissue. Healthy subjects [35] or HIV-infected patients [52] treated with atazanavir for 10 days or 48 weeks, respectively, do not develop metabolic disorders or fat tissue redistribution. Moreover, naive HIV-infected patients treated with atazanavir for 96 weeks do not suffer from late-emerging adverse effects [53], though change in fat tissue distribution has not been evaluated in this study. Up to now, treatments with second-generation NRTIs (abacavir or tenofovir), as well as non-NRTIs (nevirapine, efavirenz) or the fusion inhibitor (enfuvirtide) are considered to have a low incidence on lipodystrophy [54–57].

The pathophysiology of ART-related lipodystrophies remains not entirely understood due to their multifactorial origin. Among the numerous factors found to be concerned, drugs play the leading role, but other factors linked to the disease and to the patients themselves also have to be considered. Studies performed with cohorts of patients have outlined the importance of the severity of HIV infection, of the quality of immune restoration, as well as of age, sex, and BMI in the prevalence, type, and severity of lipodystrophy. Among the NRTIs, stavudine in particular as well as zidovudine were found to be linked to peripheral lipoatrophy and PIs to visceral fat accumulation. Their association increases their prevalence and severity [58, 59]. However, individual molecules of these two classes have different effects.

In Vitro Studies

To better understand the pathophysiology of fat alterations, studies were performed first in vitro, so as to decipher the precise role of each drug on adipocyte functions. Most of the studies concerned PIs, since lipodystrophies were diagnosed shortly after their introduction. Several studies reported that in the short term, PIs were able to inhibit the insulin-activated glucose transporter GLUT4, thereby rapidly inducing insulin resistance, which was reversible when the PI concentration was lowered [48]. In the long term (several days), most of the studies reported that some PIs, but not all, were able to greatly alter adipocyte functions by decreasing adipocyte differentiation and by inducing insulin resistance [60]. Our group and others have reported that the step of the adipogenic transcription factor SREBP-1 was specifically targeted by some but not all PIs, with a decreased level of the protein and a decreased activation of the downstream pathways. We have shown that some PIs were able to impair the nuclear location of SREBP-1 and to alter the structure and stability of the nuclear lamina, by impairing the maturation of prelamin A to lamin A [61–63]. Lamin A and lamin C are encoded by the same gene and they can combine with lamin B to form a meshwork of filamentous proteins that lines the inner nuclear membrane called lamina. Lamina interacts with the nuclear membrane and with chromatin. In particular, the C-terminal globular domain of lamin A/C can bind DNA and also SREBP-1 [64, 65]. Interestingly, mutations in this domain are responsible for a genetic form of partial lipodystrophy, Dunnigan's syndrome or FPLD, with peripheral lipoatrophy, accumulation of fat at the level of the face and neck, and major metabolic alterations with hyper-TG, diabetes, and insulin resistance. The mutations responsible for FPLD reduced the interactions of lamin with DNA and SREBP-1, which could explain the altered adipose tissue differentiation observed in these patients. The cells from these patients present nuclear alterations and altered lamina stability, similar to the alterations induced in cultured adipocytes by some PIs [66]. Thus, we can hypothesize that some PIs could alter lamina structure by comparing lamin A maturation and thereby altering the SREBP-1 normal location inside the nucleus [62]. This could impair adipocyte

differentiation and induce insulin resistance. Importantly, in vitro studies have revealed that some PI were able to increase the production of reactive oxygen species (ROS) in mitochondria leading to an increased oxidative stress which alters adipocyte function. In addition, increased ROS production induced by some PIs alters the expression of adipokines in cultured adipocytes [67–69]; they increased the expression of TNF-α and/or IL-6, the proinflammatory cytokines that could play a role in adipose tissue insulin resistance and apoptosis. They were also shown to decrease the expression of adiponectin, which could explain, at least in part, the resistance to insulin.

As regards NRTIs, only a few in vitro studies have been presented. We have observed that the thymidine analogues, stavudine and zidovudine, but not the other NRTIs, were able to induce a mitochondrial dysfunction, increase ROS production and decrease lipid content in adipocytes [69, 70]. In addition, thymidine analogues also altered the expression of adipokines in vitro, in part as results of increased ROS production [68, 69].

Taken as a whole, in the two classes of ART, some drugs modified adipocyte function. PIs altered differentiation, mitochondrial function and insulin sensitivity possibly through their effect on lamin A/C and SREBP-1 and on ROS production, while NRTIs altered lipid content and adipokine production through their effect on mitochondria and ROS. Therefore, when present together, a synergistic effect could be hypothesized (Fig. 8).

Ex Vivo and In Vivo Studies

To go further, different groups performed studies on subcutaneous adipose tissue from lipodystrophic patients, which were compared with fat from control subjects or from non-lipodystrophic patients undergo-

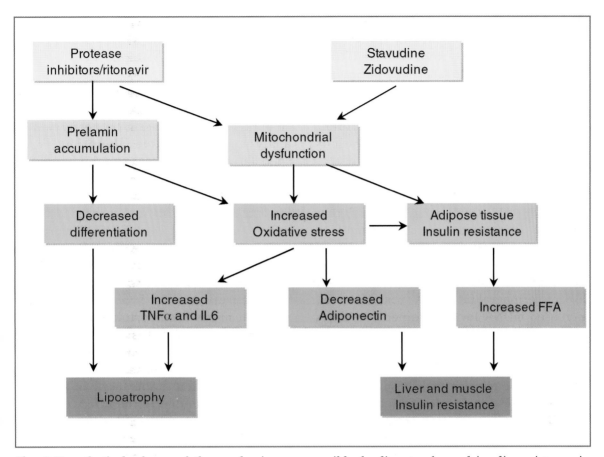

Fig. 8 Hypothetical scheme of the mechanisms responsible for lipoatrophy and insulin resistance in HAART-related lipodystrophy

ing HAART. The level of mitochondrial DNA was evaluated by several groups and consistently found to be decreased in fat from HAART-treated patients: this decrease was seen in patients undergoing stavudine treatment and to a lesser extent with zidovudine, in accordance with the hypothesis that these NRTIs can alter mitochondrial function [58]. Morphological studies revealed important morphological alterations in patients' lipoatrophic fat with adipocytes of reduced size, increased apoptosis, increased fibrosis, and mitochondria numbers [70–75]. An increased number of macrophages invading lipoatrophic adipose tissue was reported by these groups.

The expression of the transcription factors SREBP-1, PPARγ, and C/EBPα was found to be decreased in fat from lipodys-

trophic as compared to non-lipodystrophic and control subjects, indicating a state of altered differentiation and insulin resistance [71, 75, 76]. In addition, the expression of the adipokines was deeply altered in fat from lipodystrophic patients as compared to control or non-lipodystrophic patients; TNF-α and IL-6 expression was increased, while that of leptin and adiponectin was decreased [71, 75, 76]. Accordingly, the circulating levels of these cytokines were altered [42, 43].

Clinical data on the effects of individual molecules on lipodystrophy are now becoming available. A role for thymidine analogues, stavudine in particular, in peripheral lipoatrophy has been revealed by different studies, which found a strong correlation between the presence of peripheral lipoatrophy and the use of these molecules [49]. In addition, in the MITOX study, when lipoatrophic patients were switched from thymidine analogs to abacavir, peripheral fat slowly increased [51], arguing again for the implication of thymidine analogs in lipoatrophy. Other switch studies, TARHEEL or RAVE found similar results [55, 56].

Increased apoptosis was reported in fat from patients undergoing treatment with PIs and NRTIs. Domingo [77] found that when the patients were switched from PIs to nevirapine, fat-cell apoptosis persisted. Otherwise, when patients were switched from stavudine to ABC, they recovered about 20% of peripheral fat after 1 year. However, increased mDNA level remained two times lower than that of control fat and even if apoptosis was reduced, it remained higher than that observed in control fat [55]. This adipose tissue toxicity could result from the ability of these molecules to induce mitochondrial dysfunction and alter adipokine secretion. In addition, the fact that apoptosis was only partly reverted argues in favor of a role for other ART, including PIs, in lipoatrophy (Fig. 8).

We have performed a study to evaluate the specific role of the different drugs in adipose tissue alterations. To that end, we examined the reversibility of adipose tissue alterations in HIV-infected patients after a 6-month (M6) interruption of ART; A 6-month ART interruption markedly improved adipose tissue functions, although fat distribution did not visibly change. Stavudine and zidovudine were associated with marked inflammation, which improved when these drugs were withdrawn; they also had a negative impact on differentiation and mitochondrial status. PI were also associated with altered adipocyte differentiation and mitochondrial status. These data clearly show the detrimental impact of antiretroviral drugs, and particularly thymidine analogues, on adipose tissue and argue for switch strategies sparing these drugs [78].

Pathophysiology of Increased Visceral Fat in HAART-Related Lipodystrophy

While the mechanisms responsible for peripheral lipoatrophy begin to be understood, as fat biopsies can be performed to analyze adipose tissue alterations, only speculative mechanisms can be proposed for visceral fat hypertrophy, since to date no results have been presented on fat from this location. One working hypothesis could refer to the presence of 11β-HSD1 in greater amounts in visceral than in subcutaneous fat, which will result in an increased synthesis of cortisol from cortisone and an endogenous activation of fat hypertrophy. Such a mechanism has been postulated in the classic metabolic syndrome.

In addition, TNF-α has been shown to activate this enzyme. If we hypothesize that TNF-α production is increased in HAART-treated patients due to the effect of therapeutic molecules, this could lead to an even greater activation of the enzyme. Moreover, Ledru et al. has shown that CD4 and CD8 lymphocytes in HAART-treated patients produced TNF-α and were resistant to TNF-α-induced apoptosis [79], which would further increase TNF-α levels. Otherwise, in subcutaneous fat, we observed the presence of activated macrophages that release TNF-α [75, 78]. This could also be the case in visceral fat as found in animal models of obesity [26, 27]. Therefore, it could be proposed that increased TNF-α could hyperactivate 11β-HSD 1 and result in an increased synthesis of cortisol inside the adipocytes, thereby favoring their hypertrophy. In addition, other hormones could modulate this enzyme: growth hormone (GH) and testosterone were found to inactivate the enzyme. It is interesting to note that HIV-infected patients with lipodystrophy often present a relative decrease in GH [80] and testosterone levels. Moreover, when patients with visceral fat hypertrophy were treated with GH, a reduction in the amount of visceral

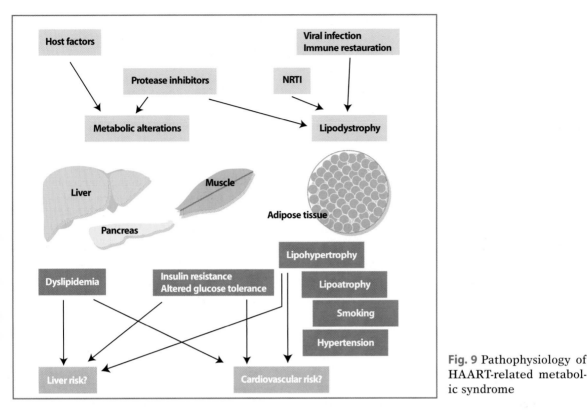

Fig. 9 Pathophysiology of HAART-related metabolic syndrome

fat was consistently reported [81] and reduced truncal adiposity has also been reported in another study with lipodystrophic HIV-infected patients [82].

Conclusion

Taken as a whole, ART-related metabolic syndrome could result from the combination of factors found in the metabolic syndrome observed in the general population and it could also result from factors related to the treatment, the infection, and the immune status specific to HIV infection. These factors will favor a proinflammatory, procoagulant, and proatherogenic state, which will worsen the situation (Fig. 9) leading to an increased occurrence of cardiovascular complications [83]. This is a major concern in patients who require continuous antiretroviral treatment to control viral infection and who can now expect prolonged life duration.

References

1. Grundy S, Cleeman JI, Daniels SR et al (2005) Diagnosis and management of the metabolic syndrome: an American heart association/national heart, lung, and blood institute scientific statement. Circulation 112:2735–2752
2. Day C (2007) Metabolic syndrome, or What you will: definitions and epidemiology. Diab Vasc Dis Res 4:32–38
3. Mondy K, Overton ET, Grubb J et al (2007) Metabolic syndrome in HIV-infected patients from an urban, midwestern US outpatient population. Clin Infect Dis 44:726–734
4. Jacobson DL, Tang AM, Spiegelman D et al (2006) Incidence of metabolic syndrome in a cohort of HIV-infected adults and prevalence relative to the US population (National Health and Nutrition Examination Survey). J Acquir Immune Defic Syndr 43:458–466
5. Bonfanti P, Ricci E, de Socio G et al; CISAI Study Group (2006) Metabolic syndrome: a real threat for HIV-positive patients?: results from the SIMONE study. J Acquir Immune Defic Syndr 42:128–131
6. Estrada V, Martinez-Larrad MT, Gonzalez-Sanchez JL et al (2006) Lipodystrophy and metabolic syndrome in HIV-infected patients

treated with antiretroviral therapy. Metabolism 55:940–945

7. Samaras K, Wand H, Law M et al (2007) Prevalence of metabolic syndrome in HIV-infected patients receiving highly active antiretroviral therapy using International Diabetes Foundation and Adult Treatment Panel III criteria: associations with insulin resistance, disturbed body fat compartmentalization, elevated C-reactive protein, and hypoadiponectinemia. Diabetes Care 30:113–119

8. Leow MK, Addy CL, Mantzoros CS (2003) Clinical review 159: Human immunodeficiency virus/highly active antiretroviral therapy-associated metabolic syndrome: clinical presentation, pathophysiology, and therapeutic strategies. J Clin Endocrinol Metab 88:1961–1976

9. Saltiel AR, Kahn CR (2001) Insulin signalling and the regulation of glucose and lipid metabolism. Nature 414:799–806

10. Randle PJ, Garland PB, Hales CN, Newsholme EA (1963) The glucose fatty-acid cycle: its role in insulin sensitivity and the metabolic disturbances of diabetes mellitus. Lancet 1:785–789

11. Perseghin G, Petersen K, Shulman GI (2003) Cellular mechanism of insulin resistance: potential links with inflammation. Int J Obes Relat Metab Disord 27(Suppl 3):S6–11

12. Fasshauer M, Paschke R (2003) Regulation of adipocytokines and insulin resistance. Diabetologia 46:1594–1603

13. Mattison RE, Jensen M (2003) The adipocyte as an endocrine cell. Curr Opin Endocrinol Diabetes 10317–10321

14. Rosen ED, Spiegelman BM (2006) Adipocytes as regulators of energy balance and glucose homeostasis. Nature 444:847–453

15. Matsuzawa Y, Funahashi T, Kihara S, Shimomura I (2004) Adiponectin and metabolic syndrome. Arterioscler Thromb Vasc Biol 24:29–33

16. Yamauchi T, Nio Y, Maki T et al (2007) Targeted disruption of AdipoR1 and AdipoR2 causes abrogation of adiponectin binding and metabolic actions. Nat Med 13:332–339

17. Ouchi N, Kihara S, Funahashi T et al (2003) Obesity, adiponectin and vascular inflammatory disease. Curr Opin Lipidol 14:561–566

18. Ruan H, Lodish HF (2003) Insulin resistance in adipose tissue: direct and indirect effects of tumor necrosis factor-alpha. Cytokine Growth Factor Rev 14:447–455

19. Lagathu C, Bastard JP, Auclair M et al (2003) Chronic interleukin-6 (IL-6) treatment increased IL-6 secretion and induced insulin resistance in adipocyte: prevention by rosiglitazone. Biochem Biophys Res Commun 311:372–379

20. Montague CT, O'Rahilly S (2000) The perils of portliness: causes and consequences of visceral adiposity. Diabetes 49:883–888

21. Lafontan M, Berlan M (2003) Do regional differences in adipocyte biology provide new pathophysiological insights? Trends Pharmacol Sci 24:276–283

22. Stulnig TM, Waldhausl W (2004) 11beta-hydroxysteroid dehydrogenase type 1 in obesity and type 2 diabetes. Diabetologia 47:1–11

23. Lewis GF, Carpentier A, Adeli K, Giacca A (2002) Disordered fat storage and mobilization in the pathogenesis of insulin resistance and type 2 diabetes. Endocr Rev 23:201–229

24. Gan SK, Kriketos AD, Poynten AM et al (2003) Insulin action, regional fat, and myocyte lipid: altered relationships with increased adiposity. Obes Res 11:1295–1305

25. Schaffer JE (2003) Lipotoxity: when tissues overeat. Curr Opin Lipidol 14:281–287

26. Wellen KE, Hotamisligil GS (2003) Obesity-induced inflammatory changes in adipose tissue. J Clin Invest 112:1785–1788

27. Weisberg SP, McCann D, Desai M et al (2003) Obesity is associated with macrophage accumulation in adipose tissue. J Clin Invest 112:1796–1808

28. Xu H, Barnes GT, Yang Q et al (2003) Chronic inflammation in fat plays a crucial role in the development of obesity-related insulin resistance. J Clin Invest 112:1821–1830

29. Cancello R, Tordjman J, Poitou C et al (2006) Increased infiltration of macrophages in omental adipose tissue is associated with marked hepatic lesions in morbid human obesity. Diabetes 55:1554–1561

30. Fernandez-Real JM, Ricart W (2003) Insulin resistance and chronic cardiovascular inflammatory syndrome. Endocr Rev 24:278–301

31. Moyle G (2007) Metabolic issues associated with protease inhibitors. J Acquir Immune Defic Syndr 45(Suppl 1):S19–26

32. Perret B, Ferrand C, Bonnet E et al (2003) Lipoprotein metabolism in HIV-positive patients. Eur J Med Res 8(Suppl II):6

33. Grinspoon SK (2005) Metabolic syndrome and cardiovascular disease in patients with human immunodeficiency virus. Am J Med 118(Suppl 2):23S–28S

34. Savès M, Raffi F, Capeau J et al (2002) Factors related to lipodystrophy and metabolic alterations in patients with human immunodeficiency virus infection receiving highly active antiretroviral therapy. Clin Infect Dis 34:1396–1405

35. Noor MA, Flint OP, Maa J et al (2006) Effects of atazanavir/ritonavir and lopinavir/ritonavir on glucose uptake on insulin sensitivity: demon-

strable differences in vitro and clinically. AIDS 20:1813–1821

36. Van der Valk M, Kastelein JJ, Murphy RL et al (2001) Nevirapine-containing antiretroviral therapy in HIV-1 infected patients results in an antiatherogenic lipid profile. AIDS 15:2407–2414

37. Carr A, Samaras K, Thorisdottir A et al (1999) Diagnosis, prediction, and natural course of HIV-1 protease-inhibitor-associated lipodystrophy, hyperlipidaemia, and diabetes mellitus: a cohort study. Lancet 353:2093–2099

38. Liang JS, Distler O, Cooper DA et al (2001) HIV protease inhibitors protect apolipoprotein B from degradation by the proteasome: a potential mechanism for protease inhibitor-induced hyperlipidemia. Nat Med 7:1327–1331

39. Lenhard JM, Croom DK et al (2000) HIV protease inhibitors stimulate hepatic triglyceride synthesis. Arterioscler Thromb Vasc Biol 20:2625–2629

40. Riddle TM, Kuhel DG, Woollett LA et al (2001) HIV protease inhibitor induces fatty acid and sterol biosynthesis in liver and adipose tissues due to the accumulation of activated sterol regulatory element-binding proteins in the nucleus. J Biol Chem 276:37514–37519

41. Bonnet E, Ruidavets JB, Tuech J et al (2001) Apoprotein c-III and E-containing lipoparticles are markedly increased in HIV-infected patients treated with protease inhibitors: association with the development of lipodystrophy. J Clin Endocrinol Metab 86:296–302

42. Lihn AS, Richelsen B, Pedersen SB et al (2003) Increased expression of TNF-alpha, IL-6, and IL-8 in HALS: implications for reduced adiponectin expression and plasma levels. Am J Physiol Endocrinol Metab 285:E1072–1080

43. Vigouroux C, Maachi M, Nguyen TH et al (2003) Serum adipocytokines are related to lipodystrophy and metabolic disorders in HIV-infected men under antiretroviral therapy. AIDS 17:1503–1511

44. Bastard JP, Pereira E, Reynes J et al (2007) Follow-up of lipodystrophy and metabolic alterations in the ANRS APROCO-COPILOTE studying HIV-infected patients initiated with protease inhibitors in 1997 and 1998: relation to adiponectin, leptin and triglycerides levels and to TNF polymorphisms. Antivir Ther L30, P-16 (abstract)

45. Ledergerber B, Furrer H, Rickenbach M et al (2007) Factors associated with the incidence of type 2 diabetes mellitus in HIV-infected participants in the Swiss HIV Cohort Study. Clin Infect Dis 45:111–119

46. Brown TT, Cole SR, Li X et al (2005) Antiretroviral therapy and the prevalence and incidence of diabetes mellitus in the multicenter AIDS cohort study. Arch Intern Med 1651179–1651184

47. Florescu D, Kotler DP (2007) Insulin resistance, glucose intolerance and diabetes mellitus in HIV-infected patients. Antivir Ther 12:149–162

48. Noor MA, Lo JC, Mulligan K et al (2001) Metabolic effects of indinavir in healthy HIV-seronegative men. AIDS 15:F11–18

49. Noor MA, Seneviratne T, Aweeka FT et al (2002) Indinavir acutely inhibits insulin-stimulated glucose disposal in humans: a randomized, placebo-controlled study. AIDS 29:F1–8

50. Bacchetti P, Gripshover B, Grunfeld C et al (2005) Fat distribution in men with HIV infection. J Acquir Immune Defic Syndr 40:121–131

51. Martin A, Smith DE, Carr A et al (2004) Reversibility of lipoatrophy in HIV-infected patients 2 years after switching from a thymidine analogue to abacavir: the MITOX Extension Study. AIDS 18:1029–1036

52. Jemsek JG, Arathoon E, Arlotti M et al (2006) Body fat and other metabolic effects of atazanavir and efavirenz, each administered in combination with zidovudine plus lamivudine, in antiretroviral-naive HIV-infected patients. Clin Infect Dis 42:273–280

53. Johnson M, Grinsztejn B, Rodriguez C et al (2006) 96-week comparison of once-daily atazanavir/ritonavir and twice-daily lopinavir/ritonavir in patients with multiple virologic failures. AIDS 20:711–718

54. Fisac C, Fumero E, Crespo M et al (2005) Metabolic benefits 24 months after replacing a protease inhibitor with abacavir, efavirenz or nevirapine. AIDS 19:917–925

55. McComsey GA, Paulsen DM, Lonergan JT et al (2005) Improvements in lipoatrophy, mitochondrial DNA levels and fat apoptosis after replacing stavudine with abacavir or zidovudine. AIDS 19:15–23

56. Moyle GJ, Sabin CA, Cartledge J et al (2006) A randomized comparative trial of tenofovir DF or abacavir as replacement for a thymidine analogue in persons with lipoatrophy. AIDS 20:2043–2050

57. Cherry CL, Lal L, Thompson KA et al (2005) Increased adipocyte apoptosis in lipoatrophy improves within 48 weeks of switching patient therapy from Stavudine to abacavir or zidovudine. J Acquir Immune Defic Syndr 38:263–267

58. Mallal SA, John M, Moore CB et al (2000) Contribution of nucleoside analogue reverse transcriptase inhibitors to subcutaneous fat wasting in patients with HIV infection. AIDS 14:1309–1316

59. Miller J, Carr A, Emery S et al (2003) HIV lipodystrophy: prevalence, severity and corre-

lates of risk in Australia. HIV Med 4:293–301

60. Gougeon M-L, Pénicaud L, Fromenty B et al (2004) Adipocytes targets and actors in the pathogenesis of HIV-associated lipodystrophy and metabolic alterations. Antivir Ther 9:161–177

61. Caron M, Auclair M, Vigouroux C et al (2001) The HIV protease inhibitor indinavir impairs sterol regulatory element-binding protein-1 intranuclear localization, inhibits preadi-pocyte differentiation, and induces insulin resistance. Diabetes 50:1378–1388

62. Caron M, Auclair M, Sterlingot H et al (2003) Some HIV protease inhibitors alter lamin A/C maturation and stability, SREBP-1 nuclear local-ization and adipocyte differentiation. AIDS 17:2437–2444

63. Caron M, Auclair M, Donadille B et al (2007) Human lipodystrophies linked to mutations in A-type lamins and to HIV protease inhibitor therapy are both associated with prelamin A accumulation, oxidative stress and premature cellular senescence. Cell Death Differ (in press)

64. Krimm I, Ostlund C, Gilquin B et al (2002)The Ig-like structure of the C-terminal domain of lamin A/C, mutated in muscular dystrophies, cardiomyopathy, and partial lipodystrophy. Structure (Camb) 10:811–823

65. Lloyd DJ, Trembath RC, Shackleton S (2002) A novel interaction between lamin A and SREBP1: implications for partial lipodystrophy and other laminopathies. Hum Mol Genet 11:769–777

66. Vigouroux C, Auclair M, Dubosclard E et al (2001) Nuclear envelope disorganization in fibroblasts from lipodystrophic patients with heterozygous R482Q/W mutations in the lamin A/C gene. J Cell Sci 114:4459–4468

67. Jones SP, Janneh O, Back DJ et al (2005) Altered adipokine response in murine 3T3-F442A adipocytes treated with protease inhibitors and nucleoside reverse transcriptase inhibitors. Antivir Ther 10:207–213

68. Lagathu C, Bastard JP, Auclair M et al (2004) Antiretroviral drugs with adverse effects on adipocyte lipid metabolism and survival alter the expression and secretion of proinflammato-ry cytokines and adiponectin in vitro. Antivir Ther 9:911–920

69. Lagathu C, Eustace B, Prot M et al (2007) Some HIV antiretrovirals increase oxidative stress and alter chemokine, cytokine or adiponectin production in human adipocytes and macrophages. Antivir Ther 12:489–500

70. Caron M, Auclair M, Lagathu C et al (2004) The HIV-1 nucleoside reverse transcriptase inhibitors stavudine and zidovudine alter adipocyte functions in vitro. AIDS 18:2127–2136

71. Bastard JP, Caron M, Vidal H et al (2002) Associ-ation between altered expression of adipogenic factor SREBP1 in lipoatrophic adipose tissue from HIV-1-infected patients and abnormal adipocyte differentiation and insulin resistance. Lancet 359:1026–1031

72. Domingo P, Matias-Guiu X, Pujol RM et al (1999) Subcutaneous adipocyte apoptosis in HIV-1 protease inhibitor-associated lipodystro-phy. AIDS 13:2261–2267

73. Nolan D, Hammond E, Martin A et al (2003) Mitochondrial DNA depletion and morphologic changes in adipocytes associated with nucleo-side reverse transcriptase inhibitor therapy. AIDS 17:1329–1338

74. Lloreta J, Domingo P, Pujol RM et al (2002) Ultrastructural features of highly active anti-retroviral therapy-associated partial lipodystro-phy. Virchows Arch 441:599–604

75. Jan V, Cervera P, Maachi M et al (2004) Altered fat differentiation and adipocytokine expres-sion are inter-related and linked to morphologi-cal changes and insulin resistance in HIV-1-infected lipodystrophic patients. Antivir Ther 9:555–564

76. Sutinen J, Korsheninnikova E, Funahashi T et al (2003) Circulating concentration of adiponectin and its expression in subcutaneous adipose tis-sue in patients with highly active antiretroviral therapy-associated lipodystrophy. J Clin Endocrinol Metab 88:1907–1910

77. Domingo P, Matias-Guiu X, Pujol RM et al (2001) Switching to nevirapine decreases insulin levels but does not improve subcuta-neous adipocyte apoptosis in patients with high-ly active antiretroviral therapy-associated lipodystrophy. J Infect Dis 184:1197–1201

78. Kim M et al (2007) A six-month interruption of antiretroviral therapy improves adipose tissue function in HIV-infected patients: the ANRS EP29 Lipostrop Study. Antivir Ther 12:1273–1283

79. Ledru E, Christeff N, Patey O et al (2000) Alter-ation of tumor necrosis factor-alpha T-cell home-ostasis following potent antiretroviral therapy: contribution to the development of human immunodeficiency virus-associated lipodystro-phy syndrome. Blood 95:3191–3198

80. Rietschel P, Hadigan C, Corcoran C et al (2001) Assessment of growth hormone dynamics in human immunodeficiency virus-related lipodys-trophy. J Clin Endocrinol Metab 86:504–510

81. Lo JC, Mulligan K, Noor MA et al (2001) The effects of recombinant human growth hormone on body composition and glucose metabolism in HIV-infected patients with fat accumulation. J Clin Endocrinol Metab 86:3480–3487

82. Luzi L, Meneghini E, Oggionni S et al (2005) GH

treatment reduces trunkal adiposity in HIV-infected patients with lipodystrophy: a randomized placebo-controlled study. Eur J Endocrinol 153:781–789

83. Friis-Møller N, Reiss P, Sabin CA et al; DAD Study Group (2007) Class of antiretroviral drugs and the risk of myocardial infarction. N Engl J Med 356:1723–1735

Chapter 4

Pathology of Cardiac Complications in HIV Infection

G. Barbaro

Pathology of the Myocardium

The prevalence of myocardial abnormalities in HIV-infected patients ranges from 25 to 75% [1]. This wide range probably reflects differences in methodology, patients' risk factors, disease stage, and environmental factors such as drug addiction or therapeutic agents. Myocardial involvement in HIV-infected patients includes dilated cardiomyopathy, myocarditis, ischemic heart disease, and neoplastic invasion from HIV-associated malignancies (e.g., non-Hodgkin's lymphoma or Kaposi's sarcoma). In addition, the right ventricle can be involved as a consequence of AIDS-related pulmonary disease.

Dilated Cardiomyopathy

The reported prevalence of this heart condition ranges between 5 and 23% of autopsy studies [1–3].

Pathologic Features

Pathologic features of AIDS-related cardiomyopathy are similar to those observed in seronegative patients. At autopsy, because of ventricular dilation and apical rounding, the heart shape is modified. Heart weight is generally increased, owing to fibrosis and myocyte hypertrophy [1]. On average, long-term survivors have significantly heavier hearts than those dying after a brief disease course. The epicardium is usually normal and coronary arteries do not show significant atherosclerosis. The myocardium is rather flabby and the ventricular wall usually collapses on section [1].

On the cut surface, the ventricles show an eccentric hypertrophy, that is, a mass increase with chamber volume enlargement. Although hypertrophy is demonstrated by the increase in cardiac weight, this is not always grossly evident owing to ventricular dilation; the free wall width may be normal, or even thinner than normal, as happens in short-term survivors. Endocardial fibrosis is a common finding, as well as mural thrombi, mainly located at the apex. Dilated cardiomyopathy can be associated with pericardial effusion or infective endocarditis, especially in intravenous drug abusers [1].

On histology, myocytes show variable degrees of hypertrophy and degenerative changes such as myofibril loss, causing hydropic changes within the myocyte. An increase in interstitial and endocardial fibrillar collagen is a constant feature in this cardiomyopathy [1–3].

Myocarditis

Myocarditis is documented at autopsy in up to 50% of AIDS patients who died from noncardiac causes [2] and in 31–83% of patients with clinical signs of congestive heart failure [1]. It can be part of a disseminated infection, resulting from opportunistic microorganisms such as *Candida albicans*, *Cryptococcus neoformans*, and *Toxoplasma gondii*. It most often shows histological features of lymphocytic myocarditis, suggestive of a viral etiology. In fact, the presence of coxsackievirus B3, cytomegalovirus, and Epstein-Barr virus has been reported from autopsy samples from HIV-infected patients [1]. In addition, HIV-1 nucleic acid sequences have been detected by in situ hybridization in autopsy samples of patients with left ventricular dysfunction [1], most of whom had active myocarditis on histology.

Pathologic Findings

On gross examination, a marked dilation of the cardiac chambers is almost always present. In most cases, owing to the focal distribution of inflammation and myocyte necrosis, the myocardium is not flabby as it is in hearts with a diffuse inflammatory response. Heart weight is within normal limits. According to the Dallas criteria [4], active myocarditis is characterized by multi-focal or diffuse interstitial inflammatory infiltrates associated with degenerative changes or frank myocyte necrosis (Fig. 1). Histological findings in HIV-infected patients with myocarditis do not substantially differ from those observed in seronegative patients. However, the degree of inflammatory infiltrate is generally milder. This is believed to result from the impaired efficiency of cell-mediated immunity [2]. In addition, the inflammatory infiltrate is mainly made by CD8+ lymphocytes, and aberrant expression of class II human leukocyte antigens (HLA) by cardiac myocytes is much rarer than in HIV-negative myocarditis [5]. The severity of clinical symptoms is not always related to the degree of myocardial inflammation and damage. Autopsy studies of AIDS patients who died of acute left ventricular dysfunction almost invariably show a marked inflammatory infiltrate [2]. However, mild and focal mononuclear infiltrates are frequently observed in hearts of AIDS patients, irrespective of the presence of cardiac symptoms.

Histology and immunohistochemistry rarely detect the presence of viruses in the myocardium. However, in situ hybridization

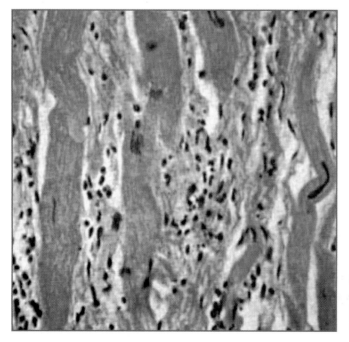

Fig. 1 AIDS-related active lymphocytic myocarditis. There is a marked interstitial lymphocytic infiltrate and myocyte necrosis. H&E, x20

or polymerase chain reaction studies reveal a high frequency of either cytomegalovirus or HIV-1, or both, in AIDS patients with lymphocytic myocarditis and severe left ventricular dysfunction [1, 6] (Fig. 2). These data support the hypothesis that, at least in a subset of patients, HIV-1 has a pathogenic action and possibly influences the clinical evolution towards dilated cardiomyopathy [2, 3].

Opportunistic myocardial infection is generally part of systemic infections. Fungal lesions are visible on gross examination as multiple, small, rounded plaques of whitish color, often hemorrhagic. On histology, the pathogens most frequently observed are protozoa such as *T. gondii*, or fungi such as *Candida albicans*, *Cryptococcus neoformans*, and *Aspergillus* spp. [2, 3]. Myocardial and cerebral toxoplasmosis are often associated; histological examination shows "pseudocysts" packed with the protozoa within cardiac myocytes [2, 3]. Bacterial myocarditis is not infrequent in HIV-infected drug addicts with infective endocarditis. It is a consequence of coronary embolization from valve vegetations [2].

Ischemic Heart Disease

The association between viral infection (cytomegalovirus or HIV-1 itself) and coronary artery lesions is not clear. HIV-1 sequences have been detected by in situ hybridization in the coronary vessels of an HIV-infected patient who died from acute myocardial infarction (Fig. 3) [7]. Potential mechanisms through which HIV-1 may damage coronary arteries include activation of cytokines and cell-adhesion molecules and alteration of major histocompatibility complex class I molecules on the surface of smooth muscle cells [7]. It is possible also that HIV-1-associated protein gp 120 may induce smooth muscle cell apoptosis through a mitochondrion-controlled pathway by activation of inflammatory cytokines (e.g., TNF-α) [8]. The incidence of ischemic heart disease is apparently increasing among HIV-infected patients receiving protease inhibitor-based highly active antiretroviral therapy (HAART), especially in those who develop HAART-associated meta-

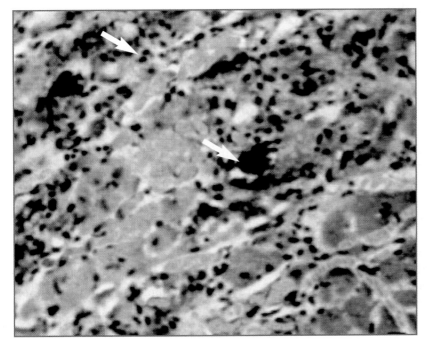

Fig. 2 In situ hybridization from an endomyocardial biopsy sample in an HIV-infected subject with echocardiographic diagnosis of dilated cardiomyopathy (left ventricular ejection fraction: 28%) and histologic diagnosis of active myocarditis. It is possible to observe two myocytes showing a positive signal for nucleic sequences of HIV-1 (*arrows*). H&E, x20

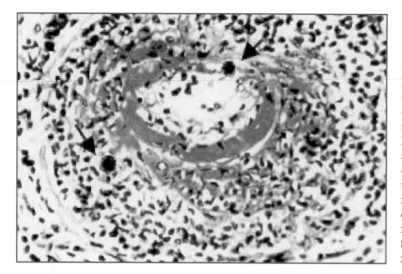

Fig. 3 In situ hybridization of an HIV-1 RNA probe in a transverse section of a branch of the anterior descending coronary artery. Intense staining indicating the presence of HIV-1 sequences within the intima and the media (*arrows*). There is a dense lymphocyte infiltrate within the media and necrosis of the intima, which is covered with swollen endothelial cells. (From [7], Copyright© 2001 Massachusetts Medical Society. All right reserved). H&E, x280

bolic syndrome during therapy [9]. However, studies on the risk of coronary heart disease in this subset of patients remain controversial [10–14].

Pathologic examination of coronary arteries generally reveals eccentric fibroatheromatous plaques with variable degrees of chronic inflammatory infiltrates. Lesions with morphologic features similar to accelerated arteriosclerosis have been described at autopsy of young HIV-infected patients [2, 3]. The pathology of coronary and peripheral vessels in HIV infection is described in detail by A. Tabib and R. Loire in a separate chapter in this volume.

Conduction System Involvement

Conduction tissue damage can be due to lymphocytic myocarditis, opportunistic infections, and drug cardiotoxicity or to the localization of HIV within the conduction system myocytes. Histological examination may reveal a lymphomonocytic infiltration, myocyte degenerative changes, and fibrosis. These changes can be associated with electrocardiographic abnormalities, most frequently first-degree atrioventricular block, left anterior hemiblock, and left bundle block [1].

Malignancies

The prevalence of cardiac Kaposi's sarcoma (KS) in AIDS patients ranged from 12 to 28% in retrospective autopsy studies in the pre-HAART period [3]. Cardiac involvement with KS usually occurs when widespread visceral organ involvement is present. The lesions are typically less than 1 cm in size and may be pericardial or, less frequently, myocardial, and are only rarely associated with obstruction, dysfunction, morbidity, or mortality [8]. Microscopically, there are atypical spindle cells lining slit-like vascular spaces (Fig. 4).

Non-Hodgkin's lymphoma (NHL) involving the heart is infrequent in AIDS [15]. Most cases are high-grade B-cell (small non-cleaved) Burkitt-like lymphomas, with the rest classified as diffuse large B-cell lymphomas (in the REAL classification; Fig. 5). Lymphomatous lesions may appear grossly as either localized or more diffuse nodular to polypoid masses [16, 17]. Most involve the pericardium, with variable myocardial infiltration [16, 17]. There is little or no accompanying inflammation and necrosis. The prognosis of patients with HIV-associated cardiac lymphoma is generally poor because of widespread organ involvement, although some patients treated with combi-

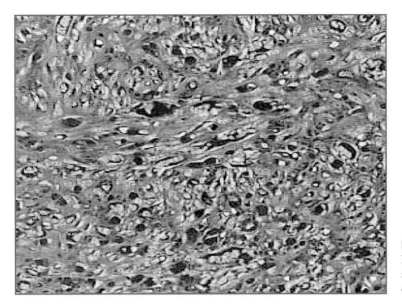

Fig. 4 Myocardial involvement by Kaposi's sarcoma. Histology shows spindle cells surrounding slit-like capillary vessels. H&E, x40

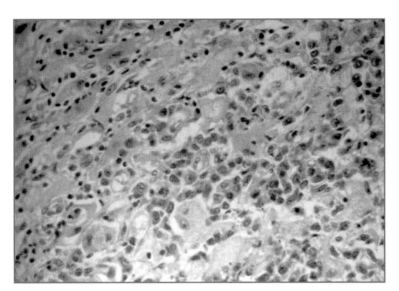

Fig. 5 Myocardial infiltration by large cell non-Hodgkin's lymphoma, associated with myocardial damage. H&E, x40

nation chemotherapy have experienced clinical remission [18].

The introduction of HAART has reduced the incidence of cardiac involvement by KS and NHL, perhaps attributable to patients' improved immunologic state and to suppression of opportunistic infections with Human Herpes Virus-8 and Epstein-Barr virus that are known to play an etiologic role in these neoplasms [18].

Isolated Right Ventricular Hypertrophy and Dilation

Right ventricular hypertrophy and/or dilation, often associated with pericardial effusion, can be observed in the clinical course of HIV infection. This finding is related to the presence of pulmonary hypertension, which can be due to pulmonary infections, to diffuse alveolar damage, or to recurrent pulmonary emboli from intravenous debris acquired through drug abuse [1]. In addition, the occurrence of right-sided infective endocarditis related to the high frequency of intravenous drug use among HIV-infected patients may explain right ventricular overload or recurrent pulmonary embolic events [2].

Pathology of the Endocardium

Non-bacterial Thrombotic Endocarditis

Non-bacterial thrombotic endocarditis has been reported with increasing frequency in HIV-infected patients in the terminal stage of the disease. This process, commonly associated with chronic severe wasting diseases, particularly malignancies, and severe inanition, was observed before the introduction of HAART in 3–5% of AIDS patients at autopsy [1–3].

Pathologic Findings

Non-bacterial thrombotic endocarditis can involve all four cardiac valves [2]. Macroscopic examination reveals thrombi adherent to the endocardial surface of the valve cusps, consisting microscopically of platelets within a fibrin mesh with few inflammatory cells. Thrombotic vegetations may be either single or multiple polypoid masses, along the cusp apposition lines. The valve often shows changes due to previous inflammatory or dystrophic lesions [3].

Thrombotic vegetations of non-bacterial thrombotic endocarditis are similar to those found in infective endocarditis; the differential diagnosis is based on the absence of the other typical features of infective endocarditis such as destruction and erosion of the cusp edges with tears and perforations through the body of the cusp itself, and valvular leaflet aneurysmal sacs [3]. Moreover, no infective pathogens are detected on histological examination. Systemic or pulmonary embolization of vegetations is usually detected at autopsy (more than 40% of patients with non-bacterial thrombotic endocarditis) and is underestimated clinically. Often, clinical symptoms of systemic thromboembolization (cerebral, pulmonary, renal, and splenic infarcts) make the valvular lesions clinically obvious. However, systemic thromboembolic disease due to non-bacterial thrombotic endocarditis is a rare cause of death (7%) in AIDS patients [1]. The vegetations in non-bacterial thrombotic endocarditis may be infected by pyogenic or fungal pathogens during a transient bacteremia, bringing about a typical infective endocarditis.

Infective Endocarditis

Infective endocarditis may be due to either pyogenic or opportunistic pathogens. In the latter case, they are often part of a systemic opportunistic infection with multiple organ localizations. Fungal endocarditis has been reported with increasing frequency as the AIDS epidemic has gained momentum, helped by the compromise of cell-mediated immunity in patients with HIV infection [2, 3].

Infective endocarditis occurs more frequently in intravenous drug users with AIDS, who comprise the second largest risk group for HIV infection after male homosexuals. These patients have frequent bacteremias, owing to the introduction of skin pathogens and talcum powder by unsterile intravenous injection, causing a higher risk of endocardial infection of right-sided cardiac valves. Infective endocarditis is higher in intravenous drug addicts who abuse multiple drugs (cocaine used intravenously in combination with heroin) in addition to alcohol.

The spectrum of pathogens responsible for endocardial infection in intravenous drug users with AIDS is not significantly different from that in HIV-uninfected drug users. However, owing to the deficit in cellular immunity, the pathogens are more virulent, leading to more significant cardiac structural damage and functional deterioration. Pyogenic bacteria more commonly causing infective endocarditis in AIDS are *Staphylococcus aureus*, *Staphylococcus epidermidis*, *Streptococcus pneumoniae*, and *Haemophilus influenzae* [2]. Infective endocarditis by Gram-negative bacteria, especially *Pseudomonas* species, has become more common in patients with AIDS, perhaps owing to the repeated hospitalizations that promote the acquisition of resistant organisms. Avirulent bacteria such as the HACEK group (*Haemophilus* species, *Actinobacillus actinomycetemcomitans*, *Cardiobacterium hominis*, *Eikenella corrodens* and *Kingella kingae*), which are often part of the endogenous flora of the mouth, can cause endocarditis in HIV-infected patients [2]. These bacteria are also difficult to culture from endocardial vegetations. Failure to obtain positive blood cultures in those patients with AIDS with strong clinical evidence for infective endocarditis should suggest prior antibiotic therapy or endocarditis by unusual bacteria (as well as HACEK organisms) or fungi.

Fungal endocarditis, especially from *Cryptococcus neoformans*, *Candida albicans*, or *Aspergillus fumigatus*, is common in AIDS, particularly in intravenous drug abusers [2, 3]. It is generally related to systemic spread of fungal infection from extracardiac foci. Candidiasis of the oropharynx and esophagus is most often the primary focus, often progressing to systemic infection. Systemic cryptococcosis is one of the most common infections in AIDS patients. Although meningitis and encephalitis are the most frequent manifestations of cryptococcosis, cardiac involvement, particularly with pericardial effusion, is common [2]. Fungal myocarditis or myocardial abscesses may also occur in association with valve destruction [2].

Pathologic Features

Infective endocarditis is an ulcerative-polypous lesion due to a destructive valve process with thrombotic stratifications (Fig. 6). Thrombotic vegetations are usually gray,

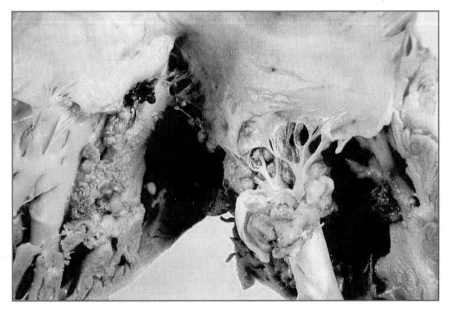

Fig. 6 *Staphylococcus aureus* endocarditis in an HIV-infected drug addicts who died of cardiogenic shock. The mitral valve shows numerous, large, grayish and friable vegetations. Involvement of the atrial endocardium is also shown. (Courtesy of Prof. D. Scevola, Department of Infectious and Parasitic Disease, University of Pavia, Italy)

but their color is highly variable depending on the pathogen involved [2]. They are generally located on the endocardial surface of valve cusps but can be found also on mural endocardium. Their consistence is variable: they are friable at first and later become compact and adherent to the endocardium, owing to their organization. The friability is increased by lithic effects of bacteria and polymorphonuclear leukocytes [2, 3]. Valvular tissue destruction may involve the tensive apparatus with chordae tendinous rupture. Endocardial ulcerations at the cusp apposition lines are frequent, resulting in leaflets with a mouth-eaten look. On histology, thrombotic vegetations consist of fibrin and agglutinated platelets with inflammatory infiltration [3]. In the acute stage of endocardial infection, there is an infiltration with polymorphonuclear leukocytes with valve tissue necrosis; later there is a chronic inflammatory infiltration, made up of macrophages, lymphocytes and plasma cells, neoformed capillary vessels, and a fibroblastic proliferation that replaces the necrotic tissue and spreads at the base of thrombotic vegetation. In fungal endocarditis, however, the vegetations are made up essentially of fungal colonies without much fibrin and they may be so bulky that they obstruct the valve ostium [2, 3].

When the left-side cardiac valves are involved, endocarditis can have a galloping course, with rapid onset of heart failure due to acute valvular insufficiency secondary to perforation of valve leaflets or a rupture of the tendinous chordae or papillary muscles [2]. Other complications are due to myocardial involvement with possible perforation of the ventricular septum or myocardial abscesses. The infection can extend to the pericardium with purulent pericarditis. The higher frequency of right-sided infectious endocarditis in HIV-infected intravenous drug users can explain the pulmonary embolic events with possible pulmonary cavitations and abscesses [2, 3]. The out-come is thrombus organization and fibrous repair. Residual bulky thrombotic polypi are often seen as calcific masses leaning out of both endocardial surfaces of the valvular leaflets [2].

Pathology of the Pericardium

Pericardial Effusions

Before the introduction of HAART, the prevalence of pericardial effusion in asymptomatic AIDS patients was estimated at 11% per year [19]. Although prospective data are lacking, retrospective data suggest that HAART has reduced the overall incidence of pericardial effusion in HIV disease by about 30% [20]. Most pericardial effusions are idiopathic. Infections, neoplasias, myocarditis, endocarditis, or myocardial infarct have been described as possible etiologies. Little is known about the pathogenesis of pericardial effusions in AIDS patients. However, in the absence of cardiac infection or malignancy, the pathogenesis is likely to be multifactorial. The causes can be metabolic or hemodynamic alterations, dysproteinemias, or pulmonary hypertension due to chronic lung disease (i.e., cytomegalovirus pneumonia). The presence of HIV-1 in macrophages inside the pericardium suggests that the virus may play a role in the pathogenesis of pericardial effusions in AIDS patients.

Pericarditis

Pericarditis is found at autopsy in 30% of AIDS patients [1]. It can be serous, fibrinous, serofibrinous, purulent, or hemorrhagic [2, 3]. Pericardial phlogosis may be caused by a wide array of pathogens, always in conjunction with disseminated infection.

Mycobacterium tuberculosis hominis and *M. avium-intracellulare*, herpes simplex (by culture only), *Actinomycetales* (*Nocardia asteroides*), and bacteria such as *Staphylococcus aureus* and *Salmonella typhimurium* may be identified in pericardial fluid, even though in a few cases no pathogens can be isolated [1]. Fungal infections by *Candida albicans*, *Cryptococcus neoformans*, and *Aspergillus fumigatus* do not often involve the pericardium [2]. The pericardium may also be involved by non-mycobacterial infections such as *Actinomycetales* (*N. asteroides* or *Streptomyces* species). Whereas pericardial disease in the immunocompetent host may be associated with a variety of viruses, most commonly coxsackievirus, pericardial involvement in AIDS is more frequently related to infection with other common viral pathogens, especially herpes simplex virus type 1 and 2 and cytomegalovirus [2].

Pathologic Features

The most common type of pericarditis is fibrinous or serofibrinous (Fig. 7). There is a variable amount of fibrin on the epicardium, while pericardial effusion may be absent or present in variable degrees [2]. Many cases of fibrinous pericarditis resolve

without residual effects. In other instances, the fibrin deposits organize and form fibrous pericardial adhesions [2, 3]. Bacterial pericarditis is characterized by a fibrinopurulent exudate. On histology, an infiltrate of polymorphonuclear leukocytes is seen in the epicardial connective tissue. Fibrous adhesions may result, leading to pericardial constriction. Hemorrhagic pericarditis shows a serofibrinous or suppurative exudate associated with the presence of serohematic fluid in the pericardium. It is typical of tuberculosis, severe bacterial infections, or pericardial malignancy [2].

Malignancies

Kaposi's Sarcoma

When Kaposi's sarcoma involves the heart, the epicardial surface is a common site of involvement. At autopsy, the pericardium and the epicardial fat show the typical nodular coalescent dark-red lesions or violaceous plaques [2, 3]. Occasionally, the myocardium may also be involved. Typically, the neoplastic infiltration then extends along the great vessels and the coronary vessels with spread of tumor through the lymph channels along the vasa vasorum [2].

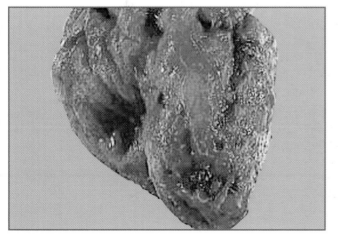

Fig. 7 Fibrinous pericarditis by *Mycobacterium avium intracellulare* in an HIV-infected subject who died of congestive heart failure. (Courtesy of Prof. D. Scevola, Department of Infectious and Parasitic Disease, University of Pavia, Italy)

Lymphomas

In contrast to non-Hodgkin's lymphomas in seronegative patients, which are epicardial or pericardial in location, in AIDS patients, the tumor is most often located within the myocardium or in the subendocardial layer [2]. There may be pericardial effusion, with a mass lesion of the heart sometimes prolapsing across the tricuspid valve or involving the inferior portions of both ventricles.

References

1. Barbaro G, Di Lorenzo G, Grisorio B, Barbarini G and the Gruppo Italiano per lo Studio Cardiologico dei pazienti affetti da AIDS Investigators (1998) Cardiac involvement in the acquired immunodeficiency syndrome: a multicenter clinical-pathological study. AIDS Res Hum Retroviruses 14:1071–7107

2. D'Amati G, Di Gioia CRT, Gallo P (2001) Pathological findings of HIV-associated cardiovascular disease. Ann NY Acad Sci 946:23–45

3. Klatt EC (2003) Cardiovascular pathology in AIDS. Adv Cardiol 40:23–48

4. Aretz HT (1987) Myocarditis: the Dallas criteria. Hum Pathol 18:619–624

5. Barbaro G, Di Lorenzo G, Soldini M et al (1999) Intensity of myocardial expression of inducible nitric oxide synthase influences the clinical course of human immunodeficiency virus-associated cardiomyopathy. Circulation 100:933–939

6. Herskowitz A, Tzyy-Choou W, Willoughby SB et al (1994) Myocarditis and cardiotropic viral infection associated with severe left ventricular dysfunction in late-stage infection with human immunodeficiency virus. J Am Coll Cardiol 24:1025–1032

7. Barbaro G, Barbarini G, Pellicelli AM (2001) HIV-associated coronary arteritis in a patient with fatal myocardial infarction. N Engl J Med 344:1799–1800

8. Twu C, Liu QN, Popik W et al (2002) Cardiomyocytes undergo apoptosis in human immunodeficiency virus cardiomyopathy through mito-

chondrion and death receptor-controlled pathways. Proc Natl Acad Sci USA 99:14386–14391

9. Barbaro G, Klatt EC (2003) Highly active antiretroviral therapy and cardiovascular complications in HIV-infected patients. Curr Pharm Des 9:1475–1481

10. Holmberg SD, Moorman AC, Williamson JM et al (2002) Protease inhibitors and cardiovascular outcomes in patients with HIV-1. Lancet 360:1747–1748

11. Barbaro G, Di Lorenzo G, Cirelli A et al (2003) An open-label, prospective, observational study of the incidence of coronary artery disease in patients with HIV receiving highly active antiretroviral therapy. Clin Ther 25:2405–2418

12. Friis-Moller N, Weber R, Reiss P et al (2003) Cardiovascular risk factors in HIV patients: association with antiretroviral therapy. Results from DAD study. AIDS 17:1179–1193

13. Bozzette SA, Ake CF, Tam HK et al (2003) Cardiovascular and cerebrovascular events in patients treated for human immunodeficiency virus infection. N Engl J Med 348:702–710

14. The Data Collection on Adverse Events of Anti-HIV Drugs (DAD) Study Group (2003). Combination antiretroviral therapy and the risk of myocardial infarction. N Engl J Med 349: 1993–2003

15. Barbaro G, Di Lorenzo G, Grisorio B, Barbarini G and the Gruppo Italiano per lo Studio Cardiologico dei pazienti affetti da AIDS investigators (1998) Cardiac involvement in the acquired immunodeficiency syndrome: a multicenter clinical-pathological study. AIDS Res Hum Retroviruses 14:1071–1077

16. Duong M, Dubois C, Buisson M et al (1997) Non-Hodgkin's lymphoma of the heart in patients infected with human immunodeficiency virus. Clin Cardiol 20:497–502

17. Sanna P, Bertoni F, Zucca E et al (1998) Cardiac involvement in HIV-related non-Hodgkin's lymphoma: a case report and short review of the literature. Ann Hematol 77:75–78

18. Dal Maso L, Serraino D, Franceschi S (2001) Epidemiology of HIV-associated malignancies. Cancer Treat Res 104:1–18

19. Heidenreich PA, Eisenberg MJ, Kee LL et al (1995) Pericardial effusion in AIDS: incidence and survival. Circulation 92:3229–3234

20. Pugliese A, Isnardi D, Saini A et al (2000) Impact of highly active antiretroviral therapy in HIV-positive patients with cardiac involvement. J Infect 40:282–284

Chapter 5

Pathology of Peripheral and Coronary Vessels in AIDS Patients

A. Tabib, R. Loire

HIV infection can provoke vascular complications, although they are not presently viewed as one of its most serious manifestations [1]. HIV vascular complications are general infective vascular diseases [2]. Most of the cases presented in this chapter occurred before the advent of highly active antiretroviral therapy (HAART) and mostly in AIDS patients because the majority of pathology examinations were done during necropsy.

Vasculitis

Microcirculation lesions are well documented by biopsies of the nervous system and muscles in AIDS peripheral neuromuscular localizations. In a cohort study published before HAART, vasculitis was present in 24% of biopsy samples from 225 patients: 12 cytomegalovirus vasculitis, 19 "micro-vasculitis," and 1 giant cells arteritis case [3]. Kieburtz et al. [4] described *Candida albicans* vasculitis with thrombosis and a cerebral infarction due to cytomegalovirus vasculitis in AIDS patients.

Peripheral Arterial Localizations

Clinical reports and systematic necropsies of AIDS patients pointed out arterial lesions. Kieburtz et al. [4] reported brain infarction in 20% of autopsies, Engstrom et al. [5] described 25 clinical cases. Joshi et al. [6] described arterial lesions in kidneys, spleen, thymus, and muscles in five children aged 1–7 years, including luminal narrowing with intima fibrosis, internal elastic lamina fragmentation, and calcifications.

Husson et al. [7] in a cohort of 250 HIV-infected children noted the appearance of two fusiform cerebral aneurysms. Rautonen et al. [8] pointed out clinical and anatomic similarities with Kawasaki's disease, which may be due to a retrovirus organism. Capron et al. [9] described toe embolism in four HIV male patients (40–56 years old) from aortic and femoral ulcerated atherosclerotic plaques. Kabus and Greco [10] described gross intimal aortic lesions at autopsy, resembling gelatiniform syphilitic ones in children with AIDS. Clinical information about vasculitis and peripheral arterial disease in HIV infection is given by P. Mercié et al. in a separate chapter in this volume.

Venous Thrombosis

Some authors described deep venous thrombosis in AIDS, an unsurprising complication in severely bedridden patients. Confusion is possible between pulmonary embolisms and opportunistic pulmonary infections, according to Pulik et al. [11]. Deep venous thrombosis and related coagulation disorder in HIV infection are described in detail by L. Drouet in a separate chapter in this volume.

Coronary Artery Lesions

It was a surprise for us to discover, during post-mortem examination, many severe latent coronary artery lesions occurring in very young (23–31 years old) AIDS patients [1]. Both hospital and forensic necropsies were performed. The death causes were not linked with coronary lesions except in one of five sudden death cases without other pathology. Clinical coronary disease symptoms were absent in all patients. The patients were homosexuals or drug addicts or both. Pathological analysis used transverse sections taken every 0.5 cm along the epicardial routes of the three main coronary trunks. Sections obtained every 1 cm were fixed in Bouin's solution, then embedded in paraffin for histopathological study, together with representative fragments of the left and right ventricular walls and interventricular septum making up the distal coronary network. Histological sections were stained with hemalum-phloxine-saffron and with Weigert's resorcin-fuchsin method. Every coronary examination of AIDS patients pointed out gross and microscopic lesions (100%), although a comparative examination of patients of the same age without AIDS showed only 14% of identical lesions.

Pathological Coronary Lesions

1. Common atherosclerotic plaques were present on the three main coronary trunks in 60% of cases, with two different patterns: either young plaques consisting in macrophages, foamy cells, and a small amount of extracellular lipid deposit (Fig. 1), or adult eccentric plaque with a lipid core surrounded by a fibrous wall consisting in macrophages, fibroblasts, smooth muscle cells, a few lymphocytes, elastic fibers, and collagenous fibers. Stenosis occluded 75% or more of the lumen (Figs. 2–4). In one case, the right coronary artery was completely occluded by a massive thrombosis (Fig. 5).

2. Uncommon intimal thickening which was diffuse, circular, and concentric throughout the whole length of every coronary trunk affected all patients, occluding over 40% of the vascular lumen. Collagenous and microelastic fibers were admixed with smooth muscle cells, macrophages, rare foam cells, and fibroblasts, without lymphocytes (Figs. 6–9).

3. Unusual and original lesions consisting in proliferation of smooth muscle cells mixed with numerous packed elastic fibers, which formed mamillated

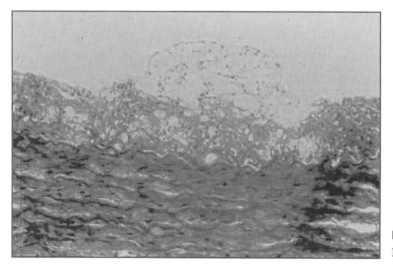

Fig. 1 Common atherosclerotic young plaque. Col HPS ×100

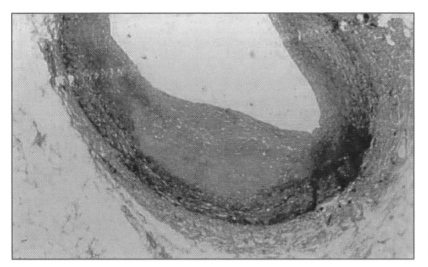

Fig. 2 Adult eccentric plaque. Col HPS, ×25

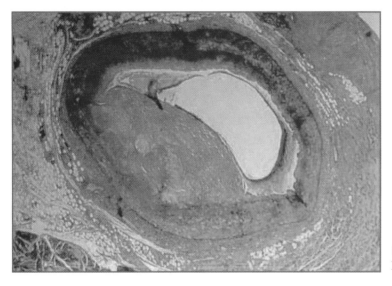

Fig. 3 Adult eccentric plaque. Col HPS, ×25

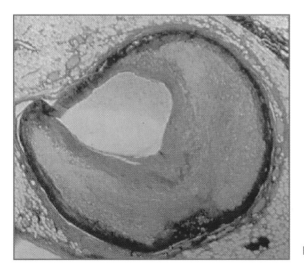

Fig. 4 Adult eccentric plaque. Col HPS, ×25

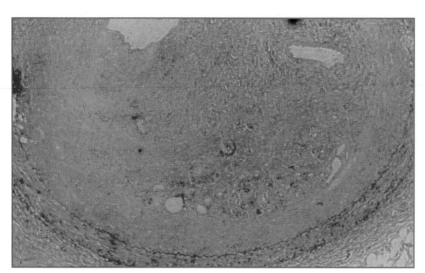

Fig. 5 Complete occlusion by fibrous organized plaque. Col HPS, ×25

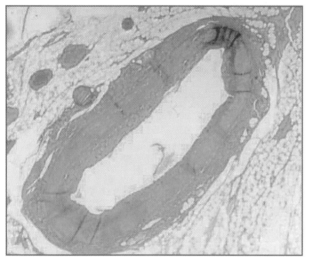

Fig. 6 Intimal diffuse and circular thickness

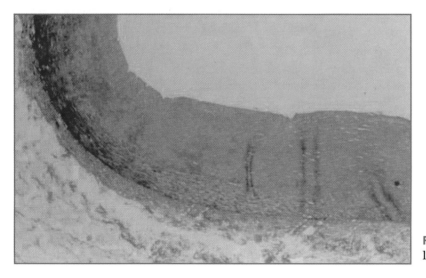

Fig. 7 Intimal diffuse and circular thickness. Col HPS, ×25

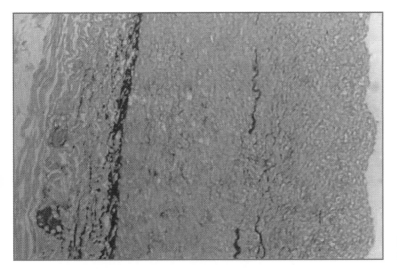

Fig. 8 Intimal diffuse and circular thickness. Col HPS, ×100

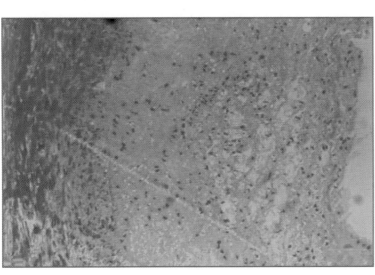

Fig. 9 Intimal diffuse and circular thickness with foamy cells. Col HPS, ×100

endoluminal protrusions resembling vegetations, were present in 40% of cases (Figs. 10–12).

The distal coronary network of intramural arterioles was also the site of a diffuse concentric intimal wall thickening occluding more than 80% of the lumen in 25% of cases (Figs. 13–15). Immunohistochemical data allowed true identification of smooth muscle cells (alpha-actin and vimentin expression) as the main elements of diffuse intimal layer thickening. The expression of tumor necrosis factor-alpha (TNF-α) and interleukin-1-alpha (IL-1α) in these cells was significantly greater than in smooth muscle cells of the underlying media. Fibrocytes and fibroblasts were scarcely disseminated on the periphery of atherosclerotic plaques, mixed with smooth muscle cells and some lymphocytes. CD68 expression identified macrophages, proving also TNF-α and IL-1 expression and Factor VIII expression appeared on endothelial cells. Coronary lesions in AIDS patients have some of the characteristics of common atherosclerosis such as eccentric fibro-lipidic plaques; however, they also present similarities with coronary lesions following heart transplantation (so-called chronic rejection) such as diffuse concentric intimal thickening occurring in coronary trucks and in the distal network [12].

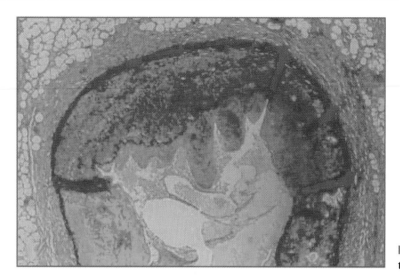

Fig. 10 Mamillated endoluminal protrusion. Col HPS, ×25

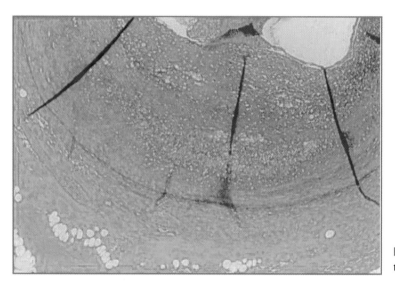

Fig. 11 Mamillated endoluminal protrusion. Col HPS, ×100

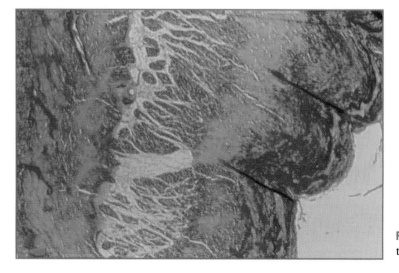

Fig. 12 Mamillated endoluminal protrusion. Col Weigert, ×25

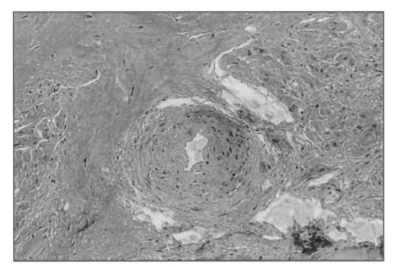

Fig. 13 Distal coronary network. Col HPS, ×25

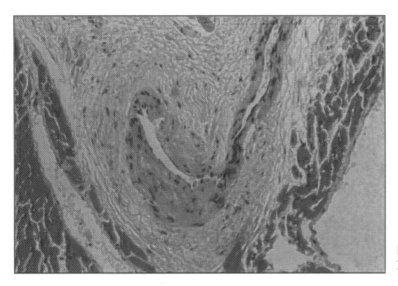

Fig. 14 Distal coronary network. Col HPS, ×100

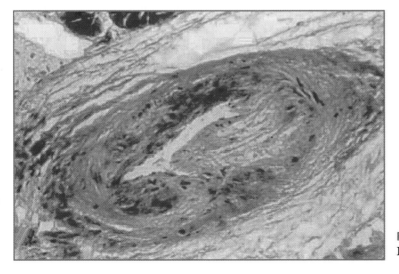

Fig. 15 Distal coronary network. Col HPS, ×100

Pathogenetic Hypotheses

Three possibilities can explain HIV-associated vascular alterations: (1) direct cellular infection by HIV (macrophages, smooth muscle cells, endothelial cells), (2) blood coagulation alterations, and (3) cellular infection by opportunistic elements [13]. Every change must naturally be mediated by numerous cytokines and adhesion molecules: today it is often possible only to demonstrate the presence or absence of these mediators, which is an indirect method that cannot indicate if cells are a source or target (or both) of the mediators.

1. Direct cellular infection by HIV-1. This phenomenon is demonstrated for macrophages, which is the first cellular target of the virus along with CD4 lymphocytes. It has not been demonstrated in vitro for endothelial cells, but some modifications are perhaps due to this alteration: von Willebrand's factor VIII, soluble thrombomodulin, E-selectin, and CD4 molecule increase [14]. These modifications involve endothelium properties–antigen presentation: IL-1; TNF-α secretion; and IL-2 production by T cells, which secondarily involve basal membrane degradation via Tat protein [15, 16]. Morphogenetic modifications of intimal intercellular matrix facilitate the penetration of lymphocytes and macrophages that are the target cells for HIV infection and replication. Infected macrophages would initiate medial smooth muscle activation and proliferation [17]. Endothelial cells seem to be heterogeneous, with discontinuous cells of sinusoid capillary cells displaying a different behavior [18]. HIV-1 sequences have been detected by in situ hybridization in the coronary vessels of an HIV-infected patient who died from acute myocardial infarction [19]. Potential mechanisms through which HIV-1 may damage coronary arteries include activa-

tion of cytokines and cell-adhesion molecules and alteration of major histocompatibility complex class I molecules on the surface of smooth muscle cells [19].

2. Hypercoagulability has been demonstrated in AIDS: von Willebrand's factor and tissular plasminogen activator increase, while there is a decrease in beta-2 microglobulin, S protein-free plasmatic fraction (protein C cofactor), and second heparin-cofactor (thrombin inhibitor). Other possible thrombogenic factors can be demonstrated: antiphospholipid antibodies (70% of AIDS cases) and lipoprotein LP(a) increase (common epitope for HIV and blood platelets), whereas hypertriglyceridemia and apolipoprotein AII decrease [20, 21].

3. Opportunistic infections demonstrate vascular tropism [22]. Viral cytolysis and endothelial necrosis favor the parietal adhesion of macrophages, an early known atherosclerotic stage. Cytomegalovirus alters endothelial cells as well as smooth muscle medial cells leading to multiplication, phenotype transformation with collagen and microelastic element synthesis and foam cells formation.

Experimental pathology studies in Macacus monkeys demonstrate a diffuse arteriopathy present in 25% of the population after simian immunodeficiency virus (SIV) infection, without a proven responsibility for either SIV or opportunistic infection [23].

Conclusion

Numerous hypotheses exist to explain AIDS vascular disorders. It is likely that the frequency of coronary lesions is high and underestimated because little attention is given during autopsy to coronary examination. Benditt's monoclonal origin of vascular lesions [24], depending on a viral cause, could provide a physiopathological answer.

References

1. Tabib A, Greenland T, Mercier I et al (1992) Coronary lesions in young HIV-positive subjects at necropsy. Lancet 340:730
2. Capron L, Loire R (1994) Passé, présent et avenir de l'infection artérielle. Rev Prat 44:906–910
3. Lacroix C, Chemoulli P, Said G (1994) Différents aspects de la pathologie neuro-musculaire chez 225 patients VIH positifs. Journées de pathologie 94:85–90
4. Kieburtz KD, Eskin TA, Ketonen I, Tuite MJ (1933) Opportunistic cerebral vasculopathy and stroke with AIDS. Arch Neurol 50:430–432
5. Engstrom JW, Lowenstein DH, Bredesen DE (1989) Cerebral infarction and transient neurologic deficits associated with AIDS. Am J Med 86:528–532
6. Joshi VV, Pawel B, Connor E et al (1987) Arteriopathy in children with AIDS. Pediatric Pathol 7:261–275
7. Husson RN, Saini R, Lewis L et al (1992) Cerebral artery aneurysm in children infected with HIV. J Pediatr 121:927–930
8. Rautonen N, White C, Martin NL et al (1994) Antibodies to HIV Tat in Kawasaki disease. Lancet 343:920–921
9. Capron L, Kim YU, Laurian C et al (1992) Atheroembolism in HIV-positive individuals. Lancet 340:1039–1040
10. Kabus D, Greco MA (1991) Arteriopathy in children with AIDS: microscopic changes in the vasa vasorum with gross irregularities of the aortic intima. Pediat Patol 11:793–795
11. Pulik M, Lionnet T, Couderc U (1993) Thromboembolic disease in HIV infection. Blood 82:2931–2937
12. Loire R, Tabib A, Dureau G, Boissonnat P (1991) Les lésions coronaires du transplanté cardiaque (rejet cardiaque chronique). Etude de 15 retransplantations. Ann Pathol 11:334–341
13. Loire R, Capron L (1995) Complications vasculaires de l'infection par le VIH. Sang-Thrombose-Vaisseaux 7:487–491
14. Lafeuillade A, Alessi MC, Poizot-Martin I et al (1992) Endothelial cell dysfunction in HIV infection. J Acq Im Def Syndromes 5:127–131
15. Teitel JM, Shore A, Read SE, Schiaron E (1989) Immune function of vascular endothelial cells is impaired by HIV. J Infect Dis 160:551–552
16. Hober D, Haque A, Watter P et al (1989) Production of tumor necrosis factor-alpha (TNF-alpha) and interleukin-1(IL-1) in patients with AIDS: enhanced level of TNF-alpha is related to a higher cytotoxic activity. Clin Experiment Immunol 78:329–333
17. Shattock RJ, Griffin G (1994) Cellular adherence enhances HIV replication in monocytic cells. Res Virol 145:139–145
18. Goerdt S, Sorg C (1992) Endothelial heterogenicity and the acquired immunodeficiency syndrome: a paradigm for the pathogenesis of vascular disorders. Clin Invest 70:89–98
19. Barbaro G, Barbarini G, Pellicelli AM (2001) HIV-associated coronary arteritis in a patient with fatal myocardial infarction. N Engl J Med 344:1799–1800
20. Toulon P, Lamine M, LedjevI et al (1993) Heparin cofactor II deficiency in patients infected with the human immunodeficiency virus. Thromb Haemost 70:730–735
21. Constans J, Pellegrin JL, Peuchant E et al (1993) High plasma lipoprotein (a) in HIV-positive patients. Lancet 341:1099–1100
22. Loire R, Bastien O, Tabib A, Vigneron M (1993) Artériolite à cytomégalovirus: gangrène des pieds et maladie coronaire précoce après transplantation cardiaque. Arch Mal Cœur 86:255–258
23. Chalifoux LV, Simon MA, Pauley DR et al (1992) Arteriopathy in macaques infected with simian immunodeficiency virus. Lab Invest 67 338–349
24. Benditt EP, Benditt JM (1973) Evidence of a monoclonal origin of human atherosclerotic plaques. Proc Nat Acad Sci USA 70:1753–1756

Chapter 6

Echocardiographic Findings in HIV-Infected Patients

S. Ederhy, C. Meuleman, N. Haddour, G. Dufaitre, F. Boccara, A. Cohen

Introduction

Echocardiography is an important imaging technique providing real-time imaging that can be performed at the bedside and easily repeated as needed (Table 1). Before the era of highly active anti-retroviral therapy (HAART), cardiac complications in HIV included pericardial effusion, dilated cardiomyopathy, myocarditis, endocarditis, pulmonary hypertension, cardiac neoplasm, coronary artery disease and drug-related cardiotoxicity [1, 2]. Cardiac abnormalities, although usually clinically silent, can be detected in necropsy series in the majority of infected HIV patients (40–60%) [3].

Due to a better prophylaxis against opportunistic infections and as a result of longer survival due to the introduction of HAART therapy, non-infectious cardiovascular manifestations are more commonly detected [4]. Echocardiography can determine left ventricular (LV), right ventricular (RV) systolic and diastolic functions, as well as the presence and severity of valvular heart disease (both stenosis and regurgitation), and pericardial disease. Doppler echocardiography can provide an accurate assessment of cardiac output, pulmonary artery pressures, resistance and filling pressures (Table 2). Echocardiography provides independent prognostic information on patients' morbidity and survival. Echocardiography is useful to detect cardiac abnormalities both in symptomatic and asymptomatic patients. The recent introduction of new technologies such as Doppler myocardial imaging, strain and strain-rate and three-dimensional echocardiography could help in identifying subtle cardiac abnormalities at an asymptomatic stage.

Table 1 Echocardiographic modalities

Modes
Two-dimensional (including hand-held)
Real time three-dimensional echocardiography
M-mode
Doppler (color, pulsed, continuous wave)
Tissue Doppler (myocardial Doppler)
Strain and strain-rate imaging
Speckle
Contrast (cavity, microcirculation)
Backscatter
Windows
Transthoracic
Transoesophageal
Epicardial (surgery, operating room)
Intracardiac (catheterization lab)
Intravascular (catheterization lab)
Modalities
Rest
Exercise
Pharmacologic (adenosine, dipyridamole, dobutamine...)
Pacing

Table 2 Main parameters derived from transthoracic echocardiography

Left ventricular dimensions and function
Left ventricular diameters and volumes (systole and diastole), wall thickness (diastole)
Left ventricular mass (indexed to BSA, height...)
Shortening fraction ($N>30\%$) and left ventricular ejection fraction ($N>60\%$)
Aortic output, Qs (N 5 at 6 l/min)
Transmitral flow
Left ventricular filling pressures (Ea and E/Ea; Vp and E/Vp; Ap–Am)
Valves
Thickness, leaflet mobility, calcifications, mass or vegetation (size, mobility)
If valvular stenosis: valvular area, maximal and mean gradient
If valvular regurgitation: mechanism, regurgitant orifice area, volume and fraction
Atria (left and right)
Size (diameters, area, volume); atrial mass or thrombus
Right ventricular dimensions and function
Right atrium and ventricle (diameter, area, volumes)
Right ventricular systolic function (fractional area, systolic velocity at tricuspid annulus)
Vena cava and hepatic veins (size, influence of respiration)
Right atrial pressure
Pulmonary pressures (systolic, diastolic, mean) and resistances
Pulmonary output, Qp (N 5 à 6 l/min)
Qp/Qs
Pericardium
Thickness, effusion, tolerance, hemodynamic consequences

Pericardial Disease

Pericardial Effusion

Pericardial effusion is the most frequent complication in HIV-infected patients. Before the introduction of HAART therapy, its frequency varied from 5 to 46% with an incidence of 11 to 17%/year and was associated with a high mortality rate [5]. Most cases remain of undetermined origin despite an extensive work-up. The cause of pericardial effusion in industrialized countries is idiopathic; in contrast, mycobacterium is the main agent involved in pericardial effusion in Africa (86%) [5] and sponta-

neous resolution could occur in 42% [6].

In the pre-HAART era, pericardial effusion was more common in patients with HIV advanced disease. Clinical manifestation of pericardial disease varies from asymptomatic pericardial effusion to cardiac tamponade.

Echocardiography is the non-invasive reference and accurate tool for the diagnosis of pericardial disease and tamponade. The echocardiographic diagnosis of pericardial effusions is usually based on visualization of a sonolucent circumcardiac space of varying width with or without hemodynamic compromise (Fig. 1).

Heidenreich et al. [6] described the incidence of pericardial effusion and its relation

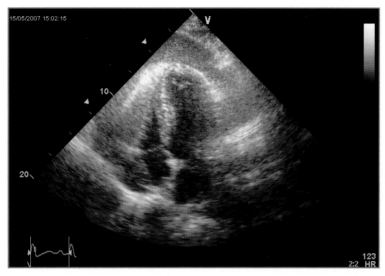

Fig. 1 Apical four-chamber view in an HIV infected patient showing a large and circumferential pericardial effusion

to mortality in HIV-positive subjects. In this study including outpatients, the prevalence of effusion in AIDS subjects was around 5%. The vast majority (80%) were small asymptomatic effusions, without any hemodynamic compromise. Survival of AIDS subjects with pericardial effusions was significantly shorter than AIDS subjects without (36 vs. 93% at 6 months, $p<0.01$). The incidence of pericardial effusion has increased as HIV infection progresses from 0% in asymptomatic HIV to 11%/year for AIDS subjects [6]. This study performed before the introduction of HAART therapy found a high prevalence and incidence of pericardial effusion in AIDS subjects, related to the stage of HIV disease. These findings are in contrast with reports evaluating hospitalized AIDS patients suggesting a high incidence of large effusions requiring pericardiocentesis. Pericardial effusion in HIV appeared as a marker of end-stage infection and was associated with decreased CD 4 count and opportunistic infections [7].

Since the introduction of HAART, the incidence of pericarditis and pericardial effusion has considerably decreased. Pugliese et al. [8] compared the incidence of cardiovascular complications during two periods (1989–1995 and 1996–1998) in 544 patients who were treated with nucleoside reverse transcriptase inhibitors (NRTI) and 498 patients treated with HAART. They reported a significant decrease of the incidence of pericarditis (13.5 vs. 3.4% $p< 0.001$).

Cardiac Tamponade

Cardiac tamponade occurs when pericardial fluids trapped in the pericardial space compress the heart and compromise heart filling and thus cardiac output. Echocardiographic findings of tamponade include significant pericardial effusion associated with right-atrial collapse, inferior vena-cava plethora, and important changes in flow velocities across the tricuspid and mitral valves [9]. Cardiac tamponade is mainly due to mycobacterium infection, malignancies and bacterial infections [10].

Pericardial Lipodystrophy

Increased visceral fat, as observed in HIV-infected patients receiving HAART, is associated with higher cardiometabolic risk and accelerated atherosclerosis. Using echocardiographic assessment of epicardial fat, Iacobellis et al. [11] found a relation between epicardial fat, an index of cardiac and visceral adiposity and carotid IMT.

Myocardial Disease

Myocarditis

Myocarditis is histologically characterized by varying degrees of myocardial necrosis, edema, apoptosis and cellular infiltration. Myocarditis may present with a wide spectrum of symptoms including chest pain, acute congestive heart failure, atrial or ventricular arrhythmias, cardiogenic shock or sudden death. Myocarditis may be associated with a number of conditions including HIV/AIDS, inflammatory states and immune disease.

Echocardiographic features of acute myocarditis are non-specific. Pinamonti et al. [12] reported echocardiographic patterns of dilated, hypertrophic, restrictive and ischemic cardiomyopathy in 41 patients with histologically proven myocarditis. Left ventricular dysfunction is common (69%), particularly in patients with congestive heart failure, often without or with minor cavity dilatation. Right ventricular dysfunction is present in 23% of patients and ventricular thrombi in 15%. In most cases, LV is typically normal sized or mildly dilated in patients with acute heart failure [13]. Transient increase in LV wall thickness due to edema has also been reported in 88% of cases in the acute phase [14]. Modifications of myocardial acoustic properties using ultrasonic backscatter have been described. The extent of edema and cell infiltration occurring in myocarditis could modify density and elasticity of myocardial tissue. Lieback [15] found significant alteration of myocardial backscatter in cases of biopsy-proven myocarditis compared to controls. Felker [16] showed that fulminant myocarditis could be distinguished from acute myocarditis by echocardiographic cri-

teria. Fulminant myocarditis had near normal LV diastolic dimension with increased septal thickness, whereas acute myocarditis was characterized by increased diastolic LV dimension but normal wall thickness [17].

Echocardiography is also useful for detecting complication of myocarditis such as LV thrombus, transient LV aneurysm, right-ventricular involvement and pericardial effusion [18]. Echocardiography could help in evaluating prognostic markers. Right ventricular function is an important independent predictor of death or cardiac transplantation in acute myocarditis. Mendes et al. [19] showed that patients with right-ventricular systolic dysfunction had a greater likelihood of death or need for cardiac transplantation during follow-up.

Dilated Cardiomyopathy

Cardiomyopathies are defined by the World Health Organization as disease of the myocardium resulting in systolic or diastolic in cardiac dysfunction [20]. Via echocardiography, dilated cardiomyopathy is characterised by the presence of a dilated left ventricle (>32 mm/m^2 in diastole) associated with impaired ventricular systolic function, assessed by impaired left ventricular ejection fraction (LVEF <45–50%) (Fig. 2). The aetiology of cardiomyopathy may be idiopathic, familial, viral, ischemic or immunological [20].

In the pre-HAART era, dilated cardiomyopathy has been described in up to 30–40% AIDS patients with an estimated annual incidence of 15.9/100 [21]. In a prospective study that included 98 HIV infected patients compared to 40 HIV seronegative patients, a depressed LVEF was noted in 32% patients and 8% had symptomatic congestive heart failure [22]. In this population, LVEF was more compromised with advanced stages of the disease.

Longo-Mbenza et al. [23] found a global incidence of dilated cardiomyopathy in 35%

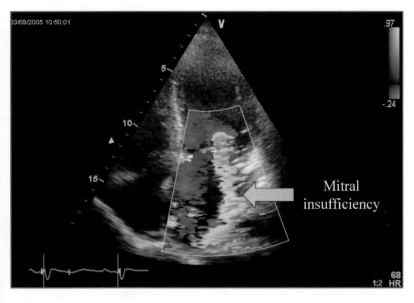

Mitral
insufficiency

Fig. 2 Apical four-chamber view plus color-Doppler in an HIV-infected patient with dilated cardiomyopathy and severe mitral insufficiency

of AIDS. According to myocardial biopsies, 83% of patients with dilated cardiomyopathies were secondary to myocarditis due to HIV or another viral agent such as Coxsackievirus (17%), Cytomegalovirus (6%) or Epstein-Barr virus (3%). This finding carries a poor prognosis with a median survival of 101 days in patients with LV dysfunction compared to 472 days in patients at a similar disease stage and no LV systolic dysfunction [21].

In sub-Saharan Africa, dilated cardiomyopathy remains an important issue. Out of 416 HIV-infected patients not receiving HAART, dilated cardiomyopathy was documented by echocardiography in 17.7% of patients. Low socio-economic status, estimated duration of HIV-1 infection, CD4 count, HIV-1 viral load, CDC stage B and C of HIV disease and low plasmatic level of selenium were significant predictors of LV systolic dysfunction [24].

Cardiomyopathy could also be secondary to drug toxicity such as zidovudine, amphotericin B or foscarnet [25]. The exact mechanism and pathogenesis of dilated cardiomyopathy in HIV patients is not unique. Nutritional disorders, direct effect of HIV on the heart, toxic effect of antiretroviral drugs, increased cytokine activity, oppor-

tunistic infection, illicit drug abuse, autoimmune reaction have been associated with dilated cardiomyopathy in HIV patients [21]. HAART has significantly decreased the incidence of dilated cardiomyopathy from 8.1 to 1.8% [8].

Pulmonary Hypertension

Pulmonary hypertension (PH) is defined by a mean pulmonary artery pressure (mPAP) >25 mmHg at rest or >30 mmHg with exercise [26]. A large case-control study, including 3,349 HIV-infected patients over a period of 5.5 years found a cumulative incidence of PH of 0.57%, resulting in an annual incidence of 0.1%, whereas its incidence in the general population is only 1–2 per 1 million people [27]. PH carries a poor and comparable prognosis in HIV-positive and seronegative patients. Mesa et al. [28] found that half of the patients died during the median follow-up of 8 months with a median time interval from the diagnosis of PH to death of 6 months. Comparing 20 HIV and PH to 93 HIV seronegative patients, Petitprez et al. [29] found a similar mortality rate. The major causes of death are right-sided heart failure, cardiogenic shock, sudden death and respiratory failure [29]. PH occurs in all stages of HIV infection without any clear relation to immune deficiency. Histologically, plexogenic pulmonary arteriopathy is the most frequent finding [29]. The pathogenesis of PH remains unclear. It has been advocated that PH might result from a genetic predisposition. An indirect role of HIV that can stimulate the production of endothelin 1, tumor necrosis factor, proteolytic enzyme and platelet derived factor has been also suggested [30, 31].

Echocardiography is a reliable tool to screen PH, rule out secondary forms and refine prognostic stratification. Echocardiography allows the estimation of pulmonary arterial systolic pressure (PASP) (Fig. 3) and provides additional information regarding the cause, consequences and prognosis of PH. A high correlation was found between transthoracic echocardiography findings and right heart catheterisation measurements [26]. Age, body mass index, systemic hypertension have been shown to increase PASP and should be taken into account when a PASP level is interpreted at an individual level [26].

Echocardiography also allows diagnosis of secondary causes of PH. It can easily recognize left heart valvular and myocardial diseases responsible for pulmonary venous hypertension, and congenital heart diseases with systemic-pulmonary shunts. The examination includes venous injection of agitated saline contrast medium to rule out atrial septal defect or patent Foramen ovale.

In the pre-HAART era and among 131 cases, the most frequent echocardiographic findings were a dilatation of right heart chambers (98%), tricuspid regurgitation (64%), and paradoxical septal motion (40%) [32]. Zuber et al. [33] suggested an indirect link between HIV, HAART and the incidence of PH. They found, in a retrospective study, an improvement of hemodynamic parameters in patients treated with HAART. In a group of 35 patients who had serial Doppler echocardiography, RV systolic pressure increased by a median of 25 mm Hg in nine patients who were not treated with HAART, decreased by a median of 3 mm Hg in nine patients who were not treated with NRTI and decreased by a median of 21 mm Hg in 14 patients who received HAART ($p<0.05$).

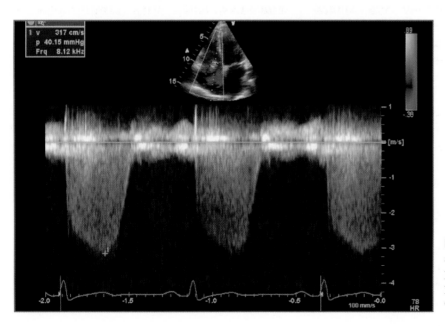

Fig. 3 Continuous Doppler allowing the evaluation of pulmonary artery systolic pressure derived from tricuspid insufficiency

Left Ventricular Mass

Left ventricular mass (LVM) can be derived from M-mode or two-dimensional echocardiographic measurements. Devereux' method allows an accurate and reproducible evaluation of LVM [34]. However, conflicting results have been reported in HIV patients. Martinez-Garcia et al. [35] found that LVM was lower in HIV infected patients. Coudray et al. [36] could not detect any difference regarding LVM in HIV patients and controls and Saman et al. [37] found a decrease in LVM in AIDS patient with associated wasting. A profound degree of immune depression, opportunistic infections, treatment with zidovudine and malnutrion were predisposing factors associated to a LVM decrease. Virus loads, CD4+ cell count, past infections were not related to left ventricular mass decrease [36].

Diastolic Function

The combination of tissue Doppler imaging and transmitral flow patterns allows a complete analysis of diastolic function. Coudray et al. [36] studied 51 HIV patients and 25 age- and sex-matched healthy controls and found that Doppler-derived parameters of diastolic function were significantly altered in the asymptomatic HIV group vs. controls. The HIV group had increased isovolumic relaxation time ($p=0.03$), early filling duration ($p<0.001$) and decreased early mitral flow peak velocity ($p=0.02$).

In 98 consecutive adults with HIV receiving antiretroviral therapy (56.1% under PIs), Meng et al. [38] found a lower ratio of early peak velocity (E wave) to late peak velocity (A wave; E/A ratio; 1.36±0.30 vs. 1.53±0.31; $p=023$) than did those who did not take PIs.

Endocardial Disease

The relation between immunosuppression and the development of infective endocarditis (IE) is not clear. In a retrospective study, Losa et al. [39] found that the prevalence of IE was 2% in HIV infected patient non-intravenous drug user, which is identical to that observed in a retrospective database from institutions in three countries in non-HIV patients. Despite the immune impairment, HIV by itself is not a sufficient risk for development of IE except in intravenous drug users. Bacterial endocarditis in HIV patients is infrequent, appearing almost exclusively in intravenous drug users with a prevalence varying from 6.3–34% with predominantly localisation on the tricuspid and pulmonary valve. *Staphylococcus aureus* is the most common organism (>75%), followed by *Streptococcous pneumoniae* and *Haemophilus influenzae* [40, 41]. The prognosis of right sided infective endocarditis is generally good [42].

Bacterial, non-bacterial thrombotic, and fungal endocarditis have been reported in HIV patients. Patients suspected of having infectious endocarditis should be screened with transthoracic echocardiography (TTE) and frequently with transesophageal echocardiography (TEE). If the first TEE examination remains negative, TEE should be repeated in case of persistent suspicion [43].

The two major criteria of IE in native valves are the finding of a vegetation which appears in echocardiography as a mobile echodense mass attached to the valvular or mural endocardium and the demonstration of abscesses or fistulas [43]. TEE overcomes the limitation of TTE and is characterized by a better sensitivity (88–100%), specificity (91–100%) and negative predictive value (68–97%) when compared to TTE in the detection of suspected vegetations [43]. Moreover, TEE allows the differential diagnosis with other valvular masses such as thrombi, papillary fibroelastomas, Lambl's excrescences and non-infected valve attached vegetation.

Cardiac Tumors

Kaposi Sarcoma

In patients with HIV infection, Kaposi sarcoma and lymphoma occur more commonly than in immunocompetent subjects. In the pre-HAART period, the cardiac Kaposi sarcoma prevalence varies from 12–8% in retrospective autopsies studies [44]. Echocardiographic findings in this setting found pericardial tamponade or pericardial constriction.

Malignant Lymphoma

Lymphomas are observed in 5–10% of patients with AIDS, which is 25–60 times higher than expected in the general population [45]. Primary cardiac lymphoma is rare [46]. Clinical presentation and echocardiographic findings include congestive heart failure, pericardial effusion or tamponade with nodular or polypoid masses involving the pericardium with variable myocardial infiltration and of the right atria. Malignant lymphoma is infrequent in HIV patients; the lesions predominantly involve the pericardium with myocardial infiltration [46]. The introduction of HAART led to the reduction in the incidence of cardiac involvement by Kaposi sarcoma and non-Hodgkin's lymphoma [8].

Conclusion

Echocardiography has an important role for HIV patients, allowing the diagnosis of cardiac abnormalities, allowing follow-up and in evaluating the prognosis. In the HAART era, the prevalence and incidence of cardiac abnormalities should be reassessed. The effect of HAART therapy on the incidence of HIV-related cardiovascular disease and manifestations should be prospectively determined. Prospective studies are needed to fully analyse the impact of HAART therapy on the development of cardiac abnormalities and to evaluate the potential complications due to their administration. Echocardiography with the development of new technologies such as myocardial Doppler imaging, strain-rate imaging, three-dimensional and contrast echocardiography, should be useful in this respect.

References

1. Barbaro G (2002) Cardiovascular manifestations of HIV infection. Circulation 106:1420–5
2. Fisher SD, Lipshultz SE (2001) Epidemiology of cardiovascular involvement in HIV disease and AIDS. Ann NY Acad Sci 946:13–22
3. Barbaro G (2003) Evolution of the involvement of the cardiovascular system in HIV infection. Adv Cardiol 40:15–22
4. Barbarini G, Barbaro G (2003) Incidence of the involvement of the cardiovascular system in HIV infection. AIDS 17:S46–50
5. Reuter H, Burgess LJ, Doubell AF (2005) Epidemiology of pericardial effusions at a large academic hospital in South Africa. Epidemiol Infect 133:393–399
6. Heidenreich PA, Eisenberg MJ, Kee LL et al (1995) Pericardial effusion in AIDS: incidence and survival. Circulation 92: 3229–3234
7. Chen Y, Brennessel D, Walters J et al (1999) Immunodeficiency virus-associated pericardial effusion: report of 40 cases and review of the literature. Am Heart J 137:516–521
8. Pugliese A, Isnardi D, Saini A et al (2000) Impact of highly active antiretroviral therapy in HIV-positive patients with cardiac involvement. J Infect 40: 282–284
9. Roy CL, Minor MA, Brookhart MA, Choudhry NK (2007) Does this patient with a pericardial effusion have cardiac tamponade? JAMA 297:1810–1818
10. Gowda RM, Khan IA, Sacchi TJ, Vasavada BC (2003) Cardiac tamponade in acquired immun-

odeficiency syndrome. Int J Cardiol 88:313–314

11. Iacobellis G, Pellicelli AM, Sharma AM et al (2007)Relation of subepicardial adipose tissue to carotid intima-media thickness in patients with human immunodeficiency virus. Am J Cardiol 99:1470–1472

12. Pinamonti B, Alberti E, Cigalotto A et al (1988) Echocardiographic findings in myocarditis. Am J Cardiol 62:285–289

13. Camerini F, Bussani R, Lenarda D et al (1991) Clinical aspects and haemodynamics in the follow-up of dilated cardiomyopathy and myocarditis. Eur Heart J 12(Suppl D):193–196

14. Hiramitsu S, Morimoto S, Kato S et al (2001) Transient ventricular wall thickening in acute myocarditis: a serial echocardiographic and histopathologic study. Jpn Circ 65:863–866

15. Lieback E, Hardouin I, Meyer R et al (1996) Clinical value of echocardiographic tissue characterization in the diagnosis of myocarditis. Eur Heart J 17:135–142

16. Felker GM, Boehmer JP, Hruban RH et al (2000) Echocardiographic findings in fulminant and acute myocarditis. J Am Coll Cardiol 36:227–232

17. Mendes LA, Picard MH, Dec GW et al (1999) Ventricular remodeling in active myocarditis: myocarditis treatment trial. Am Heart J 138:303–308

18. Thuny F, Avierinos JF, Jop B et al (2006) Images in cardiovascular medicine: massive biventricular thrombosis as a consequence of myocarditis: findings from 2-dimensional and real-time 3-dimensional echocardiography. Circulation 113:e932–933

19. Mendes LA, Dec GW, Picard MH et al (1994) Right ventricular dysfunction: an independent predictor of adverse outcome in patients with myocarditis. Am Heart J 128:301–307

20. Swedberg K, Cleland J, Dargie H et al (2005) Task Force for the Diagnosis and Treatment of Chronic Heart Failure of the European Society of Cardiology Eur Heart J 26:1115–1140

21. Barbaro G, Di Lorenzo G, Grisorio B, Barbarini G (1998) Incidence of dilated cardiomyopathy and detection of HIV in myocardial cells of HIV-positive patients. Gruppo Italiano per lo Studio Cardiologico dei Pazienti Affetti da AIDS. N Engl J Med 339:1093–1099

22. Cardoso JS, Moura B, Martins L et al (1998) Left ventricular dysfunction in human immunodeficiency virus (HIV) infected patients. Int J Cardiol 63:37–45

23. Longo-Mbenza B, Seghers KV, Phuati M et al (1998) Heart involvement and HIV infection in African patients: determinants of survival. Int J Cardiol 64:63–73

24. Twagirumukiza M, Nkeramihigo E, Seminega B et al (2007) Prevalence of dilated cardiomyopathy in HIV-infected African patients not receiving HAART: a multicenter, observational, prospective, cohort study in Rwanda. Curr HIV Res 5:129–137

25. Brown DL, Sather S, Cheitlin MD (1993)Reversible cardiac dysfunction associated with foscarnet therapy for cytomegalovirus esophagitis in an AIDS patient. Am Heart J 125:1439–1441

26. Galia N, Torbicki A, Barst R et al (2004) Guidelines on diagnosis and treatment of pulmonary arterial hypertension: The Task Force on Diagnosis and Treatment of Pulmonary Arterial Hypertension of the European Society of Cardiology. Eur Heart J 25:2243–2278

27. Opravil M, Pechere M, Speich R et al (1997) HIV-associated primary pulmonary hypertension: a case control study. Swiss HIV Cohort Study. Am J Respir Crit Care Med 155:990–995

28. Mesa RA, Edell ES, Dunn WF, Edwards WD (1988) Human immunodeficiency virus infection and pulmonary hypertension: two new cases and a review of 86 reported cases. Mayo Clin Proc 73:37–45

29. Petitpretz P, Brenot F, Azarian R et al (1994) Pulmonary hypertension in patients with human immunodeficiency virus infection: comparison with primary pulmonary hypertension. Circulation 89:2722–2727

30. Ehrenreich H, Rieckmann P, Sinowatz F et al (1993) Potent stimulation of monocytic endothelin-1 production by HIV-1 glycoprotein 120. J Immunol 150:4601–4609

31. Humbert M, Monti G, Fartoukh M et al (1998) Platelet-derived growth factor expression in primary pulmonary hypertension: comparison of HIV seropositive and HIV seronegative patients. Eur Respir J 11:554–559

32. Mehta NJ, Khan IA, Mehta RN, Sepkowitz DA (2000) HIV-related pulmonary hypertension: analytic review of 131 cases. Chest 118:1133–1141

33. Zuber JP, Calmy A, Evison JM et al; Swiss HIV Cohort Study Group (2004) Pulmonary arterial hypertension related to HIV infection: improved hemodynamics and survival associated with antiretroviral therapy. Clin Infect Dis 38:1178–1185

34. Lang RM, Bierig M, Devereux RB et al (2005) Recommendations for chamber quantification: a report from the American Society of Echocardiography's Guidelines and Standards Committee and the Chamber Quantification. J Am Soc Echocardiogr 18:1440–1463

35. Martinez-Garcia T, Sobrino JM, Pujol E et al (2000) Ventricular mass and diastolic function in patients infected by the humanimmuno defi-

ciency virus. Heart 84:620–624

36. Coudray N, de Zuttere D, Force G et al (1995) Ventricular diastolic function in asymptomatic and symptomatic human immunodeficiency virus carriers: an echocardiographic study. Eur Heart J 16:61–67

37. Samaan SA, Foster A, Raizada V et al (1995) Myocardial atrophy in acquired immunodeficiency syndrome: associated wasting. Am Heart J 130:823–827

38. Meng Q, Lima JA, Lai H, Vlahov D et al (2002) HIV protease inhibitors is associated with left ventricular morphologic changes and diastolic dysfunction. J Acquir Immune Defic Syndr 30:306–310

39. Losa JE, Miro JM, Del Rio A et al (2003) Endocarditis not related to intravenous drug abuse in HIV-1-infected patients: report of eight cases and review of the literature. Clin Microbiol Infect 9:45–54

40. De Rosa FG, Cicalini S, Canta F et al (2007) Infective endocarditis in intravenous drug users from Italy: the increasing importance in HIV-infected patients. Infection 35:154–160

41. Gebo KA, Burkey MD, Lucas GM et al (2006) Incidence of, risk factors for, clinical presentation, and 1-year outcomes of infective endocarditis in an urban HIV cohort. J Acquir Immune Defic Syndr 43:426–432

42. Valencia E, Miro J (2004) Endocarditis in the setting of HIV infection. AIDS Rev 6:97–106

43. Horstkotte D, Follath F, Gutschik E et al (2004) Guidelines on prevention, diagnosis and treatment of infective endocarditis executive summary: the task force on infective endocarditis of the European society of cardiology. Eur Heart J 25:267–276

44. Biggar RJ, Chaturvedi AK, Goedert JJ, Engels EA; HIV/AIDS Cancer Match Study (2007) AIDS-related cancer and severity of immunosuppression in persons with AIDS. J Natl Cancer Inst 99:962–972

45. Khan NU, Ahmed S, Wagner P et al (2004)Cardiac involvement in non-Hodgkin's lymphoma: with and without HIV infection. Int J Cardiovasc Imaging 20:477–481

46. Iwahashi N, Nakatani S, Kakuchi H et al (2005) Cardiac tumor as an initial manifestation of acquired immunodeficiency syndrome. Circ J 69:243–245

Chapter 7

Cardiac MRI in Diagnosis of Myocardial Disease in HIV-Infected Patients

J. Garot

Introduction

The heart and great vessels are not the sites most frequently affected by opportunistic infections or tumors in patients with AIDS. However, cardiovascular complications are relatively common and may be responsible for sudden death. A wide spectrum of cardiovascular complications have been reported in HIV infection and AIDS, which may be depicted at imaging, including pericardial disease with effusion and tamponade, non-specific or infectious myocarditis, dilated cardiomyopathy with global left ventricular dysfunction, endocardial valvular disease due to marantic or infective endocarditis, arrhythmias, human immunodeficiency virus-associated pulmonary hypertension, thrombosis, embolism, vasculitis, coronary artery disease, aneurysm, and cardiac involvement in AIDS-related tumors. However, more specifically, myocardial involvement in HIV seropositive patients is multifactorial and associated with increased morbidity and mortality. Classically, a variety of potential aetiologies have been postulated in HIV-related myocardial diseases, ultimately leading to cardiomyopathy, which include myocardial infection with HIV itself, opportunistic infections, viral infections, autoimmune response to viral infection, drug-related cardiotoxicity, ischemic myocardial damage, nutritional deficiencies, and prolonged immunosuppression. Of note, the epidemiology has changed dramatically since the introduction of highly active antiretroviral therapy (HAART). Coronary artery disease and dyslipidaemia, drug-related cardiotoxicity and cardiac autonomic dysfunction are becoming increasingly prevalent.

Recent developments of cardiac magnetic resonance (CMR) imaging have led to tremendous breakthrough in functional imaging and tissue characterization of the left (LV) and right (RV) ventricular myocardium. Advances in hardware, acquisition sequences and coil technology have greatly contributed to the improvement of image quality while simplifying cardiac examinations, thereby offering new possibilities for the characterization of myocardial diseases. Cine-CMR allows for accurate time-resolved imaging of global and segmental LV and RV function with high spatial resolution. Dynamic multislice CMR of myocardial perfusion is very useful for diagnosis of coronary artery disease (CAD). In addition, gadolinium-based contrast CMR with the so-called late enhancement technique has shown great value for non-invasive imaging of myocardial infarction and myocarditis. According to reports of clinical and autopsy studies, the prevalence of myocardial abnormalities in HIV-positive patients ranges from 25 to 75% [1, 2].

In this chapter, we will review myocardial diseases that may occur in HIV-positive patients, focusing on dilated cardiomyopathy, ischemic heart disease, and myocarditis, while excluding endocardial, pericardial and pericardiac diseases. We will not address non-invasive coronary MR angiography that is currently not a routine tool for imaging of the coronary arteries and there is no data on the particular coronary disease of HIV patients. Also, myocardial involvement in Kaposi sarcoma or lymphoma, as well as the hypertrophy of the right ventricle in response to AIDS-related pulmonary disease will not be detailed [2].

CMR of Myocardial Infarction

Coronary artery disease and ischemic heart disease are relatively common in patients with HIV infection [3, 4]. The prevalence of ischemic heart disease and its related mortality are increasing among HIV-positive patients [5,6]. The increased prevalence could be, at least in part, related to an improvement in the overall survival of HIV-positive patients, especially since the introduction of HAART. The origins of the disease appear to be multifactorial and related to the higher incidence of infection with herpesvirus, cytomegalovirus, or HIV-1, as well as to the inclusion of protease inhibitors, which have been reported to produce lipodystrophy, hyperlipidaemia, and hyperglycaemia [6–8]. In a retrospective analysis of data from the Frankfurt HIV cohort, which included almost 5,000 patients, a fourfold increase in the annual incidence of myocardial infarction (MI) among HIV-infected patients was found after the establishment of HAART with protease inhibitors, compared with the incidence among patients who underwent treatment before the institution of HAART [6]. Histopathologic examination of coronary arteries generally reveals eccentric atheromatous and fibrous plaques, with variable degrees of chronic inflammation and accelerated atherosclerosis. Unusual proliferation of smooth muscle cells with abundant elastic fibers, as well as diffuse and circumferential involvement of the coronary arteries have been reported [1, 9, 10]. Investigators in the Data Collection on Adverse Events of Anti-HIV Drugs Study, a prospective observational study of a cohort of 23,468 HIV-positive patients, found that the incidence of MI increased by an average of 26% per year of therapy with combined antiretroviral agents [11]. Not surprisingly, a further analysis of data from the same population indicated that these patients experienced an increased incidence and higher risk of other cardiac and cerebrovascular events (e.g. stroke; death from end-stage ischemic heart disease other than MI; and invasive cardiovascular procedures such as angioplasty, coronary bypass grafts, and carotid endarterectomy) [12]. Therefore, the diagnosis of cardiovascular disease by noninvasive imaging is increasingly required in the HIV-infected population.

Cine-CMR with steady-state free precession allows for accurate assessment of LV global and regional LV and RV function. Myocardial infarction appears as hypokinesia or akinesia during systole, which occurs in a myocardial wall supplied by an epicardial coronary artery (Fig. 1). Myocardial thinning may occur during systole. Besides rapid imaging of cardiac morphology, cine-CMR also permits the assessment of mitral valve regurgitation. Mechanical complications occurring after acute MI may be depicted by CMR in the cine mode. They include pericardial effusion, LV aneurysm, intracavitary thrombus, and mitral regurgitation (Fig. 2). Acute infarcts may be recognized as hyperintense signal on breath-hold ECG-gated T2-weighted black-blood fast spin-echo CMR images during the first days after the onset of MI (Fig. 3) [13]. This technique, however, does not identify chronic infarcts and may overestimate infarct size by including area at risk. In addition, T2-weighted images often have a low signal-to-noise ratio. Dynamic ultrafast multislice CMR of myocardial perfusion allows for the detection of microvascular obstruction after MI (Fig. 4) [14], or may add significant diagnostic value over usual clinical and biological markers after non-

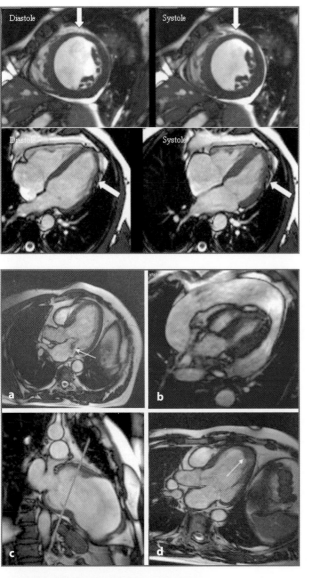

Fig. 1 HIV-infected 36-year old male with HAART who suffered a first recent anterior acute MI. Still images extracted from a cine-CMR sequence, performed at day 3, in the short axis (*upper panel*) and 4-chamber views (*lower panel*), at end-diastole (*left*) and end-systole (*right*), showing a segmental akinesia in the mid-anterior (*upper panel, arrows*) and apicolateral walls (*lower panel, arrows*), corresponding to the left anterior descending coronary territory

Fig. 2a-d Still frames extracted from cine-CMR in four different patients who presented with MI. **a** 3-chamber-view during systole, showing mitral regurgitation as a dark jet (*arrow*). **b** abundant pericardial effusion and cardiac tamponade. **c** Chronic MI, old apical aneurysm. **d** apical thrombus (*arrow*) complicating the course of anterior acute MI

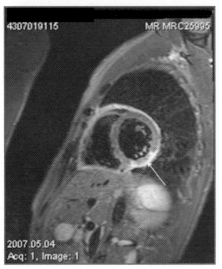

Fig. 3 42-year-old male with HIV and HAART. Pre-contrast T2-weighted black-blood fast spin-echo CMR image in the short-axis view showing a hypersignal in the inferolateral wall (*arrow*) 2 days after the onset of acute MI

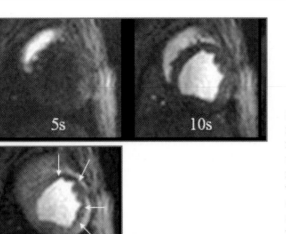

Fig. 4 Still frames in the short-axis view extracted from dynamic first-pass myocardial perfusion imaging, acquired 5,10 and 15 s after gadolinium injection, showing the distribution of contrast agent from RV (5 s) to LV cavity (10 s) and ultimately within the myocardium (15 s). Microvascular obstruction is displayed as hyposignal in the anterolateral wall (*arrows*) in this 53-year-old male who suffered acute MI and underwent successful angioplasty of the left anterior descending 48 hours before

ST elevation acute coronary syndromes [15]. Direct high-resolution CMR imaging of MI with the so-called "delayed-enhancement technique" after Gadolinium contrast injection is well standardized and carries important clinical implications for the diagnosis of myocardial viability [16]. With this imaging sequence, Gadolinium-DTPA enhanced imaging provides great contrast and high resolution images in which the infarct appears as a hyperenhanced region relative to noninfarcted tissue on inversion-recovery images acquired 10–15 min after contrast injection (Fig. 5). Indeed, the differences observed after MI in myocardial wash-in/wash-out kinetics of Gadolinium enable to differentiate three patterns [14]: normal nonischemic myocardium is characterized by rapid wash-in of the contrast agent on first-pass images (<30 s) with progressive wash-out over the following minutes. Conversely, infarcted myocardi-

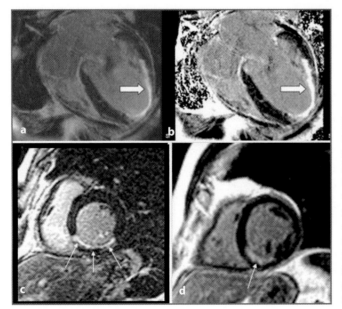

Fig. 5a-d Late inversion-recovery Gadolinium-enhanced CMR images in the four-chamber view (a–b) showing late hyperenhancement of the apex and apical septum (*arrows*) at day 3 in a HIV infected patient who presented acute anterior MI. The infarct is transmural at the apex and subendocardial at mid-septum. c–d Late inversion-recovery Gadolinium-enhanced CMR images in the short axis view in a HIV infected patient who presented inferior MI, showing subendocardial late hyperenhancement in the posterior wall (*arrows*) at day 2

um is characterized by a slower wash-in but more importantly by a delayed wash-out (>30 min) due in a large part to an increase of the distribution volume. Therefore, and because of greater Gadolinium content, the signal is enhanced (bright) on delayed images as compared to noninfarcted tissue.

The third pattern corresponds to microvascular obstruction when perfusion is not adequate at the tissue level despite reopening of the culprit coronary artery. In this case, gadolinium wash-in is dramatically delayed and the signal is very low (black) on first-pass myocardial perfusion images relative to noninschemic or necrotic but reperfused myocardium. It is well established from contrast-echocardiography and contrast-enhanced CMR that microvascular obstruction identified at the tissue level during the days following MI is a predictor of poor outcome and adverse LV remodelling [17, 18]. Delayed-enhanced CMR has important clinical implications for detection of infarct size, which is the strongest determinant of prognosis in these patients, and for detection of myocardial viability [16]. Infarct imaging by CMR is very sensitive and can depict subtle non-transmural infarcts or even infarctlets [19, 20]. The method has been validated against PET for detection of viability and has been recognized as the standard of reference for viability detection by the ESC Consensus Panel report [21, 22].

Finally, common features of infarct imaging by CMR are characterized by the presence of delayed enhancement of the infarcted tissue, which occurs in a specific coronary territory and predominates in the subendocardium. The delayed-enhancement within the infarcted myocardium corresponds typically to a single area of hypersignal that extends towards the subepicardium as a wavefront. These patterns are observed in recent, as soon as a few hours after the onset of MI, and in chronic MI. The transmural extent of MI serves as an index of tissue viability, with graded probability of subsequent recovery after revascularization for a given myocardial segment that is inversely proportional to the initial transmural extent [16].

CMR of Myocarditis

Histopathologic evidence of myocarditis has been found in more than one-third of AIDS patients at autopsy, but no specific cause was identified in more than 80% of the cases [23]. Common pathogens found in patients with AIDS-related myocarditis include *Toxoplasma gondii*, *Mycobacterium tuberculosis*, and *Cryptococcus neoformans*. Other infective agents that have been reported are *M. avium-intracellulare* complex, *Aspergillus fumigatus*, *Candida albicans*, *Coccidioides immitis*, cytomegalovirus, herpesvirus types 1 and 2 [24, 25], and Chagas disease in South America. HIV itself has been implicated as a cause of myocarditis. Since cardiac myocytes do not possess CD4 receptors that would allow a virus to enter the cell, it is not clear how a virus gets into the myocytes. Reservoir cells (dendritic cells), along with infection and injury of myocytes by cardiotropic viruses, may facilitate the entry of HIV into CD4 receptor–negative cells [26–28]. Lymphocytic myocarditis was present in almost 50% of patients who died of AIDS [23], and it is frequent in patients with LV dysfunction [29, 30]. Autoimmune abnormalities and nutritional deficiencies have been implicated in AIDS-related myocardial disease, and cardiac-specific autoantibodies such as antimyosin, have been found in 30% of patients with HIV-associated cardiomyopathy [31]. An association between the use of zidovudine and cardiomyopathy also has been reported [32]. Myocarditis corresponds to an acute aggression of the myocardium, resulting in various degrees of myocyte necrosis associated with cellular infiltration, inflammation, and edema [33–35].

In contrast to MI, myocyte necrosis preferentially occurs in the subepicardial layers and tends to diffuse inward transmurally during the course of the disease. The myocardial areas involved by the pathologic process do not correspond to any predefined coronary territory. In approximately 10% of the cases, acute myocarditis can lead to acute heart failure. It may also have subacute course such as rapidly progressive dilated cardiomyopathy with subsequent heart failure. The disease can evolve to chronic features and persistent dilated cardiomyopathy. Acute myocarditis can also be revealed by an acute chest pain mimicking ST-elevation or non-ST-elevation acute coronary syndrome. In both cases, troponin I measurements may be increased. The presumed diagnosis of myocarditis is often difficult to confirm. The clinical presentations, ECG, laboratory tests, and echocardiography are not specific. Coronary angiography may serve to eliminate an unstable coronary stenosis. Endomyocardial biopsy is the most specific examination and has been considered as the method of reference. In clinical practice, it is often skipped because of its invasive property and low sensitivity, estimated in the range of 50–65%, due to the patchy and heterogeneous distribution of myocardial tissue damage [35, 36]. The sensitivity of [67]Gallium myocardial scintigraphy is relatively poor [35, 37]. Myocardial scintigraphy with [111]Indium-labelled antimyosine monoclonal antibodies, which are fixed specifically to intracellular myosine within the damaged cells, carries higher sensitivity but low specificity [36, 38]. Therefore, the need for a reliable diagnostic tool is of great importance.

Several preliminary studies have shown the capability of CMR to image myocardial damage during the course of acute myocarditis [39, 40]. One of the main interests of this technique relies on its sensitivity to rapid changes in tissue composition and its ability to visualize the entire myocardium, which is required for the accu-

rate detection of a patchy and sometime diffuse inflammatory pathologic process [33, 41]. The comprehensive CMR examination is well standardized and quite similar to that used in particular for the evaluation of ischemic cardiomyopathy and viability assessment [42, 43]. It includes steady-state free precession cine-CMR for assessment of LV function, pre-contrast breath-hold ECG-gated black-blood T2-weighted sequence, dynamic first-pass perfusion myocardial imaging during the minute following 0.05–0.1 mmol.kg^{-1} Gadolinium chelate injection, and delayed-enhanced T1-weighted imaging with inversion-recuperation 10 min after injection.

CMR features vary according to the time elapsed from the onset of symptoms to the time of the CMR study. Although still debated, one can schematically distinguish a focal form of acute myocarditis within the first 5 days that may evolve towards a more diffuse process [33, 44, 45]. CMR is able to detect ongoing inflammation, its extent and severity, and to differentiate myocardial involvement from that of acute or chronic MI [46, 47]. It may also depict myocardial damage as sequelae of a previous episode of myocarditis when fibrotic scar tissue is present. During the first days of the disease, myocardial edema is present in about 30% of cases and appears as a hypersignal on T2-weighted images (Fig. 6). Edema involves predominantly the inferolateral wall with or without increased wall thickening. Pericardial effusion is noted in approximately 20% of cases and generally moderate. Cine-CMR may reveal wall motion abnormalities that may be segmental or more diffuse. In the most severe forms (fulminant myocarditis), LV ejection fraction is severely depressed without LV dilation. Segmental wall-motion abnormality may be present in myocardial segments that can be different from those exhibiting myocardial damage on delayed enhancement sequence.

In contrast to microvascular obstruction frequently observed after acute MI, there is

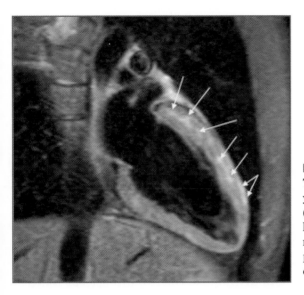

Fig. 6 Non-contrast black-blood ultrafast spin echo T2-weighted image in the 2-chamber view, in a 31-year-old HIV-infected male with acute myocarditis (day 2), showing multiple nodular and linear foci of hypersignal in the anterior wall that predominate at midwall and in the subepicardium (*arrows*). These patterns that occur most frequently in the inferolateral wall are very specific of viral acute myocarditis

no perfusion defect on contrast-enhanced first-pass perfusion imaging [47, 48]. Conversely, areas of delayed contrast-enhancement are frequent, either nodular predominating in the subepicardium or showing up as linear bands preferentially at mid-wall (Fig. 7). Myocyte membrane rupture leading to increased extracellular space, edema related to the inflammatory phenomenon with capillary compression, increased vascular permeability responsible for an increased distribution volume, along with decreased Gadolinium clearance may explain Gadolinium accumulation in regions involved in the pathologic process of acute myocarditis. These lesions occur in the same territory as edema and do not correspond to a specific coronary territory. These abnormal areas of delayed-enhancement are very often localized in the inferolateral wall.

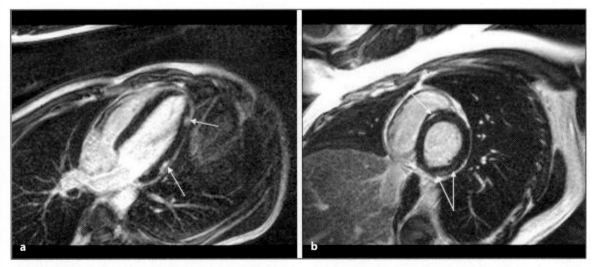

Fig. 7a, b Delayed contrast-enhancement CMR images obtained in the four-chamber (**a**) and the short-axis views (**b**) in a 34-year-old male with HIV infection, presenting with acute myocarditis at day 3, and showing nodular foci of hyperenhancement in the subepicardium of the lateral wall (**a**, *arrows*) and linear bands at mid-wall in the inferolateral and anteroseptal walls (**b**, *arrows*)

More subtle patterns such as micronodular lesions can be observed. These abnormal delayed-enhancement patterns have low sensitivity (around 60%) but a high specificity (97–100%), underlining the crucial need of performing a comprehensive CMR examination using a combination of different imaging sequences to improve diagnostic accuracy [43, 47, 48]. After 10 days, subacute forms are more difficult to pick by CMR because of the diffusion of the viral process in the myocardium [33, 39, 44, 45]. The edema is less important and more diffuse such as wall-motion abnormality. Delayed-enhancement may be difficult to highlight because of a more diffuse process. Specific outcome data in HIV infected patients are missing. Several longitudinal studies have followed non-HIV patients up to 3 months [39, 44, 49]. A favourable outcome was observed when LV contractile function improved and paralleled a significant decrease or involution of damaged delayed-enhanced myocardial tissue. Although still controversial, early hyperenhancement occurring a few minutes after gadolinium injection at the acute phase and persisting up to 1 month after the onset of symptoms could be indicative of poor outcome.

Myocarditis or Acute Coronary Syndrome?

It is well known that acute myocarditis can clinically masquerade as acute MI. In the setting of acute chest pain with concomitant ST-segment elevation on at least two contiguous ECG leads, guidelines for therapeutic management of ST-segment elevation MI should be applied. We suggest that invasive coronary angiography should be the preferred method when rapidly available in order to avoid inappropriate thrombolytic therapy. CMR should play an important role when coronary angiography rules out significant coronary stenosis in these cases and

has the potential to confirm the diagnosis of myocarditis. On the other hand, in the setting of acute chest pain without ST-segment elevation, CMR if rapidly available may become the first line imaging study, especially in those patients with low risk profile and/or recent history of flu.

Myocardial edema may be depicted on T2-weighted black-blood spin echo CMR during the acute phase of MI. Although myocardial distribution of edema is theoretically different, it is often difficult to distinguish between myocarditis and acute MI based on T2-weighted CMR images. First-pass myocardial perfusion imaging may help distinguish the two diseases as there is no early subendocardial defect in myocarditis, whereas it is very common in acute MI despite prompt reopening of the infarct-related-artery (60% of cases). As previously described, patterns of delayed hyperenhancement are very distinct and the most useful to discriminate between acute MI and acute myocarditis (Table 1).

Dilated Cardiomyopathy in Patients with HIV Infection: Is there a Role for CMR?

HIV-related disease is recognized as an important cause of dilated cardiomyopathy, with a prevalence of 8–30% [23, 27, 50, 51]. Prior to the introduction of HAART, the annual incidence of dilated cardiomyopathy was estimated at 15.9 per 1,000 patients with HIV infection [27]. Usually observed at the late stage of AIDS, dilated cardiomyopathy is associated with a low CD4 count (<400 cells/ml) [1, 24, 27]. At gross pathology, hearts with AIDS-related dilated cardiomyopathy reveal a great variety of findings. The LV myocardium may show eccentric hypertrophy with increased wall thickness and chamber dilatation.

Conversely, there may be thinning of the ventricular wall. In this setting, endocardial

Table 1 Differentiation between myocardial infarction and myocarditis from comprehensive CMR

CMR patterns	Myocardial infarction	Myocarditis
Wall motion abnormality on cine-CMR	Segmental	More diffuse
Edema on T2-weighted images	Discrete	More pronounced
Early hyposignal on first-pass perfusion imaging	Often present in acute MI	Absent

Late hyperenhancement
  Type
  Shape
  Contrast
  Topography
  LV distribution
	One focus
	Linear
	High
	Coronary territory
	Depends on infarct related artery
		Multiple foci, patchy
		Nodular or bands
		Moderate
		Non coronary territory
		Predominates in inferolateral wall
		Subepicardium, mid-wall

Transmural distribution Extension	Subendocardium Towards subepicardium	Towards mid-wall and subendo-cardium
Evolution	Persistent, shrinkage	Less visible after 10 days.

fibroelastosis and apical mural thrombi are frequent. Pericardial effusion or infective endocarditis may be present, especially in intravenous drug users [1]. Dilated cardiomyopathy with depressed LV function is the common joint manifestation of end-stage heart diseases that are caused by three main aetiologies: idiopathic, ischemic, and myocarditis.

Myocarditis due to HIV or other viral agents such as a group B coxsackievirus (17%), cytomegalovirus (6%), or Epstein-Barr virus (3%), has been found in 83% of HIV patients with dilated cardiomyopathy on the basis of histopathology [27]. However, the implication of these viruses in the course of the disease has not been formally demonstrated. Various studies have shown a clear correlation between dilated cardiomyopathy and poor prognosis in HIV infected patients. Cine-CMR is the most accurate imaging technique for measurement of LV dimensions, shape, mass and function. LV ejection fraction may be determined precisely as regional LV wall motion. RV function may also be measured with accuracy and is frequently impaired in AIDS patients. Anatomic and functional abnormalities found in RV and pulmonary artery parameters suggest a systolic overload on RV. Besides myocardial damage itself, pulmonary circulation abnormalities may influence RV structure and function in AIDS patients.

A Role in Diagnosis

As dilated cardiomyopathy may be the final pathway of several cardiac diseases, the most important role of CMR in this setting is to provide insights into the aetiology of dilated LV dysfunction. Although the data are available in non-HIV-infected patients, it is important to note that late-enhanced contrast CMR is very useful for differentiating idiopathic from ischemic dilated cardiomyopathy. Mc Crohon et al. have studied 90 patients with heart failure and low LV ejection fraction (EF <35%) by CMR [52]. All patients underwent invasive coronary angiography as a reference for diagnosis of

CAD. All patients with CAD have typical patterns of late enhancement corresponding to MI, predominating in the subendocardium and extending transmurally, in a specific coronary territory. Among patients without coronary stenosis on angiography, 60% have no late enhancement on CMR, and 30% have either linear hyperenhanced bands at midwall that are quite distinct from infarct features and correspond to fibrosis, or myocarditis-like subepicardial nodular foci of hyperenhancement in a non-coronary territory (Fig. 8). Only 10% of these patients have a late hyperenhancement on CMR that is difficult to distinguish with that of MI. The authors speculate that it may correspond to MI followed by spontaneous reopening of the culprit coronary artery. Thus, in the setting of dilated cardiomyopathy with LV dysfunction, the distinction between ischemic, nonischemic and viral cardiomyopathy may be further refined based on contrast-enhanced CMR.

A Role in Prognosis

Recently, Assomull et al. have studied the prognostic value of the presence of linear hyperenhancement at midwall on contrast

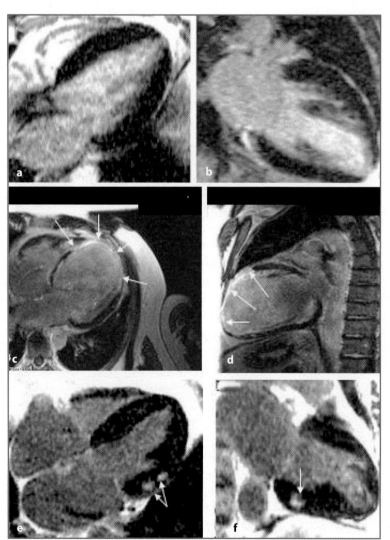

Fig. 8a-f Delayed Gadolinium-enhanced CMR images in the four-chamber (*left*) and 2-chamber views (*right*) in 3 different patients with HIV infection. The first pattern shows no late hyperenhancement suggestive of idiopathic cardiomyopathy (**a, b**). The second pattern shows late hyperenhancement that predominates in the subendocardium in the left anterior descending coronary, indicative of ischemic cardiomyopathy (**c, d**; *arrows*). The third pattern is highly suggestive of viral infection with nodular foci of hyperehnancement in the subepicardium, predominating in the inferolateral wall (**e, f**; *arrows*)

CMR in patients with dilated cardiomyopathy [53]. Overall, a cohort of 101 patients with nonischemic cardiomyopathy has been followed over a period of 2 years. Linear hyperehnancement at midwall has been observed in 35% of patients, and is associated with a higher incidence of clinical events, including all-cause mortality and cardiovascular hospitalization (RR 3.4, $p<0.001$). In multivariate analysis, the presence of fibrosis at midwall is the only independent predictor of death and hospitalization. Importantly, it is also predictive of the occurrence of sudden death or ventricular tachycardia (RR 5.2, $p<0.001$).

Similarly, late gadolinium enhancement was recently shown to be the most important independent predictor of major cardiac events over other clinical predictors, including ejection fraction, in a cohort of 195 patients who underwent CMR to evaluate for ischemia in the setting of CAD [54]. Even the smallest amount of LGE was predictive of an adverse outcome. Thus, in ischemic and nonischemic myocardial disease, fibrosis is a marker of poor outcome over and above standard clinical markers, including EF. In ischemic cardiomyopathies, it is likely a marker of the burden of CAD and its activity. The extent of infarct scar by CMR is also a better marker of inducible ventricular tachycardia than EF [55]. The presence of fibrosis is more characteristic of nonischemic cardiomyopathy and is thought to be at the root of myocardial re-entry leading to ventricular tachycardia [56]. Fibrosis may also involve the conduction system and lead to dyssynchrony and worsening congestive heart failure. Risk stratification in patients with congestive heart failure is a growing necessity in patients with HIV-related cardiomyopathy. It is becoming increasingly apparent that fibrosis may be an important prognostic marker and may identify patients at higher risk of ventricular arrhythmias and cardiac death. CMR has the unique feature of providing a coalescence of the ability to image fibrosis by late gadolinium-enhanced CMR with an enhanced understanding of its aetiology and prognostic implications.

Cardiovascular Manifestations in Children

Cardiac manifestations and complications of HIV infection in children are common. They include cardiac dysfunction, arrhythmias, cardiac arrest, myocarditis, pericardial disease, cardiac tumors, aortic root dilatation, and cerebral aneurysmal arteriopathy [57–59]. Serious cardiac events and cardiac death are common among children with AIDS, since 28% experience serious cardiac events after AIDS is diagnosed [60]. Pericardial effusion in children is commonly associated with pleural fluid and ascites [57]. CMR has great imaging diagnostic capabilities for most of these diseases without radiation and exposure to iodinated contrast. It may be performed in children with no hazard, but it requires patient cooperation for breath-holds and limitation of motion artefacts. In younger children and infants, when cooperation is poor and when CMR is required for diagnosis, particular anaesthetic procedures are mandatory in order to obtain sufficient image quality for diagnosis.

Conclusion

In conclusion, cardiac involvement and cardiovascular complications are common in HIV-infected patients. As the epidemic progresses and new treatments help increase the long-term survival of affected individuals, cardiovascular complications will become more common. The spectrum of disease is broad, but myocardial diseases are mainly represented by myocarditis, dilated cardiomyopathy, CAD, and cardiac tumors. The risk of CAD has dramatically increased in these patients. Many HIV-infected patients have dyslipidemia and other cardiovascular risk factors prior to acquiring infection. HIV infection itself and antiretroviral therapy can cause or worsen lipid abnormalities. Increased risk of CAD may be of special concern in the selection of HAART therapy, because differences in potential CAD risk have been reported for different regimens. Functional comprehensive CMR has routine clinical applications in the setting of myocardial ischaemia and infarction. Besides accurate assessment of LV function and cardiac anatomy with cine-CMR, the study of myocardial perfusion permits the detection of microvascular obstruction after MI that carries important prognostic implications. Contrast-enhanced CMR has become the clinical reference method for detection of myocardial viability after MI or in chronic ischemic LV dysfunction. In addition, CMR is also becoming a reference diagnostic tool in suspected myocarditis. The evolution of CMR patterns during the course of myocarditis may be of great interest for the establishment of prognosis especially in patients with initial LV dysfunction, heart failure, or with familial history of cardiomyopathy. Finally, CMR has the unique capability of discriminating between ischemic or nonischemic disease in HIV-infected patients with dilated cardiomyopathy, and providing important prognostic information in this setting.

References

1. d'Amati G, di Gioia CR, Gallo P (2001) Pathological findings of HIV-associated cardiovascular disease. Ann N Y Acad Sci 946:23–45
2. Lewis W (1989) AIDS: cardiac findings from 115 autopsies. Prog Cardiovasc Dis 32:207–215
3. Paton P, Tabib A, Loire R, Tete R (1993) Coronary artery lesions and human immunodeficiency virus infection. Res Virol 144:225–231
4. Tabib A, Greenland T, Mercier I et al (1992) Coronary lesions in young HIV-positive subjects at necropsy [letter]. Lancet 340:730
5. Louie JK, Hsu LC, Osmond DH et al (2002) Trends in causes of death among persons with acquired immunodeficiency syndrome in the era of highly active antiretroviral therapy, San Francisco, 1994–1998. J Infect Dis 186:1023–1027
6. Rickerts V, Brodt H, Staszewski S, Stille W (2001) Incidence of myocardial infarctions in HIV-infected patients between 1983 and 1998: the Frankfurt HIV-cohort study. Eur J Med Res 5:329–333
7. Barbaro G, Barbarini G, Pellicelli AM (2001) HIV-associated coronary arteritis in a patient with fatal myocardial infarction. N Engl J Med 344:1799–1800
8. Periard D, Telenti A, Sudre P et al (1999) Atherogenic dyslipidemia in HIV-infected individuals treated with protease inhibitors: the Swiss HIV cohort study. Circulation 100:700–705
9. Mehta NJ, Khan IA (2003) HIV-associated coronary artery disease. Angiology 54:269–275
10. Tabib A, Leroux C, Mornex JF, Loire R (2000) Accelerated coronary atherosclerosis and arteriosclerosis in young human-immunodeficiency-virus-positive patients. Coron Artery Dis 11:41–46
11. Friis-Moller N, Sabin CA, Weber R et al (2003) Combination antiretroviral therapy and the risk of myocardial infarction. N Engl J Med 349:1993–2003
12. d'Arminio A, Sabin CA, Phillips AN et al (2004) Cardio- and cerebrovascular events in HIV-infected persons. AIDS 18:1811–1817
13. Gerber BL, Lima JA, Garot J, Bluemke DA (2000) Magnetic resonance imaging of myocardial infarct. Top Magn Reson Imaging 11:372–382
14. Lima JA, Judd RM, Bazille A et al (1995) Regional heterogeneity of human myocardial infarcts demonstrated by contras-enhanced MRI: potential mechanisms. Circulation 92:1117–1125
15. Kwong RY, Schussheim AE, Rekhraj S et al (2003) Detecting acute coronary syndrome in the emergency department with cardiac magnetic resonance imaging. Circulation 107:531–537
16. Kim RJ, Wu E, Rafael A et al (2000) The use of contrast-enhanced MRI to identify reversible myocardial dysfunction. N Engl J Med 343:1445–1453
17. Wu KC, Zerhouni EA, Judd RM et al (1998) The prognostic significance of microvascular obstruction by magnetic resonance imaging in patients with acute myocardial infarction. Circulation 97:765–772
18. Gerber BL, Garot J, Bluemke DA et al (2002) Accuracy of contrast-enhanced magnetic resonance imaging in predicting improvement of regional myocardial function in patients after acute myocardial infarction. Circulation 106:1083–1089

19. Wagner A, Mahrholdt H, Holly TA et al (2003) Contrast-enhanced MRI and routine single photon emission computed tomography (SPECT) perfusion imaging for detection of subendocardial myocardial infarcts: an imaging study. Lancet 361:374–379

20. Ricciardi MJ, Wu E, Davidson CJ et al (2001) Visualization of discrete microinfarction after percutaneous coronary intervention associated with mild creatine kinase-MB elevation. Circulation 103:27802783

21. Kuhl HP, Beek AM, van der Weerdt AP et al (2003) Myocardial viability in chronic ischemic heart disease: comparison of contrast-enhanced magnetic resonance imaging with (18)F-fluorodeoxyglucose positron emission tomography. J Am Coll Cardiol 41:1341–1348

22. Pennell DJ, Sechtem UP, Higgins CB et al (2004) Clinical indications for cardiovascular magnetic resonance: consensus panel report. Eur Heart J 25:1940–1965

23. Anderson DW, Virmani R, Reilly JM et al (1988) Prevalent myocarditis at necropsy in the acquired immunodeficiency syndrome. J Am Coll Cardiol 11:792–799

24. Rerkpattanapipat P, Wongpraparut N, Jacobs LE, Kotler MN (2000) Cardiac manifestations of acquired immunodeficiency syndrome. Arch Intern Med 160:602–608

25. Kaul S, Fishbein MC, Siegel RJ (1991) Cardiac manifestations of acquired immune deficiency syndrome: a 1991 update. Am Heart J 122:535–544

26. Ippolito G, Galati V, Serraino D, Girardi E (2001) The changing picture of the HIV/AIDS epidemic. Ann N Y Acad Sci 946:1–12

27. Barbaro G, Di Lorenzo G, Grisorio B, Barbarini G for the Gruppo Italiano per lo Studio Cardiologico dei Pazienti Affetti da AIDS (1998) Incidence of dilated cardiomyopathy and detection of HIV in myocardial cells of HIV-positive patients. N Engl J Med 339:1093–1099

28. Grody WW, Cheng L, Lewis W (1990) Infection of the heart by the human immunodeficiency virus. Am J Cardiol 66:203–206

29. Baroldi G, Corallo S, Moroni M et al (1988) Focal lymphocytic myocarditis in acquired immunodeficiency syndrome (AIDS): a correlative morphologic and clinical study in 26 consecutive fatal cases. J Am Coll Cardiol 12:463–469

30. Reilly JM, Cunnion RE, Anderson DW et al (1988) Frequency of myocarditis, left ventricular dysfunction and ventricular tachycardia in the acquired immune deficiency syndrome. Am J Cardiol 62:789–793

31. Currie PF, Goldman JH, Caforio AL et al (1998) Cardiac autoimmunity in HIV related heart muscle disease. Heart 79:599–604

32. Herskowitz A, Willoughby SB, Baughman KL et al (1992) Cardiomyopathy associated with antiretroviral therapy in patients with HIV infection: a report of six cases. Ann Intern Med 116:311–313

33. Feldman AM, McNamara D (1987) Myocarditis. New Engl J Med 343:1388–1398

34. Aretz HT, Billingham ME, Edwards WD et al (1987) Myocarditis: a histopathologic definition and classification. Am J Cardiovasc Pathol 1:3–14

35. Magnani JW, Dec GW (2006) Myocarditis: current trends in diagnosis and treatment. Circulation 113:876–890

36. Kuhl U, Lauer B, Souvatzoglu M et al (1998) Antimyosin scintigraphy and immunohistologic analysis of endomyocardial biopsy in patients with clinically suspected myocarditis: evidence of myocardial cell damage and inflammation in the absence of histologic signs of myocarditis. J Am Coll Cardiol 32:1371–1376

37. Veluvolu P, Balian AA, Goldsmith R et al (1992) Lyme carditis: evaluation by Ga-67 and MRI. Clin Nuclear Med 17:823–827

38. Sarda L, Colin P, Boccara F et al (2001) Myocarditis in patients with clinical presentation of myocardial infarction and normal coronary angiograms. J Am Coll Cardiol 37:786–792

39. Friedrich MG, Strohm O, Schulz-Menger J et al (1998) Contrast media-enhanced magnetic resonance imaging visualizes myocardial changes in the course of viral myocarditis. Circulation 97:1802–1809

40. Lie JT (1998) Detection of acute myocarditis using nuclear magnetic resonance imaging. Am J Med 85:282–283

41. Liu PP, Yan AT (2005) Cardiovascular magnetic resonance for the diagnosis of acute myocarditis: prospects for detecting myocardial inflammation. J Am Coll Cardiol 45:1823–1825

42. Edelman RR (2004) Contrast-enhanced MR imaging of the heart: overview of the literature. Radiology 232:653–668

43. Laissy JP, Messin B, Varenne O et al (2002) MR imaging of acute myocarditis: a comprehensive approach based on various imaging sequences. Chest 122:1638–1648

44. Gagliardi MG, Polletta B, Di Renzi P (1999) MRI for the diagnosis and follow-up of myocarditis. Circulation 99:458–459

45. Billingham ME, Tazelaar MD (1986) The morphological progression of viral myocarditis. Postgrad Med J 62:581–584

46. Hunold P, Schlosser T, Vogt FM et al (2005) Myocardial late enhancement in contrast-enhanced cardiac MRI: distinction between infarction scar and non-infarction-related disease. AJR Am J Roentgenol 184:1420–6

47. Laissy JP, Hyafil F, Feldman LJ et al (2005) Dif-

ferentiating acute myocardial infarction from myocarditis: diagnostic value of early- and delayed-perfusion cardiac MR imaging. Radiology 237:75–82

48. Abdel-Aty H, Boye P, Zagrosek A et al (2005) Diagnostic performance of cardiovascular magnetic resonance in patients with suspected acute myocarditis: comparison of different approaches. J Am Coll Cardiol 45:181522

49. Wagner A, Schulz-Menger J, Dietz R, Friedrich MG (2003) Long-term follow-up of patients with acute myocarditis by magnetic resonance imaging. Magma 16:17–20

50. Himelman RB, Chung WS, Chernoff DN et al (1989) Cardiac manifestations of human immunodeficiency virus infection: a two-dimensional echocardiographic study. J Am Coll Cardiol 13:1030–1036

51. Levy WS, Simon GL, Rios JC et al (1989) Prevalence of cardiac abnormalities in human immunodeficiency virus infection. Am J Cardiol 63:86–89

52. McCrohon JA, Moon JC, Prasad SK et al (2003) Differentiation of heart failure related to dilated cardiomyopathy and coronary artery disease using gadolinium-enhanced cardiovascular magnetic resonance. Circulation 108:54–59

53. Assomull RG, Prasad SK, Lyne J et al (2006) Cardiovascular magnetic resonance, fibrosis, and prognosis in dilated cardiomyopathy. J Am Coll Cardiol 48:1977–1985

54. Kwong RY, Chan AK, Brown KA et al (2006) Impact of unrecognized myocardial scar detected by cardiac magnetic resonance imaging on event-free survival in patients presenting with signs or symptoms of coronary artery disease. Circulation 113:2733–2743

55. Bello D, Fieno DS, Kim RJ et al (2005) Infarct morphology identifies patients with substrate for sustained ventricular tachycardia. J Am Coll Cardiol 45:1104–1108

56. Hsia HH, Marchlinski FE (2002) Characterization of the electroanatomic substrate for monomorphic ventricular tachycardia in patients with nonischemic cardiomyopathy. Pacing Clin Electrophysiol 25:1114–1127

57. Mast HL, Haller JO, Schiller MS, Anderson VM (1992) Pericardial effusion and its relationship to cardiac disease in children with acquired immunodeficiency syndrome. Pediatr Radiol 22:548–551

58. Dubrovsky T, Curless R, Scott G et al (1998) Cerebral aneurysmal arteriopathy in childhood AIDS. Neurology 51:560–565

59. Keesler MJ, Fisher SD, Lipshultz SE (2001) Cardiac manifestations of HIV infection in infants and children. Ann N Y Acad Sci 946:169–178

60. Al-Attar I, Orav EJ, Exil V et al (2003) Predictors of cardiac morbidity and related mortality in children with acquired immunodeficiency syndrome. J Am Coll Cardiol 41:1598–1605

Chapter 8

Coronary Heart Disease in HIV-Infected Patients: Epidemiology

M. Mary-Krause, D. Costagliola

Cardiovascular disease continues to be the leading cause of death among the general population of industrialized countries. It is also the main reason for hospitalization. But what about HIV-infected subjects? With the advent of combination antiretroviral therapy (cART) for HIV infection, including protease inhibitors (PIs), in April 1996 in France, the morbidity of AIDS-defining illnesses has been reduced and HIV-infected patients are living longer [1, 2]. Thus, the spectrum of diseases related to HIV is shifting from opportunistic diseases towards long-term complications such as cancers, co-infection with other viruses such as hepatitis C virus, and the metabolic effects of cART. Some of these disorders are potential risk factors for cardiovascular diseases and so could lead to cardiovascular over-mortality and over-morbidity. Cardiovascular diseases currently account for 7% of deaths among HIV-infected subjects in France, for 14% of non-HIV-related deaths [3], and about 16% of deaths among subjects with a good immunovirologic response to cART [4].

Defined as any combination of at least three antiretroviral drugs –usually two nucleoside analog reverse transcriptase inhibitors (NRTI) and either a PI or a non-nucleoside reverse transcriptase inhibitor (NNRTI)– cART is the current reference standard of antiretroviral treatment [5, 6]. The adverse effects of cART have received much attention in recent years. Although lipid disorders were described in HIV-infected patients before the advent of cART [7, 8], several class-specific metabolic effects of cART may have a deleterious impact on the heart, including increased insulin resistance, hypercholesterolemia and/or hypertriglyceridemia, and lipodystrophy syndromes [9–12]. Likewise, although coronary lesions were described well before the advent of PIs [13, 14], cART has been implicated in the aggravation of coronary heart diseases (CHD) and in other vascular complications [15–20]. However, even if most of studies were in favor of the impact of the PIs, especially myocardial infarction (MI), concerning the risk of CHD, this impact remains controversial. The increased rate of MI has been linked to PI by some studies, others have shown a link to HIV disease with limited data on treatment.

Estimation of the Coronary Risk

The two traditional components of epidemiological research (descriptive/analytical) contribute to improve our knowledge of diseases. Analysis of incidence and mortality data, which provides a description of a given disease at the population level, and knowledge of general characteristics (age, sex, transmission group, etc.) that are associated with a higher risk, also contribute towards identifying areas for improvement in access to care and generate etiologic assumptions. Analytical studies are designed to test these hypotheses and to characterize risk factors (i.e., any attribute, characteristic, or exposure of an individual which increases the likelihood of a disease or injury). However, epidemiological studies (descriptive or analytical) are solely observational: they describe what is happening in the "real world" and may suggest causality; the level of causal presumption depends on the strength of the association, its consistency (observed repeatedly by different persons, in different circumstances and times), specificity (limited to specific sets of characteristics), relationship in time, biological gradient (dose response), biological plausibility (the weakest link, depending on the current state of knowledge), and coherence.

However, epidemiological studies have important implications for prevention, early detection, diagnosis, and access to care. The importance of a phenomenon can be characterized by the use of crude numbers (frequency) or rates and ratios. The numerator is included in the denominator of the incidence or prevalence rate; however, rates, as opposed to frequencies, imply an element of time. With incidence rates, for example, only new cases of the disease occurring during a defined time period (e.g., 1 year) are taken into account, being divided by the average size of the population exposed during the same period. If the observation period is not a 1-year period, the denominator is usually expressed as the amount of "person-time" per observation. Person-time is calculated as the sum total of the time all individuals remain in the study without developing the outcome of interest (the total amount of time that the study members are at risk of developing the outcome of interest). Person-time can be measured in days, months, or years (1,000 subjects followed for 2 years = 2,000 person-years). The incidence or death rate definitions correspond to a "dynamic" dimension of the rate, which is the rapidity of occurrence of disease or death in the population. These rates can be used to assess the risk of disease or death, but such health indicators (expressed per unit time) are not, strictly speaking, probabilities.

To quantify the association between a disease and a risk factor, one generally uses relative risk (RR), R1/R0, where R1 is the risk of disease or death among the population exposed to the risk factor and R0 is the risk among unexposed subjects. Usually, RR above 1 denotes a deleterious effect of the risk factor, while an RR below 1 suggests a beneficial effect. An RR of 1 suggests that there is no correlation. Another index is the odds ratio (OR), defined as [R1/(1-R1))/(R0/(1-R0)].

When comparing morbidity rates in a cohort with those of the general population, for example, direct comparison of crude rates can lead to erroneous conclusions. Indeed, it is known, for example, that the risk of almost all diseases, and particularly cardiovascular diseases, increases with age. If the age distribution is different between the two populations, the comparison of the risk will be affected by this confounding bias. Standardization appears the best way to avoid this kind of bias, and is based on the crude disease rate that would be observed in the cohort if its age distribution were the same as that of the comparator population. Thus, the standardized morbidity or mortality ratio compares the observed number of cases of disease or death in the cohort with an expected number of cases. The expected number is calculated by (1) classifying the study group in terms of demographic variables such as age and sex; (2) computing the expected number of cases or deaths for each class (by multiplying the number of individuals in the study group in that class by the class-specific death rate in a standard reference population); and (3) adding together the expected cases or deaths in all classes.

Impact of Antiretroviral Treatments on Coronary Heart Disease

Although it is now clearly established that cART is linked to metabolic disorders, the long-term impact of these disorders is still being discussed. The first questions concerning an increase in the risk of CHD and the possible responsibility of PIs were raised in May 1998. Henry et al. [15] described two cases of coronary artery disease in HIV-infected patients treated with PIs. One of the subjects had lipodystrophy and hypercholesterolemia with no other known risk factors, while the second patient had traditional risk factors such as smoking and cocaine use. Similar series of cases were reported in the medical literature in subsequent months [16–19, 21–23]. Gallet et al. [17] reported the cases of three patients with ischemic cardiopathy, including two with MI. All were being treated with PIs, and two had high lipid levels that were not present before antiretroviral treatment. Similarly, Vittecoq et al. [24] described four young patients with ischemic coronary events (MI in three cases). Three subjects were being treated with PIs, and three had major lipid disorders, associated with smoking and familial factors in two cases. Passalaris et al. [25] described six subjects with coronary artery disease who were receiving PI-containing combinations of antiretroviral drugs; four of these patients had acute MI. Coronary angiography revealed thrombotic lesions in two subjects, atheromatous lesions in two subjects, and both types of lesions in one subject. Friedl et al. [20] later described 14 coronary events in 11 subjects treated with PIs or NNRTIs. However, none of these studies proved a link between CHD and antiretroviral treatment.

Some studies [26–32], but not others [33–36, 37], have shown a link between the risk of CHD and exposure to PIs (Table 1). Some suffered from methodological problems such as small sample size, median PI treatment periods of less than 12 months (two studies), and likely underreporting relative to the general population. Some studies used different endpoints. In addition, the incidence of MI in people under 50 years of age is very low, meaning that lengthy follow-up of large populations (person-years) is necessary to observe a small

difference between the HIV-infected population and the general population, or between two HIV-infected populations treated/not treated with cART.

Far from increasing the incidence of cardiovascular events, a study from a database on administrative data [36] showed that cART tended to reduce the short-term risk in a population of more than 36,000 HIV-infected U.S. army veterans. Between 1995 and 2001, the rate of hospital admission for cardiovascular or cerebrovascular disease fell from 1.7 to 0.9 per 100 person-years (PY), while the overall mortality rate fell from 21.3 to 5.0 per 100 PY during the same period.

A study based on the French Hospital Database on HIV (FHDH) using DMI2 software (property of the French Ministry of Health) included 34,976 men with a total follow-up of 88,029 PY between 1996 and 1999 [31]. There were 49 cases of MI during 39,023 PI-exposed PY. The incidence rate of MI among subjects exposed to PIs between 1996 and 1999 was estimated according to the duration of PI therapy, based on three periods: <18 months (group 1), 18–29 months (group 2), and ≥30 months (group 3). The authors compared the 1996–1999 MI incidence rates estimated from the FHDH dataset with the 1997–1998 incidence rates estimated from the French general male population of the same age, obtained from three French regional registries (Lille, Strasbourg, and Toulouse) [41]. This analysis accounted only for age and sex. Then, in order to take into account potential differences in other CHD risk factors (family history, smoking, hypertension, and diabetes mellitus) between the general population and the HIV-infected population [42–45], the authors compared the MI incidence rates in groups 2 and 3 with those in group 1. There were 21 cases of MI among patients exposed to PIs for less than 18 months (25,734 PY), 15 cases among subjects exposed for 18–29 months (9,440 PY), and 13 among patients exposed for 30 months or more (3,849 PY).

Table 1 Risk of coronary heart disease among HIV-infected subjects treated with cART

Studies	Study design	Studied event	Study period	Number of subjects	Number of coronary events	Number of subjects exposed to HAART	Duration of follow-up with HAART	Results
Jütte, 1999 [26]	Database on medical records No validation of cases	Myocardial infarction	Between January 1990 and August 1998	1324 subjects 1911 PY	8	373 subjects 469 PY	10 months (med)	Incidence of 0.21 per 100 PY in non PI group and of 1.06 per 100 PY in PI group
Rickerts, 2000 [27]	Database on medical records Validation of cases	Myocardial infarction	From 1st January 1983 to 31 December 1998	4993 subjects 16 478 PY	29	1572 subjects		OR=2.61 (1.19-5.66) HAART vs non HAART
David, 2002 [33]	Database on medical records Case-control analysis No validation of cases	Ischemic cardiovascular diseases	From 1st April 1999 through 25 April 2000	48 subjects	16	34 subjects	27 months for cases (med) 14 months for controls (med)	PI not directly associated with greater risk of ischemic CVD
Holmberg, 2002 [28]	Database on medical records Validation of cases	Myocardial infarction	Between January 1993 and January 2002	5672 subjects 17 712 PY	21	3247 subjects	49 months (mean)	Higher risk HR=6.5 (0.9-47.8) PI vs non PI
Bozzette, 2003 [36]	Database on administrative data No validation of cases	Cardiovascular and cerebrovascular diseases	Between 1st January 1993 and 30 June 2001	36 766 subjects 121 935 PY	1207	15 296 subjects 26957 PY	16 months (med)	HR=1.23 (0.78-1.93) 24 months of PI exposure vs 0 months
Klein, 2003 [34, 35]	Database on administrative data No validation of cases	Myocardial infarction	Between 1st January 1996 and 31 December 2002	4408 subjects 18792 PY	65	2860 subjects 10 686 PY	47 months (med)	4.0 cases/1000 PY if no PI vs 3.9/1000 PY if PI

Study	Design	Event	Period	Subjects/PY	Cases		Follow-up	Results
Friis-Moller, 2003 [29]	Specifically designed cohort / Validation of cases	Myocardial infarction	Between December 1999 and February 2002	23 468 subjects 36199 PY	126			RR=1.26 per year of combination antiretroviral treatment exposure
Moore, 2003 [30]	Database on medical records / Case-control analysis / No validation of cases	Myocardial infarction + unstable angina	After 1st January 1996	2671 subjects 7330 PY	43			Observed incidence of 5.9 events/1000 PY vs expected incidence of 2/1000 PY / PI as independent factor
Mary-Krause, 2003 [31]	Database on medical records / Validation of cases	Myocardial infarction	Between 1st January 1996 and 31 December 1999	34 976 men 88 029 PY	60 / 49 treated with PI	21 906 subjects 39 023 PY	34 months (med)	Higher risk SMR=3.6 (1.8-6.2) = 30 months of PI exposure vs <18 months
D'Arminio Monforte, 2004 [38]	Specifically designed cohort / Validation of cases	Cardio- and cerebro-vascular events	Between December 1999 and July 2002	36 145 PY	207			RR=1.26 per year of combination antiretroviral treatment exposure
Friis-Moller, 2007 [32]	Specifically designed cohort / Validation of cases	Myocardial infarction	Between December 1999 and February 2005	23 437 subjects 94 469 PY	345			RR=1.16 (1.09-1.23) per year of cART exposure / RR=1.16 (1.10-1.23) per year of PI exposure / RR=1.05 (0.98-1.13) per year of NNRTI exposure
Bozette, 2008 [37]	Database on administrative data / No validation of cases	Serious cardiovascular diseases, stroke or death	Between 1st January 1993 and 31 December 2003	41 213 subjects 168 213 PY	Inpatient stays for serious CV events	42 406 PY		HR=1.28 (0.71-2.30) 72 months of PI exposure vs 0 months
Sabin, 2008 [39, 40]	Specifically designed cohort / Validation of cases	Myocardial infarction	Between December 1999 and January 2007	33 347 subjects 157 912 PY	517			RR=1.90 (1.47-2.45) recent use abacavir vs no recent use / RR=1.49 (1.14-1.95) recent use didanosine vs no recent use

PY, person-years; *med*, median

The expected incidence of MI in the general male population with the same age distribution was 10.8 cases per 10,000 PY. The estimated incidence of MI was 8.2 per 10,000 PY (95% CI=4.7–11.7) in group 1, 15.9 (95% CI=7.9–23.9) in group 2, and 33.8 (95% CI=15.4–52.1) in group 3 (Fig. 1). No significant difference was observed between the general male population of the same age and the patients treated with PIs for less than 18 months. Although not significantly so, the risk of MI increased among patients treated with PIs for 18–29 months. In contrast, the risk of MI among patients exposed to PIs for 30 months or more was three times that of the general population (standardized morbidity ratio, SMR=2.9, 95% CI=1.5–5.0). Compared to patients exposed to PIs for less than 18 months, those treated for 18 months or more were at an increased risk of MI (SMR=1.9, 95% CI=1.0–3.1 for group 2 and SMR=3.6, 95% CI=1.8–6.2 for group 3). These results show that the risk of MI in HIV-infected men increases with the dura-

tion of PI treatment, while other antiretroviral classes are not associated with an increased risk of MI.

How can this discordance between the results of Bozzette et al. [36] and Mary-Krause et al. [31] be explained? A direct comparison of the results of the two studies is impossible because they did not examine the same types of event. Mary-Krause et al. [31] examined admissions for and deaths from MI, whereas Bozzette et al. [36] only looked at admissions for cardiovascular disease, without taking deaths into account (especially deaths occurring outside hospital), probably leading to an underestimation of the number of cases. Also, this latter study grouped together deaths and admissions for cardiovascular and cerebrovascular disease. Holmberg et al. [28], who found an effect of PIs regarding the risk of MI, did not observe an increased risk of cerebrovascular disease. Results from the published DAD study (Data Collection on Adverse Events of Anti-HIV Drugs) indicated that there is an increasing

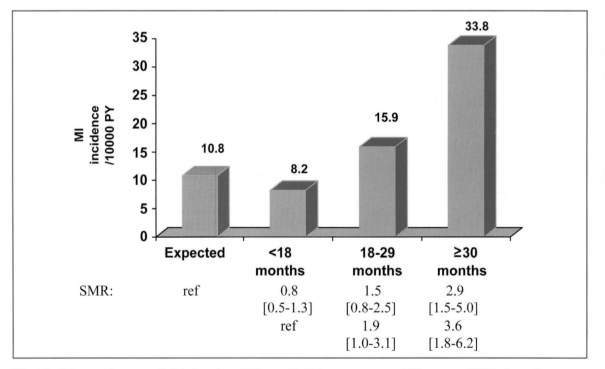

Fig. 1 Incidence of myocardial infarction (*MI*) per 10,000 person-years (*PY*) among HIV-infected men according to the duration of PI exposure (in months) compared to the incidence of MI among the general male population of the same age. The standardized morbidity ratios (*SMR*) with their 95% confidence intervals in brackets were used to test the differences between incidence rates. (From [31], with permission)

risk of first cardio- and cerebrovascular events with longer exposure to combination antiretroviral treatment [38]. The ninth version of the international classification of diseases [46], used by Bozzette et al. [36], includes codes 410 (acute MI), 411 (other acute and subacute forms of ischemic heart disease), 413 (angina pectoris), and 414 (other forms of chronic ischemic heart disease), whereas Mary-Krause et al. [31] used only code 410. It would be interesting to study the impact of PIs on each pathology separately. It should be noted that, although not significant, Bozzette et al. observed a higher risk of admission for cardiovascular diseases [36] among subjects exposed to PIs for 24 months as compared with 0 months (RR=1.23). It is surprising that the incidence of admissions for cardiovascular disease–more than 10 cases per 1,000 PY–observed in the study by Bozette et al. [36] was much higher than the incidence rates of CHD observed among seropositive American subjects exposed to PIs in other studies (5.9–6.6 events per 1,000 PY) [30, 35]. It is also surprising that Bozzette et al. found that the rate of CHD fell with time despite the increasing age of HIV-infected subjects.

A recent update of the study of Bozette et al [37] continues to find hazards for serious cardiovascular events near 1.0 for exposure to cART. Nevertheless, the HR of cART that includes an NNRTI or a PI, even non significant, is equal to 1.22 (95% CI=0.77-1.92) and the HR of cART that includes a PI only is equal to 1.28 (95% CI=0.71-2.30).

The DAD study [29], a prospective observational study of 23,468 patients enrolled in 11 cohorts on 3 continents from December 1999 to July 2002, showed a similar relationship between exposure to combination antiretroviral therapy (including PIs or NNRTIs) and the risk of MI to that found by Mary-Krause et al. [31], the risk increasing with the duration of cART. In the same way, Moore et al. [30] reported a study of 2,671 subjects followed up after 1 January 1996, in which the risk of cardiovascular events was higher among subjects exposed to PIs. Of 3,083,209 individuals analyzed among them, 28,513 were HIV-infected. Currier et al. [44] found a higher incidence of CHD among young men and women with HIV infection than that among non-HIV-infected individuals. Their results also suggest that any exposure to potent combination antiretroviral therapy may contribute to the incidence of CHD among younger individuals when controlling for certain comorbidities.

An update of the DAD study [32] on 23,437 subjects corresponding to 94,469 person-years (PY) of follow-up among them 345 MI showed an incidence of 3.7/1,000 PY with a decrease between 1999 and 2005. The incidence increased with increasing length of exposure to PI with an incidence increased from 1.5 per 1,000 PY among those not exposed to PI to 6.0 per 1,000 PY among those exposed to PI. In addition, the relative rate per year of exposure to PI was 1.16 (95% CI=1.10–1.23), result found as well by Klein et al. [47], which corresponds to a doubling of the risk over a 5-year period of exposure, whereas for non-nucleoside reverse transcriptase inhibitors it was 1.05 (95% CI=0.98–1.13).

Recent results reported by the D:A:D group at the 2008 CROI meeting [39], and published in The Lancet [40], showing that recent use of abacavir and didanosine (current use or interruption less than 6 months previously) was associated with an increased risk of myocardial infarction (MI) need to be confirmed or not by other studies.

The Strategies for Management of Antiretroviral Therapy (SMART) study [48] recently showed an increased risk of cardiovascular disease in patients whose antiretroviral therapy was interrupted when their CD4+ cell count reached a certain level as opposed to patients who received continuous treatment. This international randomized trial, conducted in 318 sites in 33 countries, had enrolled 5,472 patients when it was stopped. The HIV-infected persons who had a CD4+ cell count of more than $350/mm^3$ were randomly assigned to the continuous use of antiretroviral therapy (the viral suppression group) or the episodic use of antiretroviral therapy (the drug conservative group) until the CD4+ count decreased to less than 250/mm^3. This trial was stopped because episodic antiretroviral therapy increased the risk of opportunistic disease or death from any cause, as compared with continuous antiretroviral therapy (HR=2.6, 95% CI=1.9–3.7). The risk for major cardiovascular, renal or hepatic disease was also higher in the episodic group (HR=1.7, 95% CI=1.1–2.5). So, these drug conservative strategy guided by the CD4 is not recommended. One of the most discussed hypotheses is that treatment may contribute to atherosclerotic plaque formation and that inflammation, due to viral load replication rebond following interruption of treatment, should support the destabilization of these atherosclerotic plaques.

The increased risk of MI observed just after the advent of PI could be in part explained by a population who lived longer, and so the aging of the population which is at higher risk of cardiovascular diseases; by the chronic inflammatory state of HIV-infection, by the impact of known risk factors or CHD as smoking, and by the metabolic effects of antiretroviral treatment. Nevertheless, although today it is admitted that incidence of CHD was higher in HIV-infected patients than in the general population, links between viral infection, antiretroviral treatment, especially the impact of new antiretroviral drugs which have potentially less metabolic disturbances than PI, and the increase of MI incidence need to be precise even if we are not able to study each drug separately.

Outcome of Coronary Heart Disease in HIV-Infected Subjects

Few data have been published on the outcome of acute coronary events among HIV-infected patients compared to HIV-seronegative subjects. Compared with HIV-seronegative patients with idiopathic dilated cardiomyopathy, HIV-infected counterparts had

markedly reduced survival and a hazards ratio for death of 4.0 [49]. A study of 24 HIV-seropositive subjects with acute MI [50] showed that characteristics at hospital admission, the treatment strategy, and the relatively benign in-hospital outcome were similar to those of HIV-seronegative subjects admitted for acute MI. In contrast, after 15 months of follow-up, a higher incidence of recurrent infarction was observed among HIV-infected patients (20% vs. 4%, p=0.07), together with a higher incidence of hospitalization for other recurrent coronary events (45% vs. 11%, p=0.007). Although the TIMI risk scores of HIV-infected patients with acute coronary syndromes (ACS) are lower and these patients have less extensive coronary disease than HIV-seronegative patients with ACS, percutaneous coronary intervention in HIV-infected patients is associated with high restenosis rates [51]. Further studies are necessary to confirm this worse long-term prognosis of HIV-seropositive subjects with CHD.

Conclusion

Available data suggest that exposure to PIs increases the risk of MI to a degree that depends on the duration of exposure. However, the rate of MI remains low and the risk-benefit ratio of PIs remains positive, as the increase in life expectancy conferred by cART far outweighs the associated risk of MI. Indeed, one study showed that the 3-year risk of MI increased from 0.30% (95% CI=0.20–0.38%) in antiretroviral-naive patients to 1.07% (95% CI=0.43–1.77%) in patients receiving antiretrovirals of all three classes. The estimated 3-year risk of AIDS or death is between 6.2 and 11.1% among patients receiving antiretroviral therapy when they continue treatment, and from 22.5 to 29.4% when they stop treatment [52].

In keeping with current guidelines [5, 53, 54], the risk of CHD must be taken into account in antiretroviral treatment decisions, especially for patients with known vascular risk factors. Factors significantly associated with MI are older age, smoking either currently or formerly, previous cardiovascular disease, and male sex, but not a family history of CHD [29]. A higher total serum cholesterol level, a higher triglyceride level, and diabetes mellitus were also associated with an increased incidence of MI [29]. However, changes in lipid metabolism are different according to the different combined antiretroviral and the adverse events associated with antiretroviral treatment are different according to the drug regimen [55–58]. Thus, cholesterol, triglyceride, and blood glucose levels must be determined before and regularly during cART in order to diagnose any abnormalities as they occur and to manage the risk by following guidelines on the general population. In the DAD study, which compares the impact of two strategies of treatment, lipid lowering therapy (LTT) or switching from PI to a NNRTI (switch), versus a control group (no changes to therapy) [59], lipid changes were better with LTT or switch than the control group. LTT was better to decrease total (TC) and LDL-cholesterol, switch was better to increase HDL-cholesterol and they have similar benefits in regards to TC/HDL and triglycerides. Nevertheless, if lipid-lowering drug therapy is indicated, it should be limited to those agents with a low risk of interaction with antiretroviral drugs [60].

It is also necessary to keep in mind that the fight against CHD includes action on modifiable risk factors such as smoking, diabetes mellitus, arterial hypertension, and lipid disorders. Chiuve et al. have recently showed that 62% of CHD events were potentially preventable via adherence to healthy lifestyle practices [61]. Therefore, prevention should be promoted among patients with CHD risk factors even if it is unclear if risk will continue to rise with use of intervention. Nevertheless, in one study, time trends indicated changes in CHD risk factors, especially a decrease in the percentage of smokers and individuals with high cholesterol among HIV-seropositive patients between 2000 and 2005 [62].

Longer follow-up of PI therapy is needed in order to tell whether the risk of MI continues to increase with the duration of PI exposure. Moreover, further studies are necessary to confirm the association evidenced for abacavir and didanosine on CHD observed in the DAD study [39, 40] and to determine the impact of new therapeutic classes.

References

1. Palella FJ Jr, Delaney KM, Moorman AC et al (1998) Declining morbidity and mortality among patients with advanced human immunodeficiency virus infection: HIV Outpatient Study Investigators. N Engl J Med 338:853–860
2. The CASCADE Collaboration (2000) Survival after introduction of HAART in people with known duration of HIV-1 infection. Lancet 355:1158–1159
3. Lewden C, Salmon D, Morlat P et al (2004) Causes of death among HIV-infected adults in the era of potent antiretroviral therapy: emerging role of hepatitis and cancers, persistent role of AIDS. Int J Epidemiol 34:121–130
4. May T, Lewden C, Bonnet F et al (2004) Causes et caractéristiques des décès des patients infectés par le VIH-1, en succes immuno-virologique sous traitement antirétroviral. Presse Med 33:1487–1492
5. Delfraissy JF (2006) Prise en charge thérapeutique des personnes infectées par le HIV. Mise à jour 2006. Recommandations du groupe d'experts sous la direction du Pr P Yéni. Flammarion Médecine-Sciences, Paris
6. Hammer SM, Saag MS, Schechter M et al (2006) Treatment for adult HIV infection: 2006 recommendations of the International AIDS Society-USA Panel. JAMA 296:827–843
7. Grunfeld C, Pang M, Doerrler W et al (1992) Lipids, lipoproteins, triglyceride clearance, and cytokines in human immunodeficiency virus infection and the acquired immunodeficiency syndrome. J Clin Endocrinol Metab 74:1045–1052
8. Feingold KR, Krauss RM, Pang M et al (1993) The hypertriglyceridemia of acquired immunodeficiency syndrome is associated with an increased prevalence of low density lipoprotein

subclass pattern B. J Clin Endocrinol Metab 76:559–565

9. Carr A, Samaras K, Burton S et al (1998) A syndrome of peripheral lipodystrophy, hyperlipidaemia and insulin resistance in patients receiving HIV protease inhibitor. AIDS 12:F51–F58

10. Carr A, Samaras K, Thorisdottir A et al (1999) Diagnosis, prediction, and natural course of HIV-1 protease-inhibitor-associated lipodystrophy, hyperlipidaemia, and diabetes mellitus: a cohort study. Lancet 353:2093–2099

11. Safrin S, Grunfeld C (1999) Fat distribution and metabolic changes in patients with HIV infection. AIDS 13:2493–2505

12. Hadigan C, Meigs JB, Corcoran C et al (2001) Metabolic abnormalities and cardiovascular disease risk factors in adults with human immunodeficiency virus infection and lipodystrophy. Clin Infect Dis 32:130–139

13. Tabib A, Greenland T, Mercier I et al (1992) Coronary lesions in young HIV-positive subjects at necropsy. Lancet 340:730

14. Paton P, Tabib A, Loire R, Tete R (1993) Coronary artery lesions and human immunodeficiency virus infection. Res Virol 144:225–231

15. Henry K, Melroe H, Huebsch J et al (1998) Severe premature coronary artery disease with protease inhibitors. Lancet 351:1328

16. Behrens G, Schmidt H, Meyer D et al (1998) Vascular complications associated with use of HIV protease inhibitors. Lancet 351:1958

17. Gallet B, Pulik M, Genet P et al (1998) Vascular complications associated with use of HIV protease inhibitors. Lancet 351:1958–1959

18. Laurence J (1998) Vascular complications associated with use of HIV protease inhibitors. Lancet 351:1960

19. Flynn TE, Bricker LA (1999) Myocardial infarction in HIV-infected men receiving protease inhibitors. (letter) Ann Intern Med 131:548

20. Friedl AC, Attenhofer Jost CH, Schalcher C et al (2000) Acceleration of confirmed coronary artery disease among HIV-infected patients on potent antiretroviral therapy. AIDS 14:2790–2792

21. Karmochkine M, Raguin G (1998) Severe coronary artery disease in a young HIV-infected man with no cardiovascular risk factors who was treated with indinavir. AIDS 12:2499

22. Eriksson U, Opravil M, Amann FW, Schaffner A (1998) Is treatment with ritonavir a risk factor for myocardial infarction in HIV-infected patients? AIDS 12:2079–2080

23. Koppel K, Bratt G, Rajs J (1999) Sudden cardiac death in a patient on 2 years of highly active antiretroviral treatment: a case report. AIDS 13:1993–1994

24. Vittecoq D, Escaut J, Monsuez JJ (1998) Vascular complications associated with use of HIV protease inhibitors. Lancet 351:1959

25. Passalaris JD, Sepkowitz KA, Glesby MJ (2000) Coronary artery disease and human immunodeficiency virus infection. Clin Infect Dis 31:787–797

26. Jütte A, Schwenk A, Franzen D et al (1999) Increasing morbidity from myocardial infarction during HIV protease inhibitor treatment? (letter) AIDS 13:1796–1797

27. Rickerts V, Brodt HR, Staszewski S, Stille W (2000) Incidence of myocardial infarctions in HIV-infected patients between 1983 and 1998: The Frankfurt HIV-cohort study. Eur J Med Res 5:329–333

28. Holmberg SD, Moorman AC, Williamson JM et al (2002) Protease inhibitors and cardiovascular outcomes in patients with HIV-1. Lancet 360:1747–1748

29. Friis-Møller N, Sabin CA, Weber R et al (2003) Combination antiretroviral therapy and the risk of myocardial infarction. N Engl J Med 349:1993–2003

30. Moore RD, Keruly JC, Lucas G (2003) Increasing incidence of cardiovascular disease in HIV-infected persons in care. 10th conference on retroviruses and opportunistic infections, Boston, USA, 10–14 February 2003. Abstract no. 132

31. Mary-Krause M, Cotte L, Simon A et al (2003) Increased risk of myocardial infarction with duration of protease inhibitor therapy in HIV-infected men. AIDS 17:2479–2486

32. DAD Study Group, Friis-Møller N, Reiss P, Sabin CA et al (2007) Class of antiretroviral drugs and the risk of myocardial infarction. N Engl J Med 356:1723–1735

33. David MH, Hornung R, Fichtenbaum CJ (2002) Ischemic cardiovascular disease in persons with human immunodeficiency virus infection. Clin Infect Dis 34:98–102

34. Klein D, Hurley LB, Quesenberry CP, Sidney S (2002) Do protease inhibitors increase the risk for coronary heart disease in patients with HIV-1 infection? J Acquir Immune Defic Syndr 30:471–477

35. Klein D, Hurley M (2003) Hospitalizations for coronary heart disease and myocardial infarction among men with HIV-1 infection: additional follow-up. 10th conference on retroviruses and opportunistic infections, Boston, USA, 10–14 February 2003, Abstract no. 747

36. Bozzette SA, Ake CF, Tam HK et al (2003) Cardiovascular and cerebrovascular events in patients treated for human immunodeficiency virus infection. N Engl J Med 348:702–710

37. Bozzette SA, Ake CF, Tam HK et al (2008) Long-

term survival and serious cardiovascular events in HIV-infected patients treated with highly active antiretroviral therapy. J Acquir Immune Defic Syndr 47:338–341

38. D'Arminio Monforte A, Sabin CA, Phillips AN et al (2004) Cardio- and cerebrovascular events in HIV-infected persons. AIDS 18:1811–1817

39. Sabin CA, Worm SW, Weber R et al (2008) Recent use of Abacavir and didanosine, but not of Thymidine Analogues, is associated with risk of myocardial infarction. 15th Conference on Retroviruses and Opportunistic Infections, Boston, USA, February 3-6, 2008. Abstract n°957c.

40. DAD Study Group, Sabin CA, Worm SW, Weber R et al (2008) Use of nucleoside reverse transcriptase inhibitors and risk of myocardial infarction in HIV-infected patients enrolled in the D:A:D study: a multi-cohort collaboration. Lancet 371:1417–1426

41. Anonymous (2000) Les registres français de cardiopathies ischémiques 1997–1998. Fédération Française de cardiologie, Paris

42. Depairon M, Chessex S, Sudre P et al (2001) Premature atherosclerosis in HIV-infected individuals: focus on protease inhibitor therapy. AIDS 15:329–334

43. Savès M, Chêne G, Ducimetière P et al (2003) Risk factors for coronary heart disease in patients treated for human immunodeficiency virus infection compared with the general population. Clin Infect Dis 37:292–298

44. Currier JS, Taylor A, Boyd F et al (2003) Coronary heart disease in HIV-infected individuals. J Acquir Immune Deficit Syndr 35:506–512

45. Smith C, Levy I, Sabin C et al (2004) Cardiovascular disease risk factors and antiretroviral therapy in HIV-positive UK population. HIV Med 5:88–92

46. Anonymous (1977) Manuel de la classification statistique internationale des maladies, traumatismes et causes de décès, Révision 1975. Organisation Mondiale de la Santé, Geneva

47. Klein D, Hurley L, Silverberg M et al (2007) Surveillance data for myocardial infarction hospitalizations among HIV+ and HIV- Northern California. 14th Conference on Retroviruses and Opportunistic Infections, Los Angeles, USA, 25–28 February 2007, Abstract no. 807

48. El-Sadr WM, Lundgren JD, Neaton JD et al; Strategies for Management of Antiretroviral Therapy (SMART) Study Group (2006) CD4+ count-guided interruption of antiretroviral treatment. N Engl J Med 355:2283–2296

49. Barbaro G, Di Lorenzo G, Soldini M et al Gruppo Italiano per lo Studio Cardiologico dei pazi-enti affetti da AIDS (GISCA) (1999) Intensity of myocardial expression of inducible nitric oxide synthase influences the clinical course of human immunodeficiency virus-associated cardiomyopathy. Circulation 100:933–939

50. Matetzky S, Domingo M, Kar S et al (2003) Acute myocardial infarction in human immunodeficiency virus-infected patients. Arch Intern Med 163:457–460

51. Hsue PY, Giri K, Erickson S et al (2004) Clinical features of acute coronary syndromes in patients with human immunodeficiency virus infection. Circulation 109:316–319

52. Law M, Friis-Møller N, Weber R et al (2003) Modelling the 3-year risk of myocardial infarction among participants in the Data Collection on Adverse Events of Anti-HIV Drugs (DAD) study. HIV Med 4:1–10

53. Dube MP, Stein JH, Aberg JA et al (2003) Guidelines for the evaluation and management of dyslipidemia in human immunodeficiency virus (HIV)-infected adults receiving antiretroviral therapy: recommendations of the HIV Medical Association of the Infectious Disease Society of America and the Adult AIDS Clinical Trials Group. Clin Infect Dis 37:613–627

54. Department of Health and Human Services (2004) Guidelines for the use of antiretroviral agents in HIV-1 infected adults and adolescents. AIDSinfo, Rockville, MD, USA. http://www.AIDSinfo.nih.gov/guidelines. Cited 23 March 2004

55. Fellay J, Boubaker K, Lederberger B et al (2001) Prevalence of adverse events associated with potent antiretroviral treatment: Swiss HIV cohort Study. Lancet 358:1322–1327

56. Friis-Møller N, Weber R, Reiss P et al (2003) Cardiovascular disease risk factors in HIV patients- association with antiretroviral therapy. Results from the DAD study. AIDS 17:1179–1193

57. Fontas E, van Leth F, Sabin CA et al (2004) Lipid profiles in HIV-infected patients receiving combination antiretroviral therapy: Are different antiretroviral drugs associated with different lipid profiles? J Infect Dis 189:1056–1074

58. Haubrich RH, Riddler S, DiRienzo G et al (2007) Metabolic Outcomes of ACTG 5142: A Prospective, Randomized, Phase III Trial of NRTI-, PI-, and NNRTI-sparing Regimens for Initial Treatment of HIV-1 Infection. 14th conference on retroviruses and opportunistic infections, Los Angeles, USA, February 25–28, 2007. Abstract no. 38

59. van der Valk M, Friis-Moller N, Sabin C et al (2006) Effects of different interventions to improve ART-associated dyslipidemia. 8th inter-

national congress on drug therapy in HIV infection, Glasgow, UK, November 12–16, 2006. Abstract no. PL12.2

60. Falusi OM, Aberg JA (2001) HIV and cardiovascular risk factors. AIDS Reader 11:263–268

61. Chiuve SE, McCullough ML, Sacks FM, Rimm EB (2006) Healthy lifestyle factors in the primary prevention of coronary heart disease among men: benefits among users and nonusers of lipid-lowering and antihypertensive medications. Circulation 114:160–167

62. Glass TR, Ungsedhapand C, Wolbers M et al (2006) Prevalence and risk factors for cardiovascular disease in HIV-infected patients over time: the Swiss HIV cohort study. HIV Med 7:404–410

Coronary Artery Disease in HIV-Infected Patients: Clinical Presentation, Pathophysiology, Prognosis, Prevention, and Treatment

F. Boccara, C. Meuleman, S. Ederhy, S. Lang, S. Janower, A. Cohen, F. Raoux

Introduction

The advent of new antiretroviral agents has dramatically reduced mortality and HIV-associated morbidity. In the highly active antiretroviral therapy (HAART) era, long-term side effects have been reported such as severe metabolic disorders and related acute cardiovascular complications including myocardial infarction, peripheral vascular disease, and stroke. Prevention and therapeutics for cardiovascular complications in HIV-infected patients are a new and emerging challenge for physicians involved in HIV infection care because of the prolongation of survival and long-term complications of HAART. In the present overview, we discuss the clinical presentation, pathophysiology, prognosis, prevention, and treatment of coronary heart disease (CHD) in HIV-infected patients.

The incidence of acute myocardial infarction in HIV-infected patients (HIV+) tends to be higher than in the general population [1, 2] particularly in those undergoing HAART [3], including protease inhibitors [2, 4]. The relationship between coronary artery disease (CAD) and the use of protease inhibitors in HIV-infected patients is still under debate [5]. The epidemiology of CHD in HIV-infected patients is discussed in this volume in the chapter by M. Mary-Krause and D. Costagliola.

Clinical Presentation and Cardiovascular Risk Factors

The spectrum of CAD in HIV-infected patients is similar to non-HIV-infected patients with various clinical presentations including silent ischemia, stable angina, and acute coronary syndrome (unstable angina, non-ST elevation myocardial infarction, ST elevation myocardial infarction; Figs. 1–6). The first case of CAD in the HAART era was published in 1998 followed by several case reports and series [6–13].

Whether protease inhibitors are directly responsible for CAD remains a matter of debate [5, 14].

In our cardiology department [13], 1 female and 19 male patients (mean age, 44±8 years; range, 34–65 years), infected with HIV since 9±4 years ago, were admitted from 1996 to 2002 for acute coronary syndrome (18 had myocardial infarction and 2 had unstable angina). Tobacco consumption (80%) and dyslipidemia (65%) were the most frequent cardiovascular risk factors. The median CD4 cell count was 387±184/mm3 and the median viral load was 8,000±23,000 copies/ml. Fourteen patients were treated with protease inhibitors for a mean duration of 19±13 months. Five patients were treated with thrombolysis, three had primary angioplasty.

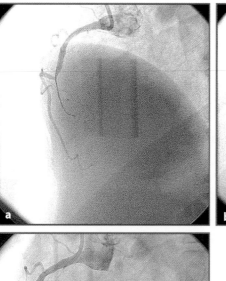

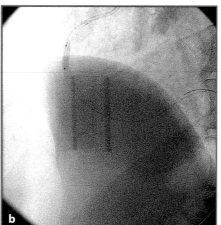

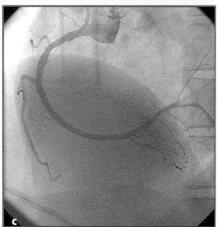

Fig. 1a-c Patient 1. a Coronary angiogram revealed an acute occlusion of the right coronary artery in a 38-year-old HIV-infected man (since 1995) during inferior acute myocardial infarction. A guide-wire is introduced into the lumen artery to pass the thrombotic occlusion. His vascular risk factors were smoking and mild dyslipidemia (high LDL cholesterol, low HDL cholesterol, and high triglyceride levels). b Balloon angioplasty performed at the site of the occlusion with 10-atmosphere expansion pressure. c Result after inflation of the balloon and implantation of a long bare stent (3.5 mm diameter, 32 mm length)

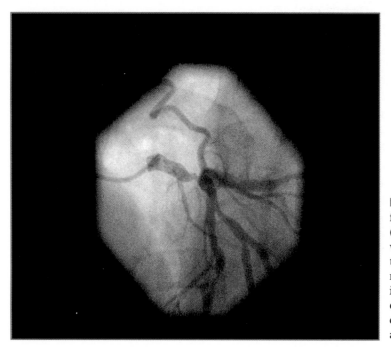

Fig. 2 Patient 2. Coronary angiogram finding a left main coronary stenosis (70%) in a 62-year-old HIV-infected woman (since 1987) who was admitted for an episode of unstable angina. Vascular risk factors were smoking and mixed dyslipidemia. She underwent a coronary artery by pass including the left internal mammary artery

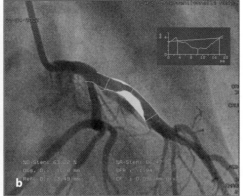

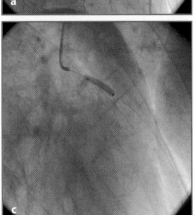

Fig. 3a-c Patient 3. a Coronary angiogram revealed a 65% diameter stenosis (eccentric) on the left anterior descending (LAD) artery in a 40-year-old HIV-infected man (since 1989) who was admitted for a non-ST elevation myocardial infarction (NSTEMI). Smoking and intravenous drug abuse were the only known vascular risk factors. b Quantitative coronary angiography revealed a 63% diameter stenosis, a 3.5-mm reference diameter and 18 mm in length. c, d Direct stenting of the lesion with a 3.5-mm diameter and 20-mm length stent. Excellent result without residual stenosis

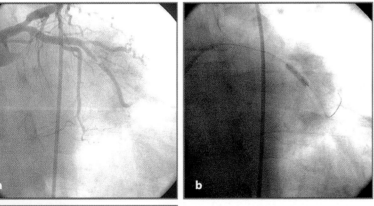

Fig. 4a-c Patient 4. a Coronary angiogram revealed a thrombotic stenosis of the first lateral artery (circumflex) in a 50-year-old HIV-infected man (since 1988) who was admitted for a NSTEMI. His only vascular risk factor was a high LDL cholesterol, a low HDL cholesterol, and mild elevated triglyceride levels. b Direct stenting (drug-eluted stent: 3 mm diameter x 13 mm length) of the lesion was performed. c Excellent result after stent implantation with TIMI 3 flow, no dissection and no residual stenosis

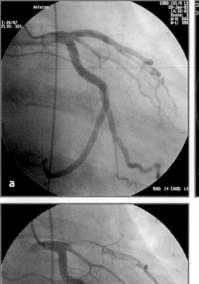

Fig. 5a-c Patient 5. a Coronary angiogram of a 35-year-old HIV-infected man (since 1992) with normal left and right coronary arteries. No atherosclerotic lesions were visualized. This examination was performed because he was admitted with congestive heart failure (NYHA class IV) and echocardiography revealed a cardiomyopathy with severe left ventricular global hypokinesia, poor ejection fraction (20%), and a suspected apical thrombus. **b** A CT scan confirmed the presence of a left ventricle apical thrombus. The patient underwent anticoagulation therapy with coumadine. **c** Three months later, he was admitted for an acute anterior myocardial infarction and the coronary angiogram revealed a long thrombus in the left anterior descending artery (TIMI flow 1). He had stopped taking coumadine 2 months earlier. After 1 month of efficient anticoagulation plus aspirin therapy, the coronary angiogram revealed no remaining thrombus and no atherosclerosis stenosis or plaque rupture. Coronary embolism from the apical left ventricle thrombus was evoked

Duong et al. [12] showed that silent myocardial ischemia (detected by treadmill test) was increased in HIV-infected patients without CHD (11%) and that age, central fat accumulation, and hypercholesterolemia were independent predictive factors. HIV-infected patients seem to be at higher risk of CAD than the general population as demonstrated by Bergersen et al. [15], who reported that compared to control subjects, twice as many HIV-infected patients on HAART had an estimated 10-year CHD Framingham risk above 20%. Neumann et al. [16], in a cohort of 309 HIV-infected patients, demonstrated that the risk of cardiovascular events is related to the age of HIV-infected patients. The overall 10-year probability for cardiovascular events was higher in the oldest group (>50 years; median, 20.5%) than in the youngest group (18–30 years; 1.9%; $p<0.01$). Therefore, an increased duration of life due to a more effective antiretroviral therapy will have a significant impact on the rate of cardiovascular events in this patient population.

Hadigan et al. [17] estimated the 10-year CHD risk among 91 HIV-infected men and women with fat redistribution and compared it with the risk estimated for 273 age-, sex-, and body mass index (BMI)-matched subjects enrolled in the Framingham Offspring Study. The 10-year CHD risk estimate was significantly elevated among HIV-infected patients with fat redistribution, particularly among men; however, when they were matched with control subjects by waist-to-hip ratio, the 10-year CHD risk estimate did not significantly differ between groups. HIV-infected patients without fat redistribution did not have a greater CHD risk estimate than did control subjects. The CHD risk estimate was greatest in HIV-infected patients who had primary lipoatrophy, compared with those who had either

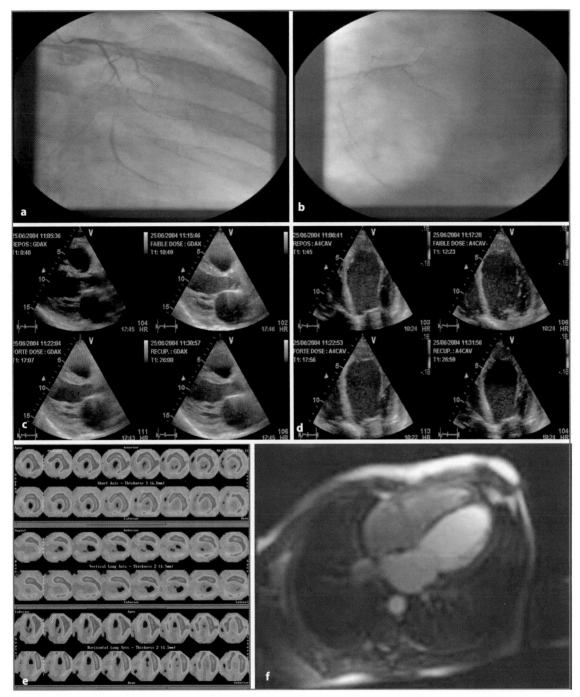

Fig. 6a-f Patient 6. a Coronary angiogram showing three-vessel CAD in a 43-year-old HIV-infected man admitted for a NSTEMI. Occlusion of proximal LAD and proximal circumflex artery. One lateral artery is visualized, but no LAD without controlateral filling. b Proximal right coronary occlusion. c-d Dobutamine stress echocardiography (c parasternal long axis, d apical four chambers) demonstrated apical viability. e Rest thallium-201 single-photon emission tomography (SPECT) finding of anterior and lateral myocardial viability. f Heart cine magnetic resonance imaging (long-axis) finding severe left ventricular dysfunction (LVEF 15%)

lipohypertrophy or mixed fat redistribution. Recently, Knobel et al. [18] described the cardiovascular risk factors in a cohort of 760 HIV-infected patients comparing three equations (Framingham, PROCAM and SCORE). They observed that the Framingham equation categorized a higher proportion of HIV-infected male patients with moderate cardiovascular risk and a lower proportion of those with low risk ($p<0.0001$) compared with PROCAM and SCORE. However, this study showed a high prevalence of HIV-infected patients at low cardiovascular risk (between 76.6 to 90.1% regardless of the equation used). However, compared with PROCAM and SCORE, Framingham risk equation in HIV-infected patients identified a higher number of male patients with moderate cardiovascular risk.

The APROCO study group (France) [19] compared the distribution of risk factors for cardiovascular disease in 227 HIV-infected patients (35–44 years) who were treated with protease inhibitors with 527 HIV-1-uninfected men from the MONICA project. HIV-infected patients had a lower prevalence of hypertension, a lower mean HDL cholesterol level, a higher prevalence of smoking, a higher mean waist-to-hip ratio, and a higher mean triglyceride level. No difference was found for total plasma or DL cholesterol levels, or for the prevalence of diabetes. The predicted risk of CHD was greater among HIV-1-infected men (RR, 1.20) and women (RR, 1.59; $p<10-6$ for both) compared with the HIV-1-uninfected cohort.

In the Swiss cohort [20] where 8,033 individuals completed at least one cardiovascular risk factors questionnaire. The most common cardiovascular risk factors were smoking (57.0%), low HDL cholesterol (37.2%), high triglycerides (35.7%), and high blood pressure (26.1%). In total, 2.7 and 13.8% of patients were categorized as being at high (>20%) and moderate (10–20%) 10-year risk for CHD, respectively. Over 6 years, the percentage of smokers decreased from 61.4 to 47.6% and the percentage of individuals with total cholesterol >6.2 mmol/L decreased from 21.1 to 12.3%. The prevalence of cardiovascular risk and CHD was higher in patients currently on antiretroviral (ART) therapy than in either pretreated or ART-naive patients.

In conclusion, HIV-infected patients undergoing HAART seem to be at a higher risk of CAD because of the higher incidence of traditional vascular risk factors [21–23] compared with same-age non-HIV-infected patients. Whether protease inhibitors have a direct impact on atherosclerosis remains hypothetical, however strong evidences now argue for a direct impact of protease inhibitors on the incidence of myocardial infarction [14, 24, 25].

Pathophysiology

Several hypotheses have been raised regarding the pathophysiology of atherosclerotic CAD in HIV-infected patients undergoing HAART. Many factors could increase the rate of cardiovascular events and accelerate atherosclerosis:

1. Insulin resistance (reported in 25–62% of HIV-infected patients), diabetes mellitus (5–10%), and lipodystrophy syndrome (20–83%) [23, 26, 27]
2. Resistant dyslipidemia–lower level of HDL cholesterol, higher level of triglycerides (50%–90%), small and dense LDL particles–with lower efficacy of lipid-lowering therapy [27–32]
3. Chronic inflammation and infection with increased cytokine levels (tumor necrosis factor-alpha, interleukin-1, interleukin-6, interleukin-10, monocyte chemoattractant protein-1) [33–37]
4. Enhanced endothelial injury due to dyslipidemia [38], oxidant stress [39], adhesion molecules [40], HIV Tat protein, related angiogenic effects [33, 41, 42] and immunological response [42]

5. A prothrombotic state linked to HIV status and/or antiretroviral therapy [43, 44]

The role of metabolic disorders (low level of HDL cholesterol and hypertriglyceridemia) is highlighted in different studies [45, 46] that included HIV+ patients with acute coronary syndrome compared with HIV+ subjects without cardiovascular manifestations. These disorders can be partly explained by HIV treatments that result in higher hypertriglyceridemia and lower levels of HDL cholesterol compared with non-infected-HIV patients. The low level of HDL cholesterol may play a major role in the pathophysiologic mechanism of atherothrombosis. Another aspect is the degree of the immunologic status reflected by the CD4 cell count level, which has been demonstrated to be lower in HIV+ patients with acute coronary syndrome compared with HIV+ patients without acute coronary syndrome [45, 46].

Direct vascular toxicity of the virus has been suggested in a report from Barbaro et al. [47]. They found HIV-1 sequences within the arterial wall in a 32-year-old man without vascular risk factors who died from an anterior myocardial infarction. In addition, Schecter et al. [34] demonstrated that HIV-envelope glycoprotein gp120 activates human arterial smooth muscle cells to express tissue factor and promote the coagulation cascade and plaque rupture, supporting the observation of a correlation between plasma HIV load, a prothrombotic state, and cellular apoptosis.

Tabib et al. [48] found that coronary artery lesions of young HIV-infected patients at autopsy, whose death was caused from other cardiovascular disease, were of an intermediate type, between those observed in coronary atherosclerosis and chronic rejection in cardiac transplant patients. Subclinical atherosclerosis in HIV-infected patients has been reported [42, 49–53] with increased intima-media thickness and atherosclerotic plaques of the carotid and femoral arteries correlated to age, dyslipidemia, and tobacco use, but not with protease inhibitor therapy. Coronary artery calcifications, another surrogate marker and prognostic factor of atherosclerosis visualized with electron beam computed tomography, are under evaluation in HIV-infected patients, with controversial results [54–56]. Coronary magnetic resonance angiography could be a further diagnostic tool for detecting infraclinic coronary atherosclerosis in the near future (Fig. 7).

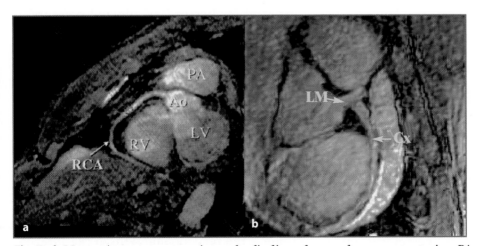

Fig. 7a,b Magnetic resonance angiography finding of normal coronary arteries. *PA*, pulmonary artery; *Ao*, aorta; *LV*, left ventricle; *RV*, right ventricle; *RCA*, right coronary artery; *LM*, left main coronary artery; *Cx*, circumflex

Prognosis

The prognosis of CAD in HIV-infected patients has been evaluated in few series [57–61]. Matetzky et al. [57] compared the characteristics and long-term course of 24 HIV-infected patients with acute myocardial infarction with matched non-HIV patients. The in-hospital course was similar without death or re-infarction. After a 15-month follow-up, HIV-infected patients had a higher incidence of re-infarction, recurrent cardiovascular event, and target vessel revascularization independently of the type of antiretroviral therapy.

Hsue et al. [58], in a case-control study, reported a higher rate of coronary restenosis after percutaneous coronary intervention (PCI) in HIV-infected patients compared with non-HIV-infected patients with acute coronary syndrome–52% (15/22 patients) vs. 14% (3/21 patients), $p = 0.032$. There was no significative difference in the subgroup of patients who had stenting (50 vs. 18%, $p=0.078$). Ambrose et al. [59] reported the outcome of 51 HIV-infected patients with acute coronary syndrome. Forty-five had coronary angiography and 25 had PCI with an excellent initial result and no hospital death in the PCI subgroup. Our group reported the results of a case-control study [61], comparing baseline characteristics, rate of procedural success and clinical outcome at 20-months (major adverse cardiac events: death from cardiac cause, myocardial infarction, target lesion or vessel revascularization) between 50 consecutive HIV+ and 50 HIV-patients matched for age and gender who underwent PCI. Procedural success rate was achieved in 98% of cases with a high rate of stenting (76 vs. 96%, $p=0.004$). In-hospital course was uneventful in both groups. Clinical restenosis including revascularization of the entire target vessel was not significantly different between HIV+ and HIV-patients (14 vs. 16%, $p=0.78$) at follow-up (20 months). Rates of occurrence of first MACE and MI at 20 months were similar in both groups (20 vs. 16%, $p=0.64$ and 8 vs. 0%, $p=0.12$). We concluded that PCI represents an adequate and safe therapeutic strategy of coronary revascularization in HIV+ patients without significant differences in term of clinical restenosis and MACE compared with control population. The prognosis of coronary revascularization in HIV-infected patients needs to be compared with a large cohort of HIV-negative subjects [62].

Prevention and Treatment

As in the general population, cardiovascular risk stratification in HIV-infected patients needs to be evaluated before and during HAART. The "traditional" cardiovascular risk factors are present in the HIV-infected population: smoking, dyslipidemia, diabetes mellitus, hypertension, premature familial cardiovascular disease, and poor physical fitness. Reducing risk factors should become a routine aspect in the care of HIV-infected patients, who now live longer because of the steep decline in morbidity and mortality as a result of HAART. Large prospective and matched control studies in HIV-infected patients in primary cardiovascular prevention are needed so as to identify specific risk factors and stratify the cardiovascular risk. Intervention studies on reducing the cardiovascular risk in HIV-infected patients, as in the general population, are needed (smoking cessation, physical activity, lipid-lowering drugs, aspirin).

The first step is to evaluate the relative risk or the absolute risk of a cardiovascular event in each patient by using the Framingham risk score (www.CHD-taskforce.com) and/or the recommendations of the International Society of Atherosclerosis (www.athero.org). The objective is to identify, in primary prevention, patients who require risk reduction by prescribing aspirin, lipid-lowering, or antihypertensive medication to decrease mortality and morbidity as proven in the general population.

Primary Prevention

Aspirin

According to the North American and European task force, aspirin should be prescribed in primary prevention using Lauer's algorithm (Fig. 8) [63] driven by the Framingham risk score, which is similar [64, 65]. Special caution should be recommended in patients with untreated or unstable hypertension because of the increased risk of

hemorrhagic stroke and in the overall population because of the risk of major gastrointestinal bleeding. For the low-risk population (<0.6% per year), the reduction of absolute risk of myocardial infarction is equivalent to the risk of gastrointestinal bleeding.

Lipid-Lowering Therapy

Serum lipid levels should be evaluated in a fasting patient (12 h), particularly for triglycerides, before HAART is started and then every 3–6 months. National Cholesterol Education Program III [66] guidelines should be applied to HIV-infected patients (Table 1), as suggested in the guidelines for the management of dyslipidemia in HIV-

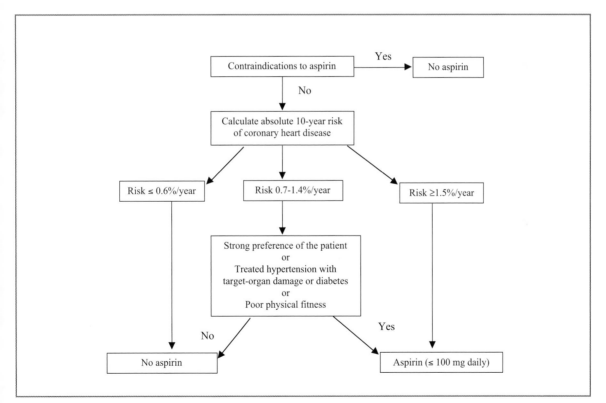

Fig. 8 Suggested algorithm for making decisions about the use of aspirin for primary prevention of CHD. Contraindications to aspirin therapy include known allergy, bleeding diathesis, platelet disorders, and active peptic ulcer disease. Relative contraindications include renal failure, concurrent use of nonsteroidal anti-inflammatory agents or anticoagulants, and uncontrolled hypertension. The risk of coronary heart disease is estimated by using the Framingham risk score. Poor physical fitness is defined as impaired exercise capacity for age and sex

Table 1 National Cholesterol Education Program treatment decisions made on the basis of LDL cholesterol levels: NCEP III guidelines [66]

Risk category	LDL goal	Initiate lifestyle changes	Initiate drug therapy
Primary prevention 0–1 Risk factor	<160 mg/dl	≥160 mg/dl	≥190 mg/dl
≥ 2 Risk factors 10-year risk 10-20%	<130 mg/dl	≥130 mg/dl	≥130 mg/dl
≥ 2 Risk factors 10-year risk <10%	<130 mg/dl	≥130 mg/dl	≥160 mg/dl
Secondary prevention CHD or 10-year risk >20 %	<100 mg/dl	≥100 mg/dl	≥130 mg/dl

Risk factors include age (men aged ≥45 years, women aged ≥55 years or who experienced premature menopause that was not being treated with estrogen replacement therapy), family history of CHD (first-degree male relative with CHD before 55 years of age or first-degree female relative with CHD before 65 years of age), current cigarette smoking, hypertension, low HDL cholesterol (<35 mg/dl), diabetes mellitus. In the presence of high HDL cholesterol (≥60 mg/dl), subtract 1 risk factor

infected patients by Dube et al. [29]. If dyslipidemia is present, secondary causes should be screened: diabetes mellitus, hypothyroidism, excessive alcohol use, obstructive liver disease, chronic renal failure, hypogonadism, and drug-induced elevated LDL cholesterol (progestins, anabolic steroids, and corticosteroids). Lipid-lowering therapy should be prescribed cautiously in HIV-infected patients because of the potentially severe interaction between statins, fibrates on the one hand and protease inhibitors on the other hand [67].

Several statins, listed in Table 2, are metabolized via the cytochrome P-450 3A4 pathway. Protease inhibitors inhibit cytochrome P-450 and could increase statin toxicity, thereby reducing the efficacy of protease inhibitors. Non-nucleoside reverse transcriptase inhibitors are inducers of cytochrome P-450 and could reduce statin efficacy. As demonstrated by Fichtenbaum et al. [67] in patients receiving ritonavir and saquinavir, the area under the curve increased about fivefold for atorvastatin, 32-fold for simvastatin, and decreased 0.5-fold for pravastatin.

Two studies have evaluated pravastatin [30] and fluvastatin [68] in the context of dyslipidemia in HIV-infected patients under antiretroviral theraphy. Stein et al. [30] demonstrated in a double-blind, placebo-controlled study, that pravastatin (40 mg/day) resulted in a 20.8% reduction in LDL particles (p=0.030), a 26.7% reduction in small LDL (p=0.100), and a 44.9% reduction in small VLDL (p=0.023). Total and non-HDL cholesterol levels decreased by 18.3% (p<0.001) and 21.7% (p<0.001), respectively. Benesic et al. [68] compared fluvastatin (40 mg daily) with pravastatin (20 mg daily) in 25 HIV-infected patients. The reduction of LDL levels was 30.2% in the fluvastatin group and 14.4% in the pravastatin group with no effect observed on triglyceride or HDL levels. Rosuvastatin, a new statin, without known interactions with protease inhibitors and more powerful compared to pravastatin seems to be promising in treating hyperlipidemia in this context [69].

Palacios et al. [70] demonstrated a significant reduction of 27% in total cholesterol, 37% in LDL cholesterol, with atorvastatin 10 mg/day. Lovastatin and simvastatin

Table 2 Different cytochrome P450 (CYP) pathways of lipid-lowering agents

	CYP	Interactions with PI	Recommendations
Statins			
Atorvastatin	3A4	Fivefold increased AUC with RITO-SAQ	Recommended at 10 mg daily
Lovastatin	3A4	High toxicity with PI	Not recommended
Simvastatin	3A4	High toxicity with PI 32-fold increased AUC with RITO-SAQ	Not recommended
Fluvastatin	2C9	Not tested	Recommended at 40 mg daily
Pravastatin	No P450 interactions	0.5-fold decreased AUC with RITO-SAQ	Recommended at 20–40 mg daily
Rosuvastatin	No	No interaction kwon but not tested	Recommended at 5-10 mg daily
Fibrates			
Bezafibrate	No P450 interactions	Not tested	Recommended at 400 mg daily
Fenofibrate	No P450 interactions	Not tested	Recommended at 200 mg daily
Gemfibrozil	No P450 interactions; interaction with simvastatin, cerivastatin, rosuvastatin but not atorvastatin	Not tested	Recommended at 900–1,200 mg daily
Ezetimibe	No	Not Tested	Recommended at 10 mg alone or with a statin

AUC, area under the curve; *RITO*, ritonavir; *SAQ*, saquinavir; *PI*, protease inhibitor

Table 3 Recommendations for the choice of drug therapy in dyslipidemia for HIV-infected patients undergoing HAART according to Dube et al. [29]

Lipid abnormalities	First choice	Second choice
Isolated high LDL cholesterol	Statin	Fibrate
Combined hyperlipidemia	Fibrate or statin	If starting fibrate, add statin
Isolated hypertriglyceridemia	Fibrate	Statin

should be avoided in patients receiving drugs that might interact with CYP-450. Bezafibrate, gemfibrozil, and fenofibrate have been tested in HIV-infected patients with isolated or combined hypertriglyceridemia and proved safe and well tolerated, whereas the efficacy seemed to be reduced in this population [71]. Fibrates have no proven interaction with the cytochrome P-450 pathway and protease inhibitors.

The use of a standard dose of rosuvastatin (5–10 mg daily) or pravastatin (20–40 mg daily) or fluvastatin (40 mg daily) seems to be the safest choice because of the lack of interaction with cytochrome P-450 in predominant hypercholesterolemia. A reduced dose of atorvastatin (10 mg daily) can be used also with monitoring of CK values because of a potential interaction with cytochrome P-450. Fibrates should be prescribed in the presence of an elevated triglyceride level (>5 g/L) with a normal or near-normal LDL cholesterol level after diet and exercise recommendations have failed.

The association of statin and fibrate should not be recommended as a first-line treatment because of their potentially high toxicity (rhabdomyolysis, hepatitis) and interaction with protease inhibitors. If necessary, in high-risk patient for CAD and uncontrolled combined dyslipidemia, this association should be used with caution: start at a low dose and titrate upward with regular control of signs of myopathy and CK plasma levels.

New lipid lowering therapies like niacin acid [72] and ezetemibe [73] may have indications in important hypertriglyceridemia and resistant dyslipidemia or hypersensitivity to statin, respectively. Table 3 indicates how lipid-lowering therapy should be prescribed, according to Dube et al. [29]. The risk–benefit ratio in treating HIV-infected patients with dyslipidemia is unknown. Male patients aged over 45 years and female patients over 55 years with hypertension and/or diabetes and/or familial premature CAD are candidates for lipid-lowering therapy. Switching from one protease inhibitor, ritonavir or indinavir to nevirapine or efavirenz to nevirapine or to atazanavir [74–77], could have beneficial effects on the reversal of dyslipidemia.

In consideration of an unlimited duration of treatment with antiretroviral drugs, it became of great importance the management or the prevention of side effects. The management of the various aspects of the tolerability of HAART, such as abnormal lipid metabolism, is one of the main topics of the studies in the field of HIV infection in industrialized Countries. The use of atazanavir, in contrast to other protease inhibitors, determines low increase of total cholesterol, LDL cholesterol and triglycerides, also in experienced patients. For a more detailed discussion of strategy will switch leads to a final algorithm.

The advent of atazanavir with a low risk of inducing dyslipidemia should be evaluated in patients with a high-risk cardiovascular profile or dyslipidemia. Switching stavudine to tenofovir demonstrated a decrease in triglyceride and total cholesterol [78]. Whether protease inhibitor therapy should be discontinued after an acute coronary syndrome and treatment switched to a nonnucleoside reverse transcriptase inhibitor (efavirenz, nevirapine) or to other nucleoside or nucleotide analogs (abacavir, tenofovir) with a better "atherogenic profile" needs further investigation.

Smoking Cessation

The prevalence of cigarette smoking among HIV-infected patients is higher compared to the general population [79]. Louie et al. [80] reported that smoking-associated pulmonary diseases such as obstructive lung disease, chronic bronchitis, and bronchiectasis were increased in the HIV-infected population. Lung cancer was the most common cause of death from non-AIDS-defining malignancies (11%) followed by Hodgkin's disease (5%), hepatocellular cancer (4%), and anal cancer (3%). Smoking cessation should be a priority for HIV-infected patients and physicians, integrated into a global risk reduction approach (dyslipidemia, diabetes mellitus, overweight, inactivity) to prevent future coronary events [81].

Exercise Training and Healthy Diet

Exercise has been shown to improve strength, cardiovascular function, psychological status, and reduce cardiovascular disease in the general population [82]. Exercise training also reduces total and abdominal fat. These changes in body composition mediate improvements in insulin sensitivity and blood pressure and may improve endothelial vasodilator function [83]. Encouraging lifestyle changes should be done as soon as possible, as HIV infection becomes a chronic disease. Various clinical interventions, including diet and exercise [84–86], switching antiretroviral agents, use of lipid-lowering and insulin-sensitizing agents, recombinant human growth hormone therapy, and plastic surgery, are under investigation in the treatment of morphologic changes (lipodystrophy syndrome).

Nutrition deficiencies (selenium, vitamin B12, carnitine, growth and thyroid hormones) should be sought because they are easily treatable and because of their great impact on ventricular function [87, 88]. Hyperhomocysteinemia is associated with an increased risk of heart and vascular diseases [89]. Vilaseca et al. [90] demonstrated that HIV-infected children undergoing protease inhibitor treatment have higher homocysteine concentrations and lower folate values compared with patients on other antiretroviral therapies, as in adults [91, 92]. In case of hyperhomocysteinemia, folic acid supplements should be prescribed.

Diabetes Mellitus

New-onset diabetes mellitus affects an increasing number of HIV-infected patients (5–10%) [93–95]. Impaired glucose tolerance and early insulin resistance are more frequent (10–25%) in HIV-infected patients mostly treated with HAART including protease inhibitors [95]. The risk factors that promote the onset of diabetes and insulin resistance are: use of certain drugs (protease inhibitors and NRTIs), ageing of the population HIV, visceral adiposity and the appearance of lipoatrophy [96].

Indinavir, lopinavir / ritonavir and ritonavir dosed, can induce, sometimes rapidly, insulin resistance [97]. Amprenavir, atazanavir, and saquinavir would seem to have a minor impact on the safety of insulin [98].

An Italian study has shown that atazanavir helps improve glucose tolerance even in pre-treated patients. From stress as all patients included in the study came from a system containing protease inhibitors and that the metabolic profile has improved after 24 weeks of therapy by the modification [99].

Insulin resistance is often accompanied by hyperinsulinemia and may predispose patients to atherosclerosis. Henry et al. [100] demonstrated that impaired fasting glucose (fasting plasma glucose 6.1–6.9 mmol/L) in seronegative patients was associated with the level of systolic blood pressure and could help predict cardiovascular mortality. Metformin increases the sensitivity of peripheral tissues to insulin and should be recommended for the treatment of type 2 diabetes mellitus in HIV-infected patients with documented insulin-resistance syndrome [93]. No cases of lactic acidosis have been reported in serial trials [101, 102], but warranted a regular follow-up.

New oral antidiabetic drugs such as thiazolidinediones (pioglitazone, rosiglitazone) could be promising therapy for lipodystrophy, metabolic syndrome, and insulin resistance in HIV-infected patients, however contradictory results have been reported [103, 104]. Thiazolidinediones reduce insulin resistance not only in type 2 diabetes but also in non-diabetic conditions associated with insulin resistance such as obesity.

Systemic Hypertension

Few data are available regarding the frequency and mechanisms of hypertension in HIV-infected patients [105]. Sattler et al. [106] showed that hypertension was more frequent in HIV-infected patients with lipodystrophy compared with HIV-infected patients without (74 vs. 48%, $p=0.01$). In a cohort of 214 HIV-1-infected patients (Frankfurt) [107], the prevalence of systemic hypertension was 29%. As in the general population, hypertensive subjects were older (49.1 ± 11.1 vs. 39.0 ± 8.1 years; $p<0.0001$) and the waist-to-hip ratio was higher than in normotensive individuals (0.99 ± 0.07 vs. 0.93 ± 0.08; $p<0.0001$). Hypertension was associated with a much higher frequency of persistent proteinuria (41.1 vs. 2.8%; $p<0.001$), CHD (16.1 vs. 1.3%; $p<0.0001$), and myocardial infarction (8.1 vs. 0.7%; $p<0.005$), whereas most cardiovascular risk factors were similar in both groups. Crane et al. [108] reported in an observational cohort study the effects of antiretrovirals on blood pressure (before and after initiating) in 444 patients. They found that treatment with lopinavir/ritonavir was significantly associated with elevated BP, an effect that appears to be mediated through an increase in BMI. Patients receiving atazanavir were least likely to develop elevated blood pressure in this cohort. Physicians should follow the current guidelines recommended for the general population by the Joint National Committee (JNC VII) [109] when treating hypertension in HIV-

infected patients and potential interactions between anti-hypertenisve agents and protease inhibitors.

Secondary Prevention

Acute coronary syndromes in HIV-infected patients with or without ST-segment elevation should be managed as recommended by international guidelines for the general population [110–112]. There are no specific recommendations for acute coronary syndrome occurring in HIV-infected patients concerning thrombolytic, antithrombotic therapy, and coronary revascularization modalities. Medical treatment should include β-blockers, aspirin, ACE inhibitors, lipid-lowering therapy, and management of other cardiovascular risk factors (tobacco, diabetes mellitus, hypertension, obesity). Coronary revascularization modalities (PCI, stenting, and coronary artery bypass graft) have not been specifically studied in HIV-infected patients. Few series of coronary artery bypass graft, valve replacement [113], and PCI [22, 57–61] have been reported in HIV-infected patients. Large controlled trials of coronary revascularization after acute coronary syndromes in HIV-infected patients in comparison with non-HIV-infected patients are needed to develop specific recommendations. Concerning heart transplantation in HIV-infected patients with severe left ventricular dysfunction, few data are available [114–116]. Cardiopulmonary bypass has no immunosuppressive effects and does not worsen the prognosis of HIV disease.

Conclusion

Multifactorial causes of atherosclerosis and thrombosis are involved in HIV-infected patients, which might be accelerated with HAART including protease inhibitors. Further experimental and clinical studies are required to understand whether this accumulation of cardiovascular risk factors promotes acute coronary syndrome so as to develop appropriate new strategies for HIV patients. It is necessary to focus on primary preventive campaigns, mainly against tobacco addiction and hyperlipidemia, in order to reduce the frequency of acute coronary syndromes in this population. Although HAART increases the risk of metabolic complications, this does not outweigh the benefits in terms of survival.

References

1. Klein D, Hurley LB, Quesenberry CP J, Sidney S (2002) Do protease inhibitors increase the risk for coronary heart disease in patients with HIV-1 infection? J Acquir Immune Defic Synd 30:471–477
2. Mary-Krause M, Cotte L, Simon A, Partisani M, Costagliola D and the Clinical Epidemiology Group from the French Hospital Database (2003) Increased risk of myocardial infarction with duration of protease inhibitor therapy in HIV-infected men. AIDS 17:2479–2486
3. Friis-Moller N, Sabin CA, Weber R et al (2003) Data Collection on Adverse Events of Anti-HIV Drugs (DAD) Study Group. Combination antiretroviral therapy and the risk of myocardial infarction. N Engl J Med 349:1993–2003
4. Holmberg SD, Hamburger ME, Moorman AC et al (2002) HIV Outpatient Study (HOPS) investigators: protease inhibitors and cardiovascular outcomes in patients with HIV-1. Lancet 360:1747–1748
5. Bozzette SA, Ake CF, Tam HK et al (2003) Cardiovascular and cerebrovascular events in patients treated for human immunodeficiency virus infection. N Engl J Med 348:702–710
6. Henry K, Melroe H, Huebsch J et al (1998) Severe premature coronary artery disease with protease inhibitors. Lancet 351:1328
7. Berhens G, Schmidt H, Meyer D et al (1998) Vascular complications associated with use of HIV protease inhibitors. Lancet 351:1958
8. Gallet B, Pulik M, Genet P et al (1998) Vascular complications associated with use of HIV protease inhibitors. Lancet 351:1958–1959
9. Vittecoq D, Escaut L, Monsuez JJ (1998) Vascular complications associated with use of HIV protease inhibitors. Lancet 351:1959
10. Jutte A, Schwenk A, Franzen C et al (1999) Increasing morbidity from myocardial infarction during HIV protease inhibitor treatment? AIDS 13:1796–1797
11. Rickerts V, Brodt H-R, Staszewski S, Stille W (2000) Incidence of myocardial infarction in HIV-infected patients between 1983 and 1998: the Frankfurt HIV-cohort study. Eur J Med Res 5:329–333
12. Duong M, Cottin Y, Piroth L et al (2002) Exercise stress testing for detection of silent myocardial ischemia in human immunodeficiency virus-infected patients receiving antiretroviral therapy. Clin Infect Dis 34:523–528
13. Boccara F, Ederhy S, Janower S et al (2005) Clinical characteristics and mid-term prognosis of acute coronary syndrome in HIV-infected patients on antiretroviral therapy. HIV Med 6:240–244
14. Friis-Moller N, Reiss P, Sabin CA et al; DAD Study Group,(2007) Class of antiretroviral drugs and the risk of myocardial infarction. N Engl J Med 356:1723–1735
15. Bergersen BM, Sandvik L, Bruun JN, Tonstad S (2004) Elevated Framingham risk score in HIV-positive patients on highly active antiretroviral therapy: results from a Norwegian study of 721 subjects. Eur J Clin Microbiol Infect Dis 23:625–630
16. Neumann T, Woiwod T, Neumann A et al (2004) Cardiovascular risk factors and probability for cardiovascular events in HIV-infected patients, part III: age differences. Eur J Med Res 9:267–272
17. Hadigan C, Meigs JB, Wilson PW et al (2003) Prediction of coronary heart disease risk in HIV-infected patients with fat redistribution. Clin Infect Dis 36:909–916
18. Knobel H, Jerico C, Montero M et al (2007) Global cardiovascular risk in patients with HIV infection: concordance and differences in estimates according to three risk equations (Framingham, SCORE, and PROCAM). AIDS Patient Care STDS 21:452–457
19. Saves M, Chene G, Ducimetiere P et al (2003) French WHO MONICA Project and the APROCO (ANRS EP11) Study Group: risk factors for coronary heart disease in patients treated for human immunodeficiency virus infection compared with the general population. Clin Infect Dis 37:292–298
20. Glass TR, Ungsedhapand C, Wolbers M et al; Swiss HIV Cohort Study (2006) Prevalence of risk factors for cardiovascular disease in HIV-infected patients over time: the Swiss HIV Cohort Study. HIV Med. 7:404–410
21. Sterne JA, May M, Bucher HC et al; Swiss HIV Cohort (2007) HAART and the heart: changes in coronary risk factors and implications for coronary risk in men starting antiretroviral therapy.

J Intern Med 261:255–267

22. Bergersen BM (2006) Cardiovascular risk in patients with HIV Infection: impact of antiretroviral therapy. Drugs 66:1971–1987

23. Grinspoon S, Carr A (2005) Cardiovascular risk and body-fat abnormalities in HIV-infected adults. N Engl J Med 352:48–62

24. Sudano I, Spieker LE, Noll G et al (2006) Cardiovascular disease in HIV infection. Am Heart J 151:1147–1155

25. Triant VA, Lee H, Hadigan C, Grinspoon SK (2007) Increased acute myocardial infarction rates and cardiovascular risk factors among patients with human immunodeficiency virus disease. J Clin Endocrinol Metab 92:2506–2512

26. Carr A, Samaras K, Thorisdottir A et al (1999) Diagnosis, prediction, and natural course of HIV-1 protease-inhibitor-associated lipodystrophy, hyperlipidaemia, and diabetes mellitus: a cohort study. Lancet 353:2093–2099

27. Piériard D, Telenti A, Sudre P et al (1999) Atherogenic dyslipidemia in HIV-infected individuals treated with protease inhibitors: the Swiss HIV Cohort Study. Circulation 100:700–705

28. Fichtenbaum CJ, Gerber JG, Rosenkranz SL et al (2002) NIAID AIDS Clinical Trials Group. Pharmacokinetic interactions between protease inhibitors and statins in HIV seronegative volunteers: ACTG Study A5047. AIDS 16:569–577

29. Dube MP, Stein JH, Aberg JA et al; Adult AIDS Clinical Trials Group Cardiovascular Subcommittee (2003) Guidelines for the evaluation and management of dyslipidemia in human immunodeficiency virus (HIV)-infected adults receiving antiretroviral therapy: recommendations of the HIV Medical Association of the Infectious Disease Society of America and the Adult AIDS Clinical Trials Group. Clin Infect Dis 37:613–627

30. Stein JH, Merwood MA, Bellehumeur JL et al (2004) Effects of pravastatin on lipoproteins and endothelial function in patients receiving human immunodeficiency virus protease inhibitors. Am Heart J 147:713

31. Asztalos BF, Schaefer EJ, Horvath KV et al (2006) Protease inhibitor-based HAART, HDL, and CHD-risk in HIV-infected patients. Atherosclerosis 184:72–77

32. Grinspoon SK (2005) Metabolic syndrome and cardiovascular disease in patients with human immunodeficiency virus. Am J Med 118(Suppl 2):23S–28S

33. Khan NA, Di Cello F, Nath A, Kim KS (2003) Human immunodeficiency virus type 1 Tat-mediated cytotoxicity of human brain microvascular endothelial cells. J Neurovirol 9:584–593

34. Schecter AD, Berman AB, Yi L, Mosoian A et al (2001) HIV envelope gp120 activates human arterial smooth muscle cells. Proc Natl Acad Sci 98:10142–10147

35. Coll B, Parra S, Alonso-Villaverde C et al (2006) HIV-infected patients with lipodystrophy have higher rates of carotid atherosclerosis: the role of monocyte chemoattractant protein-1. Cytokine 34:51–55

36. de Larranaga GF, Petroni A, Deluchi G et al (2003) Viral load and disease progression as responsible for endothelial activation and/or injury in human immunodeficiency virus-1-infected patients. Blood Coagul Fibrinolysis 14:15–18

37. Fisher SD, Miller TL, Lipshultz SE (2006) Impact of HIV and highly active antiretroviral therapy on leukocyte adhesion molecules, arterial inflammation, dyslipidemia, and atherosclerosis. Atherosclerosis 185:1–11

38. Stein JH, Klein MA, Bellehumeur JL et al (2001) Use of human immunodeficiency virus-1 protease inhibitors is associated with atherogenic lipoprotein changes and endothelial dysfunction. Circulation 104:257–262

39. Hulgan T, Morrow J, D'Aquila RT et al (2003) Oxidant stress is increased during treatment of human immunodeficiency virus infection. Clin Infect Dis 37:1711–1717

40. de Gaetano Donati K, Rabagliati R, Iacoviello L, Cauda R (2004) HIV infection, HAART, and endothelial adhesion molecules: current perspectives. Lancet Infect Dis 4:213–222

41. Wu RF, Gu Y, Xu YC et al (2004) Human immunodeficiency virus type 1 Tat regulates endothelial cell actin cytoskeletal dynamics through PAK1 activation and oxidant production. J Virol 78:779–789

42. Hsue PY, Hunt PW, Sinclair E et al (2006) Increased carotid intima-media thickness in HIV patients is associated with increased cytomegalovirus-specific T-cell responses. AIDS 20:2275–2283

43. Zandman-Goddard G, Shoenfeld Y (2002) HIV and autoimmunity. Autoimmun Rev 1:329–337

44. Karmochkine M, Ankri A, Calvez V et al (1998) Plasma hypercoagulability is correlated to plasma HIV load. Thromb Haemost 80:208–209

45. Escaut L, Monsuez JJ, Chironi G et al (2003) Coronary artery disease in HIV infected patients. Intensive Care Med 29:969–973

46. David MH, Hornung R, Fichtenbaum CJ (2002) Ischemic cardiovascular disease in persons with human immunodeficiency virus infection. Clin Infect Dis 34:98–102

47. Barbaro G, Barbarini G, Pellicelli AM (2001) HIV-associated coronary arteritis in a patient with fatal myocardial infarction. N Engl J Med 344:1799-1800

48. Tabib A, Leroux C, Mornex JF, Loire R (2000) Ac-

celerated coronary atherosclerosis and arteriosclerosis in young human-immunodeficiency-virus-positive patients. Coron Artery Dis 11:41–46

49. Hsue PY, Lo JC, Franklin A et al (2004) Progression of atherosclerosis as assessed by carotid intima-media thickness in patients with HIV infection. Circulation 109:1603–1608

50. Mercie P, Thiebaut R, Lavignolle V et al (2002) Evaluation of cardiovascular risk factors in HIV-1 infected patients using carotid intima-media thickness measurement. Ann Med 34:55–63

51. Depairon M, Chessex S, Sudre P et al (2001) Premature atherosclerosis in HIV-infected individuals: focus on protease inhibitor therapy. AIDS 15:329–334

52. Maggi P, Serio G, Epifani G et al (2000) Premature lesions of the carotid vessels in HIV-1-infected patients treated with protease inhibitors. AIDS 14:F123–128

53. Seminari E, Pan A, Voltini G et al (2002) Assessment of atherosclerosis using carotid ultrasonography in a cohort of HIV-positive patients treated with protease inhibitors. Atherosclerosis 162:433–438

54. Jerico C, Knobel H, Calvo N et al (2006) Subclinical carotid atherosclerosis in HIV-infected patients: role of combination antiretroviral therapy. Stroke 37:812–817

55. de Saint Martin L, Vandhuick O, Guillo P et al (2006) Premature atherosclerosis in HIV positive patients and cumulated time of exposure to antiretroviral therapy (SHIVA study). Atherosclerosis 185:361–367

56. Mangili A, Gerrior J, Tang AM et al (2006) Risk of cardiovascular disease in a cohort of HIV-infected adults: a study using carotid intima-media thickness and coronary artery calcium score. Clin Infect Dis 43:1482–1489

57. Matetzky S, Domingo M, Kar S et al (2003) Acute myocardial infarction in human immunodeficiency virus-infected patients. Arch Intern Med 163:457–460

58. Hsue PY, Giri K, Erickson S et al (2004) Clinical features of acute coronary syndromes in patients with human immunodeficiency virus infection. Circulation 109:316–319

59. Ambrose JA, Gould RB, Kurian DC et al (2003) Frequency of and outcome of acute coronary syndromes in patients with human immunodeficiency virus infection. Am J Cardiol 92:301–303

60. Varriale P, Saravi G, Hernandez E, Carbon F (2004) Acute myocardial infarction in patients infected with human immunodeficiency virus. Am Heart J 147:55–59

61. Boccara F, Teiger E, Cohen A et al (2006) Percutaneous coronary intervention in HIV infected patients: immediate results and long term prog-

nosis. Heart 92:543–544

62. Boccara F, Mary-Krause M, Teiger E et al (2007) Clinical and angiographic features of acute coronary syndromes in HIV-infected compared with non-HIV-infected patients. 14th Conference on Retroviruses and Opportunistic Infectious, Los Angeles, Feb 2007, Abstract no. 811

63. Lauer MS (2002) Aspirin for primary prevention of coronary events. N Engl J Med 346:1468–1474

64. Preventive services task force (2002) Aspirin for the primary prevention of cardiovascular events: recommendation and rationale. Ann Intern Med 136:157–160

65. Wood D, De Backer G, Faergeman O et al (1998) Prevention of coronary heart disease in clinical practice: recommendations of the Second Joint Task Force of European and other Societies on Coronary Prevention. Atherosclerosis 140:199–270

66. Expert Panel on Detection, Evaluation and Treatment of High Blood Cholesterol in Adults (2001) Executive summary of the third report of the National Cholesterol Education Program (NCEP) expert panel on detection, evaluation and treatment of high blood cholesterol in adults (adults treatment panel III). JAMA 285:2486–2497

67. Fichtenbaum CJ, Gerber JG, Rosenkranz SL et al (2002) Pharmacokinetic interactions between protease inhibitors and statins in HIV seronegative volunteers: ACTG Study A5047. AIDS 16:569–577

68. Benesic A, Zilly M, Kluge F et al (2004) Lipid lowering therapy with fluvastatin and pravastatin in patients with HIV infection and antiretroviral therapy: comparison of efficacy and interaction with indinavir. Infection 32:229–333

69. Calza L, Colangeli V, Manfredi R et al (2005) Rosuvastatin for the treatment of hyperlipidaemia in HIV-infected patients receiving protease inhibitors: a pilot study. AIDS 19:1103–1105

70. Palacios R, Santos J, Gonzalez M et al (2002) Efficacy and safety of atorvastatin in the treatment of hypercholesterolemia associated with antiretroviral therapy. J Acquir Immune Defic Syndr 30:536–537

71. Calza L, Manfredi R, Chiodo F (2002) Use of fibrates in the management of hyperlipidemia in HIV-infected patients receiving HAART. Infection 30:26–31

72. Dube MP, Wu JW, Aberg JA et al; AIDS Clinical Trials Group A5148 Study Team (2006) Safety and efficacy of extended-release niacin for the treatment of dyslipidaemia in patients with HIV infection: AIDS Clinical Trials Group Study A5148. Antivir Ther 11:1081–1089

73. Negredo E, Molto J, Puig J et al (2006) Ezetimibe, a promising lipid-lowering agent for the treatment of dyslipidaemia in HIV-infected patients

with poor response to statins. AIDS 20:2159–2164

74. Van der Valk M, Kastelein JJ, Murphy RL et al (2001) Nevirapine-containing antiretroviral therapy in HIV-1 infected patients results in an antiatherogenic lipid profile. AIDS 15:2407–2414

75. Negredo E, Ribalta J, Paredes R et al (2002) Reversal of atherogenic lipoprotein profile in HIV-1 infected patients with lipodystrophy after replacing protease inhibitors by nevirapine. AIDS 16:1383–1389

76. Parienti JJ, Massari V, Rey D et al; SIROCCO study team (2007) Efavirenz to nevirapine switch in HIV-1-infected patients with dyslipidemia: a randomized, controlled study. Clin Infect Dis 45:263–266

77. Mobius U, Lubach-Ruitman M, Castro-Frenzel B et al (2005) Switching to atazanavir improves metabolic disorders in antiretroviral-experienced patients with severe hyperlipidemia. J Acquir Immune Defic Syndr 39:174–180

78. Llibre JM, Domingo P, Palacios R et al; Lipo-Rec Study Group (2006) Sustained improvement of dyslipidaemia in HAART-treated patients replacing stavudine with tenofovir. AIDS 20:1407–1414

79. Niaura R, Shadel WG, Morrow K et al (2000) Human immunodeficiency virus infection, AIDS, and smoking cessation: the time is now. Clin Infect Dis 31:808–812

80. Louie JK, Hsu LC, Osmond DH et al (2002) Trends in causes of death among persons with acquired immunodeficiency syndrome in the era of highly active antiretroviral therapy, San Francisco, 1994–1998. J Infect Dis 186:1023–1027

81. Elzi L, Spoerl D, Voggensperger J et al; Swiss HIV Cohort Study (2006) A smoking cessation programme in HIV-infected individuals: a pilot study. Antivir Ther 11:787–1795

82. The Writing Group for the Activity Counseling Trial Research Group (2001) Effects of physical activity counseling in primary care: the Activity Counseling Trial: a randomized controlled trial. JAMA 286:677–687

83. Stewart KJ (2002) Exercise training and the cardiovascular consequences of type 2 diabetes and hypertension: plausible mechanisms for improving cardiovascular health. JAMA 288:1622–1631

84. Roubenoff R, Schmitz H, Bairos L et al (2002) Reduction of abdominal obesity in lipodystrophy associated with human immunodeficiency virus infection by means of diet and exercise: case report and proof of principle. Clin Infect Dis 34:390–393

85. Moyle G, Baldwin C, Phillpot M (2001) Managing metabolic disturbances and lipodystrophy: diet, exercise, and smoking advice. AIDS Read 11:589–592

86. Thoni GJ, Fedou C, Brun JF et al (2002) Reduction of fat accumulation and lipid disorders by individualized light aerobic training in human immunodeficiency virus infected patients with lipodystrophy and/or dyslipidemia. Diabetes Metab 28:397–404

87. Barbaro G, Fisher SD, Lipshultz SE (2001) Pathogenesis of HIV-associated cardiovascular complications. Lancet Infect Dis 1:115–124

88. Lewis W (2001) AIDS cardiomyopathy: physiological, molecular, and biochemical studies in the transgenic mouse. Ann N Y Acad Sci 946:46–56

89. Nakai K, Itoh C, Nakai K et al (2001) Correlation between C677T MTHFR gene polymorphism, plasma homocysteine levels and the incidence of CAD. Am J Cardiovasc Drugs 1:353–361

90. Vilaseca MA, Sierra C, Colome C et al (2001) Hyperhomocysteinaemia and folate deficiency in human immunodeficiency virus-infected children. Eur J Clin Invest 31:992–998

91. Cohn JE (2001) Homocysteine, HIV, and heart disease. AIDS Treat News 370:5–6

92. Bernasconi E, Uhr M, Magenta L et al (2001) Swiss HIV Cohort Study: homocysteinaemia in HIV-infected patients treated with highly active antiretroviral therapy. AIDS 15:1081–1082

93. Dube MP (2003) Disorders of glucose metabolism in patients infected with human immunodeficiency virus. Clin Infect Dis 31:1467–1475

94. Walli R, Herfort O, Michl GM et al (1998) Treatment with protease inhibitors associated with peripheral insulin resistance and impaired oral glucose tolerance in HIV-1-infected patients. AIDS 12:F167–173

95. Florescu D, Kotler DP (2007) Insulin resistance, glucose intolerance and diabetes mellitus in HIV-infected patients. Antivir Ther 12:149–162

96. Carr A, Samaras K, Burton S et al (1998) A syndrome of peripheral lipodystrophy, hyperlipidaemia and insulin resistance in patients receiving HIV protease inhibitors. AIDS 12 Suppl F:51-58

97. Mallon PW, Wand H, Law M et al (2005) Buffalo hump seen in HIV-associated lipodystrophy is associated with hyperinsulinemia but not dyslipidemia. J Acquir Immune Defic Syndr 38:156-162

98. Shlay JC, Visnegarwala F, Bartsch G et al (2005) Body composition and metabolic changes in antiretroviral-naïve patients randomised to didanosine and stavudine vs abacavir and lamivudine. J Acquir Immune Defic Syndr 38:147-155

99. Guffanti M, Caumo A, Galli L et al (2007) Switching to unboosted atazanavir improves glucose tolerance in highly pretreated HIV-1 infected subjects. European Journal of Endocrinology 156:503-509

100. Henry P, Thomas F, Benetos A, Guize L (2002) Impaired fasting glucose, blood pressure and cardiovascular disease mortality. Hypertension 40:458–463

101. Hadigan C, Rabe J, Grinspoon S (2002) Sustained benefits of metformin therapy on markers of cardiovascular risk in human immunodeficiency virus-infected patients with fat redistribution and insulin resistance. J Clin Endocrinol Metab 87:4611–4615

102. Hadigan C, Corcoran C, Basgoz N et al (2000) Metformin in the treatment of HIV lipodystrophy syndrome: a randomized controlled trial. JAMA 284:472–477

103. Grinspoon S (2007) Use of thiazolidinediones in HIV-infected patients: what have we learned? J Infect Dis 195:1731–1733

104. Yki-Jarvinen H, Sutinen J, Silveira A et al (2003) Regulation of plasma PAI-1 concentrations in HAART-associated lipodystrophy during rosiglitazone therapy. Arterioscler Thromb Vasc Biol 23:688–694

105. Morse CG, Kovacs JA (2006) Metabolic and skeletal complications of HIV infection: the price of success. JAMA 296:844–854

106. Sattler FR, Qian D, Louie S et al (2001) Elevated blood pressure in subjects with lipodystrophy. AIDS 15:2001–2010

107. Jung O, Bickel M, Ditting T et al (2004) Hypertension in HIV-1-infected patients and its impact on renal and cardiovascular integrity. Nephrol Dial Transplant 19:2250–2258

108. Crane HM, Van Rompaey SE, Kitahata MM (2006) Antiretroviral medications associated with elevated blood pressure among patients receiving highly active antiretroviral therapy. AIDS 20:1019–1026

109. Chobanian AV, Bakris GL, Black HR et al; National Heart, Lung, and Blood Institute Joint National Committee on Prevention, Detection, Evaluation, and Treatment of High Blood Pressure; National High Blood Pressure Education Program Coordinating Committee (2003) The seventh report of the Joint National Committee on Prevention, Detection, Evaluation, and Treatment of High Blood Pressure: the JNC 7 report. JAMA 289:2560–2572

110. Hamm CW, Bertrand M, Braunwald E (2001) Acute coronary syndrome without ST elevation: implementation of new guidelines. Lancet 358:1533–1538

111. Antman EM, Anbe DT, Armstrong PW et al (2004) ACC/AHA guidelines for the management of patients with ST-elevation myocardial infarction: a report of the American College of Cardiology/American Heart Association Task Force on Practice Guidelines (Committee to Revise the 1999 Guidelines for the Management of Patients with Acute Myocardial Infarction). J Am Coll Cardiol 44:671–719

112. Volberding PA, Murphy RL, Barbaro G et al (2003) The Pavia consensus statement. AIDS 17(Suppl 1):S170–S179

113. Trachiotis GD, Alexander EP, Benator D, Gharagozloo F (2003) Cardiac surgery in patients infected with the human immunodeficiency virus. Ann Thorac Surg 76:1114–1118

114. Halpern SD, Ubel PA, Caplan AL (2002) Solid-organ transplantation in HIV-infected patients. N Engl J Med 347:284–287

115. Morgan JA, Bisleri G, Mancini DM (2003) Cardiac transplantation in an HIV-1-infected patient. N Engl J Med 349:1388–1389

116. Bisleri G, Morgan JA, Deng MC et al (2003) Should HIV-positive recipients undergo heart transplantation? J Thorac Cardiovasc Surg 126:1639–1640

Chapter 10

Cerebrovascular Disease in HIV-Infected Patients

A. Moulignier

Neurological complications of HIV-1 infection, due either to the immunosuppression (opportunistic infections and neoplasms) or the neurotropism of the virus, are common and add considerably to the morbidity and mortality of the infection. Their frequency varies according to the stage of the disease. They have been reported to represent 10–15% of symptomatic primo-infection, and are the first manifestation of AIDS in 10–20% of symptomatic HIV-1 infection cases. Their prevalence in clinical studies has been estimated to range from 40 to 70%, and a prospective study revealed that neurological findings were present in 90% of AIDS patients examined by a neurologist [1]. Some autopsy series showed brain lesions in up to 100% of patients [2, 3].

The incidence rate of HIV-1-associated neurological diseases has significantly decreased since the introduction of combined multitherapies, generally including a protease inhibitor (PI) and HAART (highly active antiretroviral therapy), and the widespread use of prophylactic medications for opportunistic infections [4]. From a neurological point of view, however, the success of HAART is tempered by the occurrence of numerous drug-related neurotoxic effects (neuropathies, seizures, mitochondrial myopathy, psychiatric disorders, etc.), the immune reconstitution's pathology [5], the sanctuary provided by the nervous system for lentiviruses, and the development of resistance mutations with subsequent decline in CD4 cell counts. The incidence of HIV-1-associated neurological complications may begin to rise again because HIV-1 infection is now becoming a chronic disease [4]. Uncommon types of brain infection and new forms of encephalopathy are arising [6] and questions are emerging about the development of some neurodegenerative diseases. For all these reasons, the nervous system is still the second most frequently affected organ in HIV infection [7].

Among neurological complications in HIV-1 infection, cerebrovascular events were described long before the HAART era [8]. Yet, little is known about their real frequency and their specific etiologies [2, 9]. Several methodological limitations in the published literature have been noted, including the definition of stroke, the unclear identification of etiologies and the potential confounders, and the small sample size of the studies [10, 11]. Moreover, the epidemiology of human immunodeficiency virus (HIV) infection has changed in recent years, especially in Western countries. New infections in persons over the age of 50 have increased and seropositive individuals are aging due to the widespread use of HAART [reviewed in 12]. HIV-1-infected patients are therefore at higher risk for cerebrovascular diseases whatever the cause.

Epidemiology

The occurrence of cerebrovascular events, either ischemic or hemorrhagic, was recognized as early as 1983 in HIV-1 infection, before any antiretroviral therapy was available [8]. Ischemic strokes are more frequent than intracerebral hemorrhages, roughly in a proportion of two thirds to one third in several former series [13]. In more recent series, cerebral infarction accounted for 90% of stroke [14, 15]. A 50% ratio has exceptionally been reported [16]. Both types of stroke are frequently asymptomatic [13].

Although studies have often reached conflicting conclusions, there is evidence for an increased general risk of cerebrovascular events during HIV-1 infection. As early as 1988, a large study of AIDS patients found that 1.6% of the subjects had cerebrovascular complications [17]. The prevalence of clinically diagnosed stroke syndrome has been reported to be between 0.5 and 3.75% in more than 2,000 patients with AIDS or AIDS-related complex from six clinical series [9]. A population-based study conducted in the USA before the HAART era showed that AIDS was strongly associated with both ischemic stroke and intracerebral hemorrhage, with a similar incidence rate of 0.2% per year [16]. After exclusion of cases with AIDS-related medical conditions or other concomitant etiologies for stroke, the adjusted relative risk was still high: 10.4 for both types of stroke (95% confidence interval, 4.9–22.0) and 9.1 for cerebral infarction (95% confidence interval, 3.4–24.6) [16]. A European study including patients treated with HAART found the same annual incidence rate for transient ischemic accident (TIA) or ischemic stroke (0.216%), five times higher than in the non-HIV-infected population of the same age and country [18]. By contrast, there was no significant overall increase in the stroke rate in HIV-1-infected patients as compared to noninfected subjects in an African-population-based case-control retrospective study performed in South Africa [19]. There was, however, a higher rate of large-vessel cryptogenic strokes in the HIV population (91%) than in age- and sex-matched HIV-seronegative control subjects (36%), suggesting a possible intrinsic predisposition to

stroke among HIV-infected patients [16, 19]. Results from the DAD (Data collection on Adverse events of anti-HIV Drugs) study, involving over 36,145 person-years of follow-up, confirm that combination antiretroviral treatment increases the risk of cardio- and cerebrovascular disease [20]. The incidence of first cardio- and cerebrovascular events was 5.7 per 1,000 person-years and increased with longer exposure to antiretroviral treatment (relative risk per year of exposure=1.26) above that which can be explained by increasing age. This study, however, had insufficient statistical power to determine whether PIs and non-nucleoside reverse transcriptase inhibitors were associated with the same vascular risk.

The majority of available clinical and autopsy series were performed before the HAART era. Nonetheless, combined therapies with PIs do not seem to modify the incidence of stroke. No significant association was found between the use of any class of antiretroviral agent and the incidence of cerebrovascular events in a retrospective study [21]. The incidence of cerebrovascular accidents was not different between patients receiving PIs and those not receiving PIs [22]. No difference in the incidence rate of stroke before and after the introduction of HAART was observed in the series of Evers et al. [18], but the sample was too small to draw firm conclusions. The atherogenic metabolic side effects of HAART are discussed further.

Due to HIV epidemiology, most stroke patients are young, and in published series the mean age varies from 33.4 years [15] to 42 years [14] and more than 90% of patients are less than 46 years. The prevalence of cerebral infarction varies in clinical series from 0.3 to 6% [8, 23–27], and in autopsy series from 2 to 34% [13, 28–35]; in radiological series, it has been reported to be 18% [36]. Engstrom et al. [27] retrospectively identified 12 cases of ischemic stroke among 1,600 AIDS patients studied over a period of 5 years. The annual risk of ischemic stroke of these patients (0.75%) was higher than that expected (0.010–0.034%) in the general population younger than 45 years of age [37–39]. In a retrospective case-control study [40], HIV-1 infection was particularly associated with the occurrence of ischemic stroke (odds ratio, 3.4; 95% confidence interval, 1.1–8.9; p=0.03) after adjustment for several cerebrovascular risk factors; however, this association was no longer statistically significant if cases with meningitis and protein S deficiency were excluded, suggesting that the excess risk of stroke in HIV-1 patients could be mediated by these two mechanisms. In a cohort study performed over a 9-year period (1993–2001), 15 patients were diagnosed with TIA (n=6) or ischemic stroke (n=9) out of 772 HIV-1-infected patients, representing a total prevalence rate of 1.9% (1.2% for ischemic stroke only) whatever the age [18]. The prevalence for juvenile ischemic strokes occurring under the age of 46 years was 1.6%, higher than in the HIV-negative population [18]. The stroke patients were older, had a lower CD4 cell count, and were in more advanced stages of the disease than infected patients without stroke. The prevalence of ischemic cerebrovascular events according to the CDC classification increased with the stage of the disease: 0.6% for stage A, 1.1% for stage B, and 3.2% for stage C [18]. However, Bajwa et al. [41] did not find differences between asymptomatic, AIDS-related-complex, or AIDS patients.

The prevalence of TIA is about 0.8–0.9% [17, 27, 42], and the annual incidence in a prospective study reached 0.8% in HIV-1-infected patients versus 0.4% in noninfected individuals [43]. Whether these attacks are truly ischemic is unknown and transient neurological deficits (TNDs) is a better definition. A local vasospasm comparable to migrainous aura is also evoked [44]. The differential diagnosis of focal TND includes a variety of nonvascular causes such as toxoplasmic abscess, primary cerebral lymphoma, and cryptococcal and cytomegalovirus infection [43, 45]. Recurrent TNDs are usually described in late stages of HIV-1 infection and have been associated with AIDS dementia complex [43]. They can, however, occur in primary infection and can be associated with a high viral load [46]. Brain infarction rarely follows TND. Only 2 of 27 patients progressed to cerebral infraction in the series of Brew and Miller [43] and none in the series of Baily and Mandal [42].

It is disputed whether hemorrhagic strokes are more frequent in the HIV-1-infected population [13, 40], but some authors have suggested that could be the case [16, 47]. A study [16] has indeed demonstrated an adjusted relative risk of 25.5 for intracerebral hemorrhage (95% confidence interval, 11.2–58.0). Moreover, the increased hepatic involvement and longer survival in HIV-1-infected patients could be responsible for prolonged hemostatic perturbations and consequently cerebral hemorrhages.

Ischemic Cerebrovascular Events

Clinicopathological Aspects

There is no peculiar clinical presentation of HIV-1-related strokes [9, 27], although they are usually asymptomatic, and not diagnosed prior time to death [13, 31]. Hemiparesis, hemiplegia, and hemianesthesia are the most common presenting signs. Encephalopathy seems more common in cerebral infarction [27], whereas headache, language disturbance, and abnormal vision are more common in TND [27, 43]. A transient chorea has exceptionally been reported as a TND [48]. TNDs can be isolated [43, 46, 49] but are more frequently recurrent [42, 44]. Their association with PIs is controversial [50]. Although rarely reported as the presenting manifestation of HIV infection

[14, 51], stroke was the first manifestation of HIV-1 in up to 40 and 50% of South African patients described by Tipping et al. [15] and Mochan et al. [52], respectively. Infarcts are usually lacunar rather than infarcts in large-vessel territories [9, 13, 31]. In a retrospective study, 19% of patients had a small vessel occlusion and 12% had large artery atherosclerosis [14]. Yet, in a prospective clinical study of black heterosexual nonintravenous drug users, 61% of ischemic strokes were large-vessel infarcts with cortical involvement and only 39% were small-vessel infarcts with subcortical involvement [52]. These findings have also been observed in another black population cohort [19]. Autopsy series confirm, however, that infarcts are usually small, located in the basal ganglia or the thalamus and the deep white matter, more rarely in the brain stem or the cerebellum, and frequently multiple [31]. Occlusion of large vessels seems to be less frequent [14, 19, 47, 52].

Mechanisms of Ischemic Stroke

The exact distribution of the different causes of strokes in HIV-1 infection cannot be determined because a thorough exploration has not always been performed in published series. For example, in the recent series of Ortiz et al. [14], brain MRI was performed in only 57% of patients and 39% underwent lumbar puncture. Even recent clinical series are not entirely comparable. In some, previous HIV infection is documented in 91% of patients, the mean CD4 count is <200/mm^3 in 85% of patients and 80% have AIDS diagnosis [14]. In others, stroke results in the first diagnosis of HIV infection in 42% of patients, CD4 counts are > 200 in 54% of patients, and opportunistic infections defining AIDS occurred in 28% of them [15]. This is partly explained by discrepancies in demographic data and availability of antiretroviral therapies. Traditional risk factors for vascular disease have rel-

atively low prevalence, and conversely, mechanisms unusual in the general population such as infection, vasculitis and hypercoagulability, play a greater role in HIV-infected patients [14, 15]. However, two causes emerge: cardioembolism and vasculitis/vasculopathy [9] (see Table 1).

Table 1 Causes of ischemic stroke in HIV-infected patients

Cardioembolism
    Infectious and noninfectious endocarditis
    Cardiomyopathy
    HIV myocarditis
    Myxoid valvular degeneration
    Arrhythmias
    Mural thrombi
    Intra-atrial septal defect
    Patent Foramen ovale

Hematological
    Protein S deficiency
    Antiphospholipid antibodies
    Disseminated intravascular coagulation
    Neoplasm
    Hyperviscosity syndrome

Vasculitis
Opportunistic infections
    Aspergillosis
    Candidiasis
    Cytomegalovirus
    Cryptococcosis
    Herpes simplex virus
    Mucormycosis
    Syphilis
    Toxoplasmosis
    Trypanosomiasis
    Tuberculosis
    Varicella-zoster virus
Neoplasm
    Non-Hodgkin's lymphoma
HIV-related vasculitis
    HIV itself
    Immune reconstitution

Premature atherosclerosis with protease inhibitors
    Dyslipidemia
    Insulin resistance
    Endothelial dysfunction
    Hyperhomocysteinemia

Drugs (especially cocaine and heroin)

Cryptogenic

Cardioembolism

Cardiac disease may be found in as many as 50% of AIDS patients [53], and is regarded as the main cause of embolic stroke (Fig. 1) in HIV-1-infected individuals [33]. It includes viral myocarditis, bacterial and nonbacterial (marantic) endocarditis (both with and without history of intravenous drug abuse), dilated cardiomyopathy, mural thrombi, myxoid degeneration of the valves, and HIV myocarditis [8, 9, 17, 27, 33, 53]. Dilated cardiomyopathy was deemed the responsible mechanism for stroke in almost 20% of patients in the series of Ortiz et al. [14]. Conversely, in another recent study [15], cardioembolism was a cause of cerebral infarction in only 10% of patients, and

appeared less common in this population than in the HIV negative patients. Aortic root dilatation associated with left ventricular dilatation, increased viral load, and lower CD4 cell count, documented in HIV-1-infected children [54], has not been described in adults.

Opportunistic/Tumoral Vasculitis/Vasculopathy

Vasculitic changes in intracerebral vessels associated with ischemic strokes can be due to opportunistic infections as diverse as tuberculosis, cytomegalovirus, varicella-zoster virus (Fig. 2), herpes simplex virus, syphilis, cryptococcosis, candidiasis,

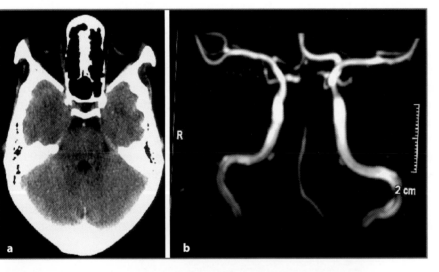

Fig. 1a, b Cardioembolic acute basilar artery occlusion. a Noncontrast CT scan shows a spontaneous hyperdensity of the basilar artery. b MR angiogram shows the acute basilar artery occlusion

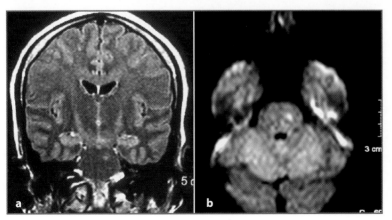

Fig. 2a, b Varicella-zoster virus-related lacunar infarct in the pons. a Fluid-attenuated inversion recovery MR image obtained in the coronal plane shows a left infarct in the pons. b Diffusion-weighted MR image shows a recent ischemic stroke in the pons

aspergillosis, mucormycosis, coccidioidomy-cosis, and trypanosomiasis (reviewed in [9, 34]). Several cases of lymphomatoid granulomatosis and malignant lymphoma have also been associated with infarcts [9, 34, 55]. Although the frequency of nervous system opportunistic infections and neoplasms has dramatically decreased with the current use of combined multitherapies in Western countries [2], infectious vasculitis remains relatively common in HIV-infected patients with stroke and advanced immunodepression and is generally predictive of poor outcome [14]. This argues for performing lumbar puncture in these cases [14].

HIV-Related Vasculitis/Vasculopathy

The frequent formation of cotton-wool spots in HIV-1-infected patients' eyes is ascribed to vasculitis-induced ischemic injury [56]. Indeed, in some cases, HIV-1 itself appears to be the cause of vasculitis [18, 36, 57–59]. As part of the immunodepression caused by the virus, a granulomatous inflammation involving small arteries and veins of the brain surface and leptomeninges, termed primary angiitis of the central nervous system (CNS), is a rare vasculitis (less than 25 cases reported, principally reviewed in [59]) usually associated with high mortality [59], although a benign course has been described [49]. Moreover, two patients in

the series of Evers et al. [18] had fluctuating intracranial stenosis which resolved within months, suggesting an inflammatory origin. It has been reported once that HIV-1 vasculitis could principally concern the cerebral posterior circulation [60]. The pathogenesis of primary angiitis of the CNS is speculative and mechanisms such as infection of endothelial cells by HIV-1, increased deposition of circulating immune complexes, and impaired regulation of cytokines and adhesion molecules have been proposed [61]. For others, cerebral vasculitis in the absence of infections or tumors is controversial [35]. Immune reconstitution promoted by HAART may exceptionally induce cerebral vasculitis (Fig. 3) in HIV-infected patients [62, 63].

Evidence supports the occurrence of a vasculopathy involving the CNS small vessels in HIV-1-infected patients free of risk factors for these vascular changes [31]. The autopsy series of the Edinburgh HIV Cohort revealed the presence of an asymptomatic vasculopathy characterized by small-vessel wall thickening, perivascular space dilatation, rarefaction and pigment deposition with vessel wall mineralization, and occasional perivascular inflammatory cell infiltrates without evidence of vasculitis [9, 35]. These patients were young (range 22–47 years) and free of vascular risk factors, although 48% of them were intravenous drug users. Features of this microvasculopa-

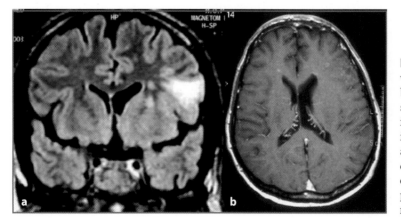

Fig. 3a, b Immune reconstitution vasculitis confirmed by brain biopsy. a Fluid-attenuated inversion recovery MR image obtained in the coronal plane shows an infarct in the left middle cerebral artery territory. b Gadolinium-enhanced T1-weighted MR image obtained in the axial plane shows punctiform bilateral enhancement

thy are similar to those observed in the brains of non-HIV aging patients with high blood pressure or diabetes mellitus [35]. Cranial nerve mononeuritis (left trochlear nerve palsy) and HIV-1 microangiopathy have been described [64]. Calcification of the vessel wall and calcium deposits occurred less often in adults than in children [31].

The alteration of the cerebral microvascularization in HIV-1-infected patients induces disturbed vasoreactivity, as demonstrated by reduced baseline cerebral flow and decreased cerebrovascular reserve capacity in response to acetazolamide challenge [65]. Abnormalities of cerebral perfusion have also been documented in the early stages of the infection and in asymptomatic HIV-1-infected patients [66]. Transcranial Doppler imaging has been used to monitor the progression of a reversible form of symptomatic cerebral vasospasm observed in two HIV-1-infected patients with presumed underlying HIV-related vasculopathy [49]. Vasoreactivity was confined to small cerebral arterioles, the same vessels showing pathologic changes in the autopsy series of Connor et al. [35]. These disturbances may represent a predisposing factor for the development of cerebral microinfarcts. Frequent in children, stroke caused by intracranial large-vessel aneurysmal HIV-associated vasculopathy has exceptionally been reported in adults [67].

Atherosclerosis and Antiretroviral Therapies

Increasingly, severe treatment-associated metabolic side effects have been observed with combined antiretroviral therapy, among them dyslipidemia, insulin resistance, and overt diabetes mellitus, which are well-known risk factors for cardiovascular disease. Endothelial dysfunction, impaired fibrinolysis, and excess inflammation may also contribute to the increased cardiovascular risk in HIV-infected individuals. Surrogate markers such as C-reactive protein (CRP), homocysteine, tissue plasminogen activator, and plasminogen activator inhibitor-1 are higher in HIV-positive than in HIV-negative subjects, are increased in patients treated with HAART in association with metabolic abnormalities and altered fat distribution [10]. The pathogenesis of atherosclerosis now includes chronic systemic inflammatory activity, and CRP is a predictor of cardiovascular mortality in HIV-infected women [68]. The results of the DAD study support the hypothesis that early atherosclerosis is a side effect of combined antiretroviral therapies [20]. The mechanism for PI-induced dyslipidemia is not yet established; direct effect of drugs themselves, interactions between antiretroviral treatment, HIV, host response to infection or genetic predisposition are hypothesized [10, 11]. The full clinical implications of vascular imaging findings are still being debated. In a recent review [69], 88% of studies measuring carotid intima thickness or atherosclerotic lesions reported worsening of these conditions in association with PIs. Several groups have examined the relationship between antiretroviral therapy, HIV, and carotid intima-media thickness in cross-sectional and longitudinal studies, with conflicting results. Some cross-sectional studies have concluded a positive correlation between PIs exposure and carotid intima-media thickness [70–72], using both presence of plaque and carotid intima-media thickness as an endpoint, while others have found that, after control for traditional cardiovascular risk factors, PIs were no longer a statistically significant predictor of plaque or carotid intima-media thickness [73, 74]. Jerico et al. [75] identified the use of combination antiretroviral therapy as a predictor of subclinical atherosclerosis independent of the Framingham risk score. Longitudinal studies of changes in carotid intima-media thickness have also produced conflicting issues. Hsue et al [76] reported rapid progression of carotid intima-media thickness. Median carotid intima-media thickness increased in the first 12 months and then decreased by month 36 for Thiébaut et al. [77]. Carotid intima-media thickness increases with age, body mass index, waist circumference, and tended to be lower in female and in subjects with higher HDL cholesterol [78]. Currier et al. [78] showed that traditional risk factors for cerebrovascular diseases can overshadow the impact of PI exposure in the development of carotid intima-media thickness. In this study, the use of PIs was not correlated with an increase of intima-media thickness [78]. The relative increase in cardiovascular disease is still small in an absolute sense, and the overwhelming effect of antiretroviral therapies is positive in terms of improvement in immune function and related morbi-mortality [10]. Yet carotid intima-media thickness appears to be a strong predictor of incident stroke, and arterial intima-media thickness per se is an important determinant of vascular disease in young HIV-negative individuals [79]. As HIV-positive individuals live longer on treatment, this risk must be evaluated, because the effectiveness of medical therapy such as antiplatelet agents or anticoagulants in the setting of HIV-associated vasculopathy is unknown. Moreover, in the light of findings suggesting that atherosclerosis, predominantly carotid atherosclerosis, is associated with an increased risk for dementia [80], an evaluation of cardiovascular risk should be offered periodically to HIV-infected subjects, especially after HAART initiation [11].

Hematological Disorders

Elevated levels of antiphospholipid IgG antibodies have been reported to occur in up to half of patients with HIV-1 infection and AIDS, and correlate highly with the presence of perfusion defects on SPECT scanning [81]. The clinical relevance of this remains uncertain. Indeed, the role of these antibodies in the pathogenesis of stroke in HIV-1/AIDS patients is not clearly understood [13], and their importance as a cardiovascular risk factor is controversial [82].

A frequent prothrombotic state in HIV-1-infected patients is protein S deficiency [40, 43, 52], also involved in ischemic stroke in noninfected individuals. However, its role in predisposing HIV-1-infected patients to cerebral infarction is not well established [40, 83]. A single retrospective case-control study showed a significant association of protein S deficiency in HIV-1-positive stroke patients compared with HIV-negative stroke patients [40]. Yet, protein S deficiency seems to be statistically related to the HIV infection rather than the stroke occurrence [84]. A high prevalence of IgG anticardiolipin antibodies and protein S deficiency was also reported in TND [43]. Disseminated intravascular coagulation [28, 29, 33] and hyperviscosity related to polyclonal hypergammaglobulinemia [85] have also been documented in rare cases.

Drugs

Associations have been reported between over-the-counter prescription and illicit drugs with sympathomimetic properties and cerebral infarction [86, 87]. Except for a few instances of vasculitis and pharmacologically induced focal vaso-spasm, the etiology of drug-related cerebrovascular accidents is often unclear. Ortiz et al. [14] found an association between recent cocaine use and non-atherothrombotic strokes. Other mechanisms are arrhythmias and foreign embolism from impurities. However, these mechanisms are not specific to HIV infection.

Unknown Mechanism

As in noninfected young individuals, the proportion of ischemic stroke whose causes remain unidentified despite complete investigations is high and varies from 24 to 40% in HIV-1-infected patients [9, 14, 27, 41, 88]. However, a thorough exploration has not always been performed in published series. In light of the increased frequency of atypical stroke mechanisms in HIV-infected patients, comprehensive diagnostic evaluations are justified [14].

Intracerebral, Subarachnoid Hemorrhages and Subdural Hematoma

Intracerebral hemorrhages are less frequent than ischemic strokes in the majority of published series, but an equivalent ratio has also been reported [16]. Mainly localized in the subtentorial regions, their localizations are various, sometimes multiple. They could be asymptomatic if of small size [31], but mortality tends to be high. The most frequent causes (Table 2) are opportunistic diseases (notably toxoplasmosis, tuberculosis, cytomegalovirus, HSV-1), mycotic aneurysms (Fig. 4), lymphoma, thrombocythemia, and metastatic Kaposi's sarcoma [9, 13, 23, 33, 67, 89]. Risk factors like alcoholism, drug abuse (especially cocaine and crack, amphetamine, phenylpropanolamine, phencyclidine), high blood pressure, or hemophilia are sometimes found [9, 32, 41, 47, 90]. Cocaine-associated intracranial hemorrhages seem to be a consequence of the pharmacodynamic effect of cocaine and not of a cocaine-induced vasculopathy [91, 92]. Other occasional causes include disseminated intravascular coagulation, ruptured mycotic aneurysms, or disruption of congenital aneurysm [8, 9, 28, 29]. Subarachnoid hemorrhage and subdural hematoma in clinical [47] and autopsy series [13, 31] are more anecdotal. A subdural hematoma was reported in an HIV-1-infected patient with an HIV-associated encephalopathy and cerebral atrophy [93]. Recently, an increased risk of intracerebral

Table 2 Causes of intracerebral hemorrhage

Thrombocythemia
  Autoimmune
  Drug-induced
  Disseminated intravascular coagulation

Hemophilia
Aneurysmal dilatation
Mycotic aneurysm
Vasculitis
  Opportunistic infections
  Drug-induced
  Neoplasms

Aspergillosis
Metastatic Kaposi's sarcoma
Alcoholism

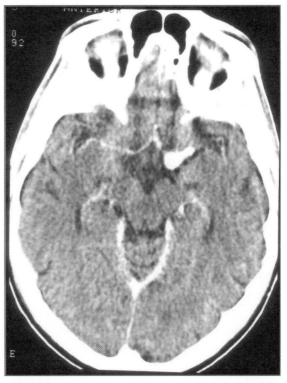

Fig. 4 Contrast-enhanced CT scan shows a mycotic aneurysm of the left middle cerebral artery

hemorrhages has been observed with tipranavir co-administrated with ritonavir. Tipranavir induces changes in coagulation parameters in rodents and may inhibit human platelet aggregation.

Cerebral Venous Thrombosis

Except for the involvement of small veins in the vasculitis process, cerebral venous thrombosis is very rare in HIV-1 infection (Fig. 5). One case of superior longitudinal sinus out of 118 patients is reported in the series of Jordan et al. [94]. The frequency is also probably underestimated because clinical and radiological diagnosis is difficult and cerebral sinuses were not always examined at autopsy. Causes include primary HIV-1 infection with concomitant cytomegalovirus infection [95], primary cerebral lymphoma, toxoplasmosis [96], cryptococcosis, protein S deficiency [97], dehydration, or cachexy [98]. Extensive intracranial sinus thrombosis was also the consequence of hypercoagulable state complicating AIDS-associated nephrotic syndrome [99].

Miscellaneous

Apart from illicit drugs, common medications have been involved in some cases of stroke in young persons. Listing them is beyond the purpose of this review. However, we want to emphasize the risk of drug interaction with antiretroviral therapies, even with a normal dosage. For instance, cerebral ergotism due to vasospasm has been described with a usual dose of ergotamine in association with ritonavir [100]. Such an association is then contraindicated. Allergic reaction with shock and low cerebral blood flow responsible for brain infarction has also been reported with rifampicin in an HIV-1-infected patient [101]. Common causes of stroke in non-HIV-infected individuals such as arterial dysplasia and carotid or vertebral artery dissection, should be also investigated in HIV-1-infected patients [102] (Fig. 6).

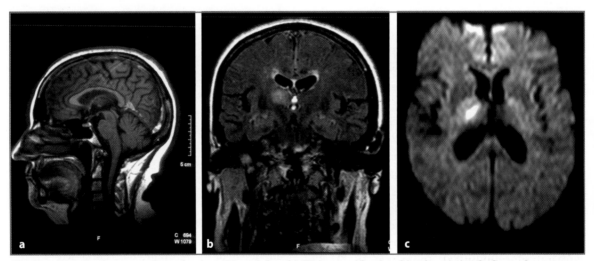

Fig. 5a-c Cerebral venous thrombosis. **a** T1-weighted MR image obtained in the sagittal plane shows superior longitudinal and rectus sinus thrombosis. **b** Fluid-attenuated inversion recovery MR image obtained in the coronal plane shows a right thalamus venous infarct. **c** Diffusion-weighted MR image confirms a recent right thalamus venous infarct

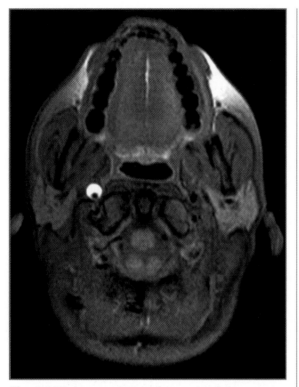

Fig. 6 MR image shows the parietal hematoma characteristic of a right carotid dissection

Ischemic Myelopathy

Ischemic myelopathy has been occasionally reported in HIV-1 infection. Brown-Sequard syndrome secondary to intravascular coagulation and ischemic lesions of the spinal cord [103] or varicella zoster virus-related necrotizing vasculitis of the CNS, predominating in the spinal cord [104, 105], have been observed.

Stroke in HIV-1-Infected Children

The clinical incidence of stroke in HIV-1-infected children has been estimated to be 1.3% in a longitudinal study [106] and 2.6% in a retrospective radiological study [107], higher than that in noninfected children [107]. At autopsy, cerebrovascular disease was documented in 25% of children, confirming that, as in adults, most strokes in children

are asymptomatic [106]. Both ischemic stroke and intracerebral hemorrhages have been described, and the reported mechanisms are similar to those reported in adults [9, 106, 107]. Strokes are principally associated with severe immunodepression and with vertically acquired HIV-1 infection or exposure to the virus in the neonatal period [106]. Cerebrovascular accident may be the initial presentation of HIV-1 infection [108]. Aneurysmal dilatation is more frequently observed in children than in adults, and infection of the parenchymal and leptomeningeal vessels by HIV-1 itself is one of the proposed mechanisms [109]. The presence of the gp41 transmembrane protein in the walls of aneurysms of the circle of Willis found by some investigators [106, 110], although not found by others [111], supports this hypothesis. Independently of exposure to antiretroviral therapy, the carotid arterial wall was also stiffer in HIV-infected children than in control subjects of the same age, but without concomitant increase of the intima-media thickness [112]. These results are of importance because antiretroviral therapy could counterbalance this possible HIV-induced vascular pathology [113]. Recently, increased carotid intima-media thickness has been reported in antiretroviral therapy-treated children by comparison to matched uninfected controls, suggesting that HIV infected children receiving combined therapies may be at increased risk for premature atherosclerosis [114]. Hyperhomocysteinemia has been observed in HIV-1-infected children on antiretroviral therapy, particularly when PIs are used [115]. Whether these children have an increased risk of premature stroke still remains unknown.

Conclusion

Some evidence shows that HIV-1 itself changes the predilection for stroke, whose causes are also related to the immunosuppression, to the risk behaviors for HIV-1 infection, and to the metabolic effects of combined therapies, especially those with PIs. In Western countries, the survival of patients infected with a neuro- and possibly vasculotrophic virus has increased considerably. Moreover, with the aging of this population, the frequency of cerebrovascular diseases in the context of immunodepression and chronic viral infection may only increase in the near future. HIV-1-infected patients presenting with a suspicion of stroke must undergo an exhaustive work-up, because therapeutic decisions in that particular situation should be rapidly individualized. If HIV-1 can indeed participate in the pathogenetic role of cerebrovascular diseases, the good blood–brain barrier penetration of new antiretroviral therapies could be a suitable therapeutic approach for this process.

References

1. Malouf R, Jacquette G, Dobkin J, Brust JCM (1990) Neurologic disease in human immunodeficiency virus-infected drug abusers. Arch Neurol 47:1002–1007
2. Moulignier A (2006) HIV and the central nervous system. Rev Neurol (Paris) 162:22–42
3. Moulignier A, Moulonguet A (2007) Complications neurologiques. In: Katalama C, Girard P-M, Pialoux G (eds) VIH 2007. Doin, Reuil Malmaison, pp 97–133
4. Sacktor N (2002) The epidemiology of human immunodeficiency virus-associated neurological disease in the era of highly active antiretroviral therapy. J Neurovirol 8(Suppl 2):115–121
5. Gray F, Bazille C, Addle-Biassette H et al (2005) Central nervous system immune reconstitution disease in AIDS patients receiving highly active antiretroviral treatment. J Neurovirol 11(Suppl 3):16–22
6. Scaravilli F, Bazille C, Gray F (2007). Neuropathologic contributions to understanding AIDS and the central nervous system. Brain Pathol 17:197–208
7. Jellinger KA, Setinek U, Drlicek M et al (2000) Neuropathology and general autopsy findings in AIDS during the last 15 years. Acta Neuropathol 100:213–220
8. Snider WD, Simpson DM, Nielsen S et al (1983) Neurological complications of acquired immune deficiency syndrome: analysis of 50 patients. Ann Neurol 14:403–418
9. Rabinstein AA (2003) Stroke in HIV-infected patients: a clinical perspective. Cerebrovasc Dis 15:37–44
10. Kamin DS, Grinspoon SK (2005) Cardiovascular disease in HIV-positive patients. AIDS 19:641–652
11. d'Arminio Monforte A, Bongiovanni M (2005) Cerebrovascular disease in highly active antiretroviral therapy-treated individuals: incidence and risk factors. J Neurovirol 11(Suppl 3):34–47
12. Moulignier A (2007) Dementia due to HIV disease and aging. Psychol Neuropsychiatr Vieil 5:1–15
13. Pinto AN (1996) AIDS and cerebrovascular disease. Stroke 27:538–543
14. Ortiz G, Koch S, Romano JG et al (2007) Mechanisms of ischemic stroke in HIV-infected patients. Neurology 68:1257–1261
15. Tipping B, de Villiers L, Wainwright H et al (2007) Stroke in patients with human immunodeficiency virus infection. J Neurol Neurosurg Psychiatry 78:1320–1324
16. Cole JW, Pinto AN, Hebel JR et al (2004) Acquired immunodeficiency syndrome and the risk of stroke. Stroke 35:51–56
17. Levy RM, Bredesen DE (1988) Central nervous system dysfunction in acquired immunodeficiency syndrome. J Acquir Immune Defic Syndr 1:41–64
18. Evers S, Nabavi D, Rahmann A et al (2003) Ischaemic cerebrovascular events in HIV infection: a cohort study. Cerebrovasc Dis 15:199–205
19. Hoffmann M, Berger JR, Nath A, Rayens (2000) Cerebrovascular disease in young, HIV-infected black Africans in the KwaZulu natal province of South Africa. J Neurovirol 6:229–236
20. d'Arminio A, Sabin CA, Phillips AN et al; Writing Committee of the DAD Study Group (2004) Cardio- and cerebrovascular events in HIV-infected persons. AIDS 18:1811–1817
21. Bozzette SA, Ake CF, Tam HK et al (2003) Cardiovascular and cerebrovascular events in patients treated for human immunodeficiency virus infection. N Engl J Med 348:702–710
22. Holmberg SD, Moorman AC, Williamson JM et al (2002) Protease inhibitors and cardiovascular outcomes in patients with HIV-1. Lancet 306:1747–1748
23. Levy RM, Bredesen DE, Rosenblum ML (1985) Neurological manifestations of the acquired immunodeficiency syndrome (AIDS): experience at UCSF and review of the literature. J Neurosurg 62:475–495
24. Koppel BS, Wormser GP, Tuchman AJ et al (1985) Central nervous system involvement in patients with acquired immunodeficiency syndrome

(AIDS). Acta Neurol Scand 71:337–353

25. Berger JR, Moskowitz L, Fischl M, Kelley RE (1987) Neurological disease as the presenting manifestation of acquired immunodeficiency syndrome. South Med J 80:683–686

26. McArthur JC (1987) Neurological manifestations of AIDS. Medicine 66:407–437

27. Engstrom JW, Lowenstein DH, Bredesen DE (1989) Cerebral infarctions and transient neurologic deficits associated with acquired immunodeficiency syndrome. Am J Med 86:528–532

28. Moskowitz LB, Hensley GT, Chan JC et al (1984) The neuropathology of acquired immunodeficiency syndrome. Arch Pathol Lab Med 108:867–872

29. Anders KH, Guerra WF, Tomiyasu U, Vinters HV (1986) The neuropathology of AIDS: UCLA experience and review. Am J Pathol 124:537–558

30. Rosemberg S, Lopes MBS, Tsanadis AM (1986) Neuropathology of acquired immunodeficiency syndrome: analysis of 22 Brazilian cases. J Neurol Sci 76:187–198

31. Mizusawa H, Hirano A, Llena SF, Shintaku M (1988) Cerebrovascular lesions of AIDS. Acta Neuropathol 76:451–457

32. Esiri MM, Scaravilli F, Millard PR, Harcourt-Webster JN (1989) Neuropathology of HIV infection in hemophiliacs: comparative necropsy study. Br Med J 299:1312–1315

33. Berger JR, Harris JO, Gragorios J, Norenberg M (1990) Cerebrovascular disease in AIDS: a case control study. AIDS 4:239–244

34. Kieburtz KD, Eskin TA, Ketonen L, Tuite MJ (1993) Opportunistic cerebral vasculopathy and stroke in patients with AIDS. Arch Neurol 50:430–432

35. Connor MD, Lammie GA, Bell JE et al (2000) Cerebral infarction in adult AIDS patients: observations from the Edinburgh HIV Autopsy Cohort. Stroke 31:2117–2126

36. Gillams AR, Allen E, Hrieb K et al (1997) Cerebral infarction in patients with AIDS. Am J Neuroradiol 18:1581–1585

37. Grindal AB, Cohen RJ, Saul RF et al (1978) Cerebral infarction in young adults. Stroke 9:39–42

38. Kristensen B, Malm J, Carlberg B et al (1997) Epidemiology and etiology of ischemic stroke in young adults aged 18 to 44 years in northern Sweden. Stroke 28:1702–1709

39. Berger K, Schulte H, Stögbauer F, Assmann G (1998) Incidence and risk factors for stroke in an occupational cohort: the PROCAM study. Stroke 29:1562–1566

40. Qureshi AI, Janssen RS, Karon JM et al (1997) Human immunodeficiency virus infection and stroke in young patients. Arch Neurol 54:1150–1153

41. Bajwa ZH, Libman R, Lipton RB et al (1991) Cerebrovascular disease in patients with HIV. Neurology 41(Suppl 1):S295

42. Baily GG, Mandal BK (1995) Recurrent transient neurological deficits in advanced HIV infection. AIDS 9:709–712

43. Brew BJ, Miller J (1996) Human immunodeficiency virus type 1-related transient neurological deficits. Am J Med 10:257–261

44. Rinaldi R, Manfredi R, Azzimondi G et al (1997) Recurrent 'migrainelike' episodes in patients with HIV disease. Headache 37:443–448

45. Klein JL, Price DA, Fisher M, Coker RJ (1996) Cytomegalovirus infection: a possible cause of recurrent transient neurological dysfunction in advanced HIV infection. AIDS 10:345–346

46. Card T, Wathen CG, Luzzi GA (1998) Primary HIV-1 infection presenting with transient neurological deficit. J Neurol Neurosurg Psychiatry 6:281–282

47. Atalaia A, Ferro J, Antunes F (1992) Stroke in an HIV-infected patient J Neurol 239:356–357

48. Bradley TP, Vas G (1997) HIV type-1-related transient neurologic deficits. Am J Med 103:250

49. Zunker P, Nabavi DG, Allardt A et al (1996) HIV-associated stroke: report of two unusual cases. Stroke 27:1694–1696

50. Vittecoq D, Escaut L, Monsuez JJ (1998) Vascular complications associated with use of HIV protease inhibitors. Lancet 351:1959

51. Casado-Naranjo I, Toledo-Santos JA, Antolin-Rodriguez MA (1992) Ischemic stroke as the sole manifestation of HIV infection. Stroke 23:117–118

52. Mochan A, Modi M, Modi G (2003) Stroke in black South African HIV-positive patients: a prospective analysis. Stroke 34:10–15

53. Roldan EO, Moskowitz L, Hensley GT (1987) Pathology of the heart in acquired immunodeficiency syndrome. Arch Pathol Lab Med 111:943–946

54. Lai WW, Colan SD, Easley KA et al (2001) Dilation of the aortic root in children infected with human immunodeficiency virus type 1: The Prospective P2C2 HIV Multicenter Study. Am Heart J 141:661–670

55. Anders KH, Latta H, Chang BS et al (1989) Lymphomatoid granulomatosis and malignant lymphoma of the central nervous system in the acquired immunodeficiency syndrome. Hum Pathol 20:326–334

56. Geier SA, Perro C, Klauss V et al (1993) HIV-related ocular microangiopathic syndrome and cognitive functioning. J Acquir Immune Defic Syndr 6:252–258

57. Scaravilli F, Daniel SE, Harcourt-Webster N, Guiloff RJ (1989) Chronic basal meningitis and vasculitis in acquired immunodeficiency syndrome: a possible role for human immunodeficiency virus. Arch Pathol Lab Med 113:192–195

58. Yankner BA, Skolnik PR, Shoukimas GM et al (1986) Cerebral granulomatous angiitis associated with isolation of human T-lymphotropic virus type III from the central nervous system. Ann Neurol 20:362–364

59. Nogueras C, Sala M, Sasal M et al (2002) Recurrent stroke as a manifestation of primary angiitis of the central nervous system in a patient infected with human immunodeficiency virus. Arch Neurol 59:468–473

60. Evidente V, Yagnik P (1995) Stroke and stroke-like syndromes in the acquired immunodeficiency syndrome. Neurology 45 (Suppl 4):A444

61. Brannagan TH (1997) Retroviral-associated vasculitis of the nervous system. Neurol Clin 15:927–944

62. van der Ven AJ, van Oostenbrugge RJ, Kubat B, Tervaert JW (2002) Cerebral vasculitis after initiation of antiretroviral therapy. AIDS 16:2362–2364

63. Dehais C, Moulignier A, Deschamps R et al (2004) Immune reconstitution vasculitis in an HIV-infected patient (abstract). Program of the Journées de Neurologie de Langue Française, Strasbourg

64. Moulignier A, Laloum L, Chauveau E et al (2003) HIV-1-related ischaemic trochlear nerve palsy. J Neurol 250:108–109

65. Brilla R, Nabavi DG, Schulte-Atedorneburg G et al (1999) Cerebral vasculopathy in HIV infection revealed by transcranial Doppler: a pilot study. Stroke 30:811–813

66. Tran Dinh YR, Mamo H, Cervoni J et al (1990) Disturbances in the cerebral perfusion of human immune deficiency virus-1 seropositive asymptomatic subjects: a quantitative tomography study of 18 cases. J Nucl Med 31:1601–1607

67. Tipping B, de Villiers L, Candy S, Wainwright H (2006) Stroke caused by human immunodeficiency virus-associated intracranial large-vessel aneurysmal vasculopathy. Arch Neurol 63:1640–1642

68. Feldman JG, Goldwasser P, Holman S et al (2003) C-reactive protein is an independent predictor of mortality in women with HIV-1 infection. J Acquir Immune Defic Syndr 32:210–214

69. Rhew DC, Bernal M, Aguilar D et al (2003) Association between protease inhibitor use and increased cardiovascular risk in patients infected with human immunodeficiency virus: a systematic review. Clin Infect Dis 31:959–972

70. Maggi P, Serio G, Epifani G et al (2000) Premature lesions of the carotid vessels in HIV-1-infected patients treated with protease inhibitors. AIDS 14:123–128

71. de Saint Martin L, Vandhuic O, Guillo P et al (2006) Premature atherosclerosis in HIV positive patients and cumulated time of exposure to antiretroviral therapy (SHIVA study). Atherosclero-

sis 185:361–367

72. Seminari E, Pan A, Voltini G et al (2002). Assessment of atherosclerosis using carotid ultrasonography in a cohort of HIV-positive patients treated with protease inhibitors. Atherosclerosis 162:433–438

73. Mercié P, Thiébaut R, Aurillac-Lavignolle V et al (2005) Carotid intima-media thickness is slightly increased over time in HIV-1-infected patients. HIV Med 6:380–387

74. Depayron M, Chessex S, Sudre P et al (2001) Premature atherosclerosis in HIV-infected individuals: focus on protease inhibitor therapy. AIDS 15:329–334

75. Jerico C, Knobel H, Calvo N et al (2006) Subclinical carotid atherosclerosis in HIV-infected patients: role of combination antiretroviral therapy. Stroke 37:812–817

76. Hsue PY, Lo JC, Franklin A et al (2004) Progression of atherosclerosis as assessed by carotid intima-media thickness in patients with HIV infection. Circulation 109:1603–1609

77. Thiébaut R, Aurillac-Lavignolle V, Bonnet F et al (2005). Change in atherosclerosis progression in HIV infected patients: ANRS Aquitaine cohort, 1999–2004. AIDS 19:729–731

78. Currier JS, Kendall MA, Henry WK et al (2007) Progression of carotid intima-media thickening in HIV-infected and uninfected adults. AIDS 21:1137–1145

79. Hollander M, Hak AE, Koudstaal PJ et al (2003) Comparison between measures of atherosclerosis and risk of stroke: the Rotterdam Study. Stroke 34:2367–2372

80. Van Oijen M, de Jong FJ, Witteman JCM et al (2007) Atherosclerosis and risk for dementia. Ann Neurol 61:403–410

81. Bock AR, Schwab J, Marienhagen J et al (1994) Anticardiolipin antibodies in HIV infection: associated with cerebral perfusion defects as detected by 99mTc-HMPAO SPECT. Clin Exp Immunol 98:361–368

82. Brey RL, Chapman J, Levine SR et al (2003) Stroke and the antiphospholipid syndrome: consensus meeting, Taormina 2002. Lupus 12:508–513

83. Hassell KL, Kressin DC, Neumann A, Ellison R, Marlar RA (1994) Correlation of antiphospholipid antibodies and protein S deficiency with thrombosis in HIV-infected men. Blood Coagul Fibrinolysis 5:455–462

84. Mochan A, Modi M, Modi G (2005) Protein S deficiency in HIV associated ischaemic stroke: an epiphenomenon of HIV infection. J Neurol Neurosurg Psychiatry 76:1455–1456

85. Martin CM, Matlow AG, Chew E et al (1989) Hyperviscosity syndrome in a patient with acquired immunodeficiency syndrome. Arch Intern Med

149:1435–1436

86. Bruno A (2003) Cerebrovascular complications of alcohol and sympathomimetic drug abuse. Curr Neurol Neurosci Rep 3:40–45

87. Hanyu S, Ikeguchi K, Imai H et al (1995) Cerebral infarction associated with 3,4-methylenedioxymethamphetamine ('ecstasy') abuse. Eur Neurol 35:173

88. Strobel M, Lamaury I, Brouzes F et al (1995) Accidents vasculaires cérébraux et sida. Rev Med Interne 16:743–746

89. Moulignier A, Baudrimont M, Martin-Negrier ML et al (1996) Fatal brain stem encephalitis due to herpes simplex virus type 1 in AIDS. J Neurol 243:491–493

90. Brust JC (2002) Neurologic complications of substance abuse. J Acquir Immune Defic Syndr 31(Suppl 2):S29–S34

91. Nolte KB, Brass LM, Fletterick CF (1996) Intracranial hemorrhage associated with cocaine abuse: a prospective autopsy study. Neurology 46:1291–1296

92. Buttner A, Mall G, Penning R, Sachs H, Weis S (2003) The neuropathology of cocaine abuse. Leg Med 5(Suppl 1):S240–242

93. Cohen JE, Eger K, Montero A, Israel Z (1998) Rapid spontaneous resolution of acute subdural hematoma and HIV related cerebral atrophy: case report. Surg Neurol 50:241–244

94. Jordan BD, Navia BA, Petito C et al (1985) Neurological syndromes complicating AIDS. Front Radiat Ther Oncol 19:82–87

95. Meyohas MC, Roullet E, Rouzioux C et al (1989) Cerebral venous thrombosis and dual primary infection with human immunodeficiency virus and cytomegalovirus. J Neurol Neurosurg Psychiatry 52:1010–1011

96. Doberson MJ, Kleinschmidt-DeMasters BK (1994) Superior sagittal sinus thrombosis in a patient with acquired immunodeficiency syndrome. Arch Pathol Lab Med 118:844–846

97. Iranzo A, Domingo P, Cadafalch J, Sambeat MA (1998) Intracranial venous and dural sinus thrombosis due to protein S deficiency in a patient with AIDS. J Neurol Neurosurg Psychiatry 64:688

98. Berger JR, Harris JO, Gregorios J, Norenberg M (1990) Cerebrovascular disease in AIDS: a case control study. AIDS 4:239–244

99. Afsari K, Frank J, Vaksman Y, Nguyen TV (2003) Intracranial venous sinus thrombosis complicating AIDS-associated nephropathy. AIDS Read 13:143–148

100. Spiegel M, Schmidauer C, Kampfl A, Sarcletti M, Poewe W (2001) Cerebral ergotism under treatment with ergotamine and ritonavir. Neurology 57:743–744

101. Martinez E, Collazos J, Mayo J (1998) Shock and cerebral infarct after rifampicin re-exposure in a patient infected with human immunodeficiency virus. Clin Infect Dis 27:1329–1330

102. Carvalho Felicio A, Sampaio G, Celso dos Santos WA et al (2006) Spontaneous artery dissection in a patient with human immunodeficiency virus infection. Arq Neuropsiquitr 64:306–308

103. Fénelon G, Gray F, Scaravilli F et al (1991) Ischemic myelopathy secondary to disseminated intravascular coagulation in AIDS. J Neurol 238:51–54

104. Gray F, Belec L, Lescs MC (1994) Varicella-zoster virus infection of the central nervous system in the acquired immune deficiency syndrome. Brain 117:987–999

105. Kenyon LC, Dulaney E, Montone KT et al (1996) Varicella-zoster ventriculo-encephalitis and spinal cord infarction in a patient with AIDS. Acta Neuropathol 92:202–205

106. Park YD, Belman AL, Kim TS et al (1990) Stroke in pediatric acquired immunodeficiency syndrome. Ann Neurol 28:303–311

107. Patsalides AD, Wood LV, Atac GK et al (2002) Cerebrovascular disease in HIV-infected pediatric patients: neuroimaging findings. Am J Roentgenol 179:999–1003

108. Visudtibhan A, Visudhiphan P, Chiemchanya S (1999) Stroke and seizures as the presenting signs of pediatric HIV infection. Pediatr Neurol 20:53–56

109. Husson RN, Saini R, Lewis LL et al (1992) Cerebral artery aneurysms in children infected with human immunodeficiency virus. J Pediatr 121:927–930

110. Kure K, Llena JF, Lyman WD et al (1991) Human immunodeficiency virus-1 infection of the nervous system: an autopsy study of 268 adult, pediatric, and fetal brains. Hum Pathol 22:700–710

111. Lang C, Jacobi G, Kreuz W et al (1992) Rapid development of giant aneurysm at the base of the brain in an 8-year-old boy with perinatal HIV infection. Acta Histochem (Suppl) 42:83–90

112. Bonnet D, Aggoun Y, Szezepanski I et al (2004) Arterial stiffness and endothelial dysfunction in HIV-infected children. AIDS 18:1037–1041

113. Mazzoni P, Chiriboga CA, Millar WS, Rogers A (2000) Intracerebral aneurysms in human immunodeficiency virus infection: case report and literature review. Pediatr Neurol 23:252–255

114. McComsey GA, O'Riordan MA, Hazen SL et al (2007) Increased carotid intima media thickness and cardiac biomarkers in HIV infected children. AIDS 21:921–927

115. Vilaseca MA, Sierra C, Colome C et al (2001) Hyperhomocysteinaemia and folate deficiency in human immunodeficiency virus-infected children. Eur J Clin Invest 31:992–998

Peripheral Arterial Disease in HIV-Infected Patients: Atherosclerosis and Vasculitic Syndromes

P. Mercié, B. Le Bail, C. Cipriano

The various cardiovascular diseases observed in HIV-infected patients and widely described in the literature have been predominantly coronary and peripheral arterial diseases (PAD) and remain poorly known. Classically, PAD is expressed as two forms: atherosclerosis, defined as an atheromatous inflammatory disease, and vasculitic syndromes, known as non-atheromatous inflammatory diseases. The prevalence and severity of peripheral arterial atherosclerosis in HIV-infected patients remain, at the moment, poorly known mostly because study protocols failed to require that it and coronary arterial disease be dissociated. Several cases of vasculitic syndromes have been reported such as pseudonecrotizing polyangiitis, Kawasaki's syndrome, Behçet's disease, Henoch-Schönlein purpura, and essential mixed cryoglobulinemia in patients co-infected with HIV and hepatitis C virus, but they remain extremely rare.

Peripheral Arterial Disease

In the retrospective and/or prospective longitudinal studies that have been published to date, symptoms suggestive of PAD, their frequency and severity, and other pertinent characteristics were not collected and reported in detail [1–5]. In the Aquitaine France Cohort, among 2,744 HIV-infected patients followed up and on file in 2002, we retrospectively identified 43 (non-coronary) peripheral arterial and/or venous PAD symptoms that had occurred in 35 patients (0.01%; P. Mercié, unpublished data from the Cohort Aquitaine Database). Although vasculitic syndromes are uncommon even in the large cohorts, several case reports and some small series have been published.

Infraclinical Atherosclerosis (Intima-Media Thickness)

Progressive atherosclerosis has been assessed using carotid or femoral intima-media thickness (IMT) measurements, and the prevalence of arterial plaques and their percentage of lumen narrowing due to stenosis have been used to estimate peripheral atherosclerosis dissemination and severity in HIV-infected patients, as shown in Figure 1.

The multicenter SUPRA study was conducted among 423 of the 2,744 HIV-infected patients in the Aquitaine Cohort [6]. Their median carotid IMT was 0.54 mm (range, 0.50–0.60). Lipodystrophy syndrome was diagnosed in 161 (38.1%) of these patients. According to univariate linear regression analysis, increased IMT was significantly associated ($p<0.05$) with older age, male gender, higher body mass index, higher waist-to-hip ratio, higher systolic blood pressure, total cholesterol, glucose disorders, elevated homocysteine level, smoking and alcohol consumption, lipodystrophy, and highly active antiretroviral therapy (HAART). After adjustment for other cardiovascular risk factors, lipodystrophy and HAART disappeared from the multivariate analysis model.

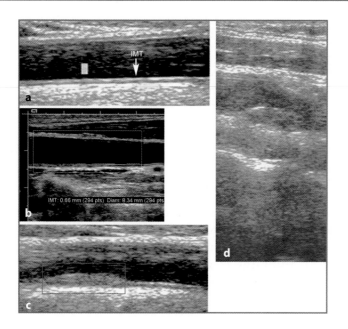

Fig. 1a-d Progressive stages of atherosclerotic plaque build-up in the carotid artery in HIV-infected patients. a An increase of the arterial intima-media thickness (IMT) is the first step of this evolution. It occurs before plaque build-up in the arterial wall. b IMT can be measured ultrasonographically using specific analytical software with a limit of detection below 1 mm. c Atherosclerotic plaque progressively accumulates and projects into the arterial lumen. d A more advanced stage of plaque build-up. The speed of plaque accumulation is not predicable. Plaque constitution can be homogeneous or heterogeneous, with a smooth or irregular surface, and be hypoechogenic or calcified. Its evolution depends on a variety of phenomena (e.g. rupture, hemorrhage, and growth)

Depairon et al. [7] reported a higher percentage of HIV-infected patients with at least one plaque compared with HIV-negative individuals (55 vs. 38%, respectively; p=0.02). Among HIV-seropositive subjects, protease inhibitor (PI) therapy was not associated with the presence of plaques.

Maggi et al. reported a color Doppler ultrasonographic study of carotid vessels in 293 HIV-infected patients. More than 52% of the patients treated with PIs presented acquired lesions of the vascular wall at ultrasonography, whereas similar lesions were found in 15.2% of PI-naive patients and 14.3% of patients treated with non-nucleoside reverse transcriptase inhibitors or naive to antiretroviral therapy. This study confirms the hypothesis of a higher prevalence of premature carotid lesions in the PI-treated patients [8], even if the definition of plaque used in this study is debatable.

In the first longitudinal study of 148 HIV-infected adults and 63 age- and sex-matched HIV-uninfected control subjects, conducted over a 12-month period, Hsue et al. reported at baseline a carotid IMT measurement of 0.91±0.33 and 0.74±0.13 mm (p=10-4), respectively. The rate of progression among 121 HIV patients with a repeated IMT measurement at 1 year was significantly increased to 0.074±0.13 mm, compared with –0.006±0.05 mm in 25 control subjects (p=0.002). Age, Latino race, and a very low CD4+ count ($\leq$200; p=0.082) were multivariable predictors of IMT progression in this cohort of HIV-infected American patients [9].

The longitudinal SUPRA study showed a significant but moderate increase in the common carotid artery (CCA) median IMT in 346 HIV-infected patients, from 0.54 to 0.56 mm ($p<10^{-4}$), i.e. an increase of 0.020 mm (95% confidence interval 0.012–0.029). There was a significant association between cross-sectional CCA IMT measures at M12 and conventional cardiovascular risk factors (higher CCA IMT with older age, $p<10^{-4}$; male gender, p=0.02; tobacco consumption, p=0.05), as well as higher CD4 cell count at M12 (>median 455 cells/ml, p=0.01). In this work, conventional cardiovascular risk factors are major determinants of IMT evolution [10]. During a 36-month period, 233 HIV-infected patients have been evaluated in the same study. Median IMT increased in the first 12 months and then decreased by month 36. The prevalence of treatment with lipid-lowering agents and protease inhibitor-free highly active antiretroviral therapy regimens increased, whereas smoking prevalence decreased. The results of this study concluded that the progression of atherosclerosis can be controlled in HIV-infected patients and the impact of individual measures to reduce the cardiovascular risk should be evaluated further [11]. More recently, Currier et al. [12] reported a prospective matched cohort study. One hundred and thirty-four individuals were enrolled in three groups: (1) HIV-infected subjects with continuous use of PI therapy ≥ 2 years; (2) HIV-infected subjects without prior PI use and (3) HIV-uninfected. There were no statistically significant differences in IMT between groups 1 and 2, or in the combined HIV groups compared with the HIV uninfected group. Significant predictors of carotid IMT in a multivariate model included high-density lipoprotein (HDL) cholesterol, the interaction of HDL cholesterol and triglycerides, age and body-mass index. In conclusion, no association between PI inhibitor exposure or HIV infection and carotid IMT was found [12].

What is the future on this topic? The utility of coronary calcium scores to quantify the amount of calcification of the coronary arteries in HIV-infected patients is not well evaluated today. Echogenicity and MRI of the atherosclerotic plaques remain to be studied. The functional indication of the endothelium may be evaluated. The most promising test is the endothelium-dependent flow-mediated vasodilatation of the brachial artery (FMD). Abnormalities of the FMD are predictive of future cardiovascular events and can be considered as a surrogate marker of the atherosclerosis progression.

Vasculitic Syndromes

Publications on vasculitic syndromes are even scarcer. The incidence of vasculitides (excluding adverse drug reactions) in HIV-infected patients has been estimated to be 1% or lower. Barbaro [13] distinguished three basic categories of vasculitides observed in HIV-infected patients.

Category 1

Vasculitides, rarely reported in HIV-infected patients, include temporal arteritis, Takayasu's arteritis [14], Behçet's syndrome [15–17], Churg-Strauss syndrome [18], Wegener's granulomatosis, essential mixed cryoglobulinemia (hepatitis C virus-related) vasculitides, and Henoch-Schönlein purpura [19, 20]. To date, the role of HIV in the development of these diseases has not yet been proven.

Category 2

This category comprises vasculitides including adverse drug reactions and diseases caused by/associated with infectious agents. Hypersensitivity reactions to drugs are common in HIV patients because of the number and types of medications they take. Directly or indirectly, microbial pathogens — cytomegalovirus, *Toxoplasma gondii* (central nervous system vasculitis), *Pneumocystis jiroveci* (ex carinii) pneumonia (pulmonary vasculitis) and hepatitis B virus — have been considered the causal agents of vasculitides, whose development may be directly influenced by preexisting HIV disease. Hepatitis B virus is a well-known cause of polyarteritis nodosa (PAN) in the HIV-negative population. Approximately 5% of PAN in HIV individuals can be attributed to hepatitis B [21, 22].

Category 3

Vasculitides with no known etiologies that appear to have a relationship with HIV disease comprise category 3. In most cases, the association is inferential, based on unusual presentations that do not fit previously defined clinical diseases or disproportionate numbers of rare illnesses among HIV-infected patients. In the absence of epidemiological studies specifically designed to collect data in this setting, it is impossible to definitively know whether these diseases are directly linked to HIV. Microscopic polyangiitis-like and PAN-like illnesses in the absence of hepatitis B virus infection have been reported in HIV patients; however, the real numbers remain unknown [23–25]. HIV patients can develop gangrene in the fingers and/or toes [23–25]. Kawasaki-like syndrome appears to be associated with HIV infection, based on 11 adult cases reported in the literature [26–33].

Case Reports

Case 1

A 49-year-old homosexual man known to be HIV-infected since 1986 (CDC-C) suddenly developed intermittent claudication within a walking distance of 100 m. His medical history associated nephrocalcinosis under indinavir and ophthalmic shingles. His weight was 58 kg and height 1.60 m; blood pressure was 130/80 mmHg and he was an active smoker (45 pack–years). Results of laboratory analyses were: hypertriglyceridemia (4.23 mmol/L), normal total cholesterol (TC; 5.40 mmol/L) and low HDL cholesterol (0.78 mmol/L) giving an increased TC/HDL ratio (6.92). Antiretroviral treatment associated stavudine, lamivudine, and indinavir. HIV viral load was undetectable (<50 copies/ml) and the CD4+ lymphocyte count was 1,086/mm^3.

Arteriography showed advanced atherosclerosis with severe aortoiliac occlusive disease (Leriche's syndrome; Fig. 2a), and the subsequent development of a collateral network arising from the inferior mesenteric artery responsible for poor irrigation of the lower limb arteries (Fig. 2b, c). He received an aortobifemoral graft.

Case 2

A 50-year-old HIV-infected homosexual man (CDC-C) had non-Hodgkin's lymphoma, treated with chemotherapy, and *Mycobacterium avium-intracellulare* septicemia. His CD4 lymphocyte count was 143/mm^3 (8.1%) and HIV viral load was 123,658 copies/ml. Erectile dysfunction became manifest several months earlier. He also had intermittent claudication within a walking distance of 250 m. Arteriography of the lower limbs showed a bilateral severe atheromatosis of the lower limb arteries associated with right external iliac stenotic narrowing evaluated at 50%, and detected thrombosis of the left external iliac at its origin with the collateral arteries arising from the internal iliac artery assuring reperfusion (Fig. 3a, b).

Case 3

In 2000, a 37-year-old HIV-infected woman, seropositive since 1988 (CDC-C), was undergoing HAART. She was treated with zidovudine, lamivudine, and invirase for the last year. Her CD4 lymphocyte count was 497/mm^3 and HIV viral load was undetectable (<50 copies/ml). She was a smoker (35 pack–years) and had an episode of tricuspid endocarditis in 1989. The month before being hospitalized, she developed numerous clinical symptoms, e.g., pyrexia, asthenia, arthralgia, myalgia, and ulceration of the left-foot toes that resolved under corticosteroids. She was admitted with acute ischemia of the left upper limb, with blue

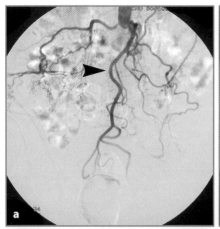

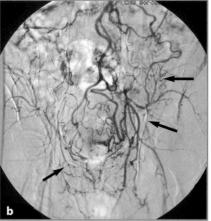

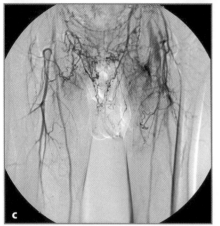

Fig. 2a-c Arteriography of the abdominal aorta and thighs of patient 1. a The aortoiliac artery is totally occluded (Leriche's syndrome; *arrow*) blocking the supply of the iliac arteries, but the inferior mesenteric artery (*arrowhead*) remains well perfused. b Aortoiliac arteriography performed at a later date. The iliac arteries are still not visualized. Note the development of a secondary vascular network arising from the inferior mesenteric artery (*arrows*). c Final arteriography of the aortoiliac junction and the thighs. The collateral network arising from the inferior mesenteric artery now assures the reperfusion of the arterial network of the thighs, bypassing the atherosclerotic lesions

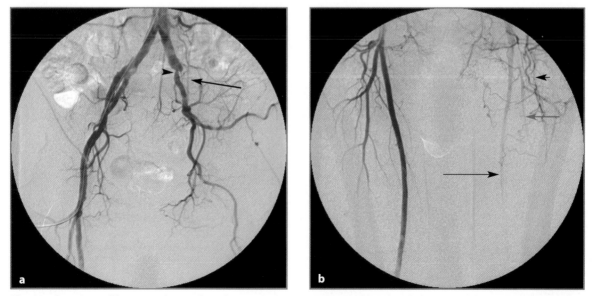

Fig. 3a, b a Aortoiliac arteriography of case 2. Severe atherosclerosis of the arterial axes. Note the left external iliac artery thrombosis (*arrow*) and the severe stenotic narrowing of the left internal iliac artery (*arrowhead*) evaluated at 50%. b Arteriography of the thighs. The occluded left deep (*red arrow*) and superficial femoral (*black arrow*) arteries are moderately reperfused by the left internal iliac artery (*arrowhead*). Contralateral arterial network is normal, showing no signs of atherosclerosis

fingers, and coldness extending into the forearm that had first manifested as intense pain in the hand followed by a drop in its temperature. Chest radiography showed cardiomegaly (Fig. 4a). Arteriography showed a thrombus in the humeral artery (Fig. 4b). Antiplatelet aggregating agents were administered and in a single night she underwent five successive thrombectomies, one each time after a new arterial thrombotic event occurred. Heparin-induced thrombocytopenia was suspected; sodium danaparoid was started then switched to antivitamin K anticoagulants. Fifteen days later, she developed a new thrombosis in her left upper arm. Doppler ultrasonography of the limb detected an occlusion of the left radial artery and a regular stenosis (Fig. 4c) in the left cubital artery, suggestive of inflammatory stenosis. The patient was given a daily intravenous infusion of corticosteroids (500 mg/day for 3 days). In January 2001, her left forearm was amputated below the elbow and corticosteroids were continued. Histopathologic examination of the amputated limb revealed many signs of atypical vasculitis evocative of necrotizing arteritis of unknown etiology associated with a leukocytoclastic vasculitis and multiple arterial thromboses (Fig. 5a–e). Two weeks later, Doppler ultrasonography showed severe stenosis of the left axillary artery consistent with a thrombotic arterial inflammatory disease. One month later the patient died, probably consecutively to an advanced dilated cardiomyopathy.

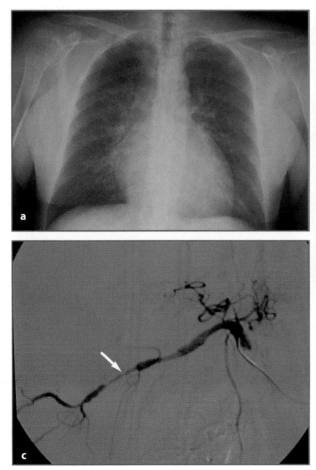

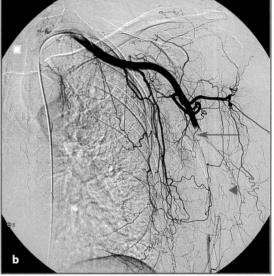

Fig. 4a-c a Chest X-ray of patient 3. Cardiomegaly in a young HIV-infected woman with peripheral vasculitis of the arms. b Arteriography of the left arm. Note the thrombosis in the left humeral artery (*arrow*) and the development of a collateral network of arteries to supply the arm (*arrowhead*). c A typical long inflammatory stenosis in the right subclavian artery (*arrow*). This image was obtained in a non-HIV-infected patient with giant-cell arteritis and is similar to that of the stenosis that developed in our case 3

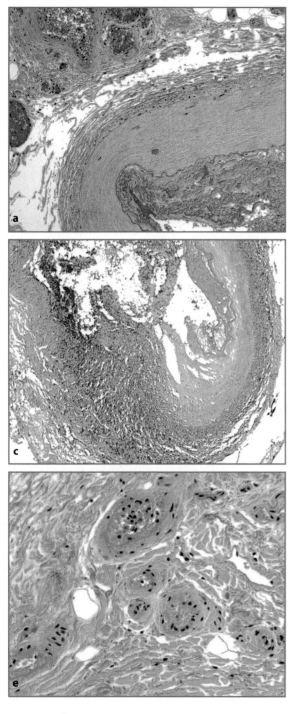
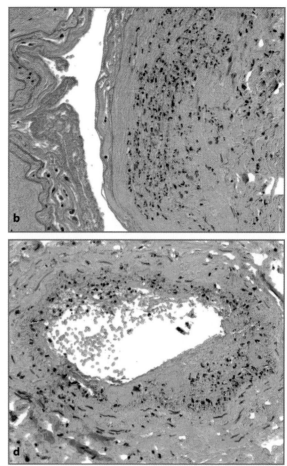

Fig. 5a-e Serial sections of radial, cubital, and palmar arteries showing alternating alternance of normal and necrotic–inflammatory aspects of the wall—hematein-eosin-saffron (HES) stain. In some segments, the entire thickness of the arterial wall contained diffuse acidophilic necrosis, and fibrinous thrombi were visible in the lumen (a original magnification ×100); in others, numerous neutrophils had infiltrated the media (b ×200) or populated the entire wall thickness (c ×50). In adjacent veins (d ×200) and capillaries (e ×200), leukocytoclasia and fibrinoid necrosis were sometimes observed. Specific stains were negative for bacteria and fungi. No viral inclusions were detected and In Situ hybridization for varicella zoster virus and cytomegalovirus were negative. Muscles were necrotic. The vascular lesions were difficult to classify, because of the diversity of types and calibers of affected vessels, the types and locations of the cellular infiltrates, and it was unknown whether the vascular necrotic-inflammatory changes were primary or secondary

Conclusion

PAD in HIV-infected patients is not well understood. So far, peripheral atherosclerosis has not been well dissociated from coronary artery disease in these patients. Vasculitides remain very rare in HIV individuals and their prevalence may be underestimated. More detailed studies are needed to improve our understanding of this particular pathology in HIV-1 infected patients.

Acknowledgements
We would like to thank all our collaborators who participated in this study: J.L. Pellegrin and J.F. Viallard, Service de Médecine Interne et Maladies Infectieuses, Hôpital Haut-Lévêque; P. Morlat and J. Beylot, F. Bonnet, D. Lacoste and N. Bernard, Service de Médecine Interne et Maladies Infectieuses, Hôpital Saint-André; J. Constans, Service de Médecine Interne et Pathologie Vasculaire, Hôpital Saint-André; H Trillaud, Service de Radiologie, Hôpital Saint-André; J.C. Baste and D. Midy, L. Besson and A. Dubourguet, Service de Chirurgie Vasculaire, Hôpital Pellegrin-Tripode; R. Thiébaut and V. Aurillac-Lavignolle, Inserm U593-ISPED, Université Victor-Segalen Bordeaux 2, France. We also thank Janet Jacobson for editing the manuscript.

References

1. Bozette SA, Ake CF, Tam HK, Chang SW, Louis TA (2003) Cardiovascular and cerebrovascular events in patients treated for human immunodeficiency virus infection. N Engl J Med 348:702–710
2. Friis-Møller N, Weber R, Reiss P et al (2003) Cardiovascular disease risk factors in HIV patients: association with antiretroviral therapy. Results from the DAD study. AIDS 17:1179–1193
3. The Data Collection on Adverse Events of Anti-HIV Drugs (DAD) Study Group (2003) Combination antiretroviral therapy and the risk of myocardial infarction. N Engl J Med 349:1993–2003
4. Mary-Krause M, Cotte L, Simon A, Partisani M, Costagliola D, and the Clinical Epidemiology Group from the French Hospital Database (2003) Increased risk of myocardial infarction with duration of protease inhibitor therapy in HIV-infected men. AIDS 17:2479–2486
5. Savès M, Chêne G, Ducimetière P et al (2003) Risk factors of coronary heart disease in patients treated for human immunodeficiency virus infection compared with the general population. Clin Infect Dis 37:292–298
6. Mercié P, Lavignolle V, Thiébaut R et al (2002) Evaluation of cardiovascular risk factors in HIV-1 infected patients using carotid intima-media thickness measurement. Ann Med 34:55–63
7. Depairon M, Chessex S, Sudre P et al (2001) Premature atherosclerosis in HIV-infected individuals focus on protease inhibitor therapy. AIDS 15:329–334
8. Maggi P, Lillo A, Perilli F et al, on behalf of the PREVALEAT Group (2004) Color Doppler ultrasonography of carotid vessels in patients treated with antiretroviral therapy: a comparative study. AIDS 18:1023–1028
9. Hsue PY, Lo JC, Franklin A (2004) Progression of atherosclerosis as assessed by carotid intima-media thickness in patients with HIV infection. Circulation 109:1603–1608
10. Mercie P, Thiebaut R, Aurillac-Lavignolle V et al (2005) Carotid intima-media thickness is slightly increased over time in HIV-1-infected patients. HIV Medicine 6:380–387
11. Thiebaut R, Aurillac-Lavignolle V, Bonnet F et al (2005) Change in atherosclerosis progression in HIV infected patients: ANRS Aquitaine Cohort, 1999–2004. AIDS 19(7):729–731
12. Currier JS, Kendall MA, Zackin R et al (2005) Carotid artery intima-media thickness and HIV infection: traditional risk factors overshadow impact of protease inhibitor exposure. AID 19:927–933
13. Barbaro G (2003) HIV infection in the cardiovascular system: vasculitic syndromes in HIV-infected patients. Adv Cardiol 40:185–196
14. Shingadia D, Das L, Klein-Gitelman M, Chadwick E (1999) Takayasu's arteritis in a human immunodeficiency virus-infected adolescent. Clin Infect Dis 29:458–459
15. Stein CM, Thomas JE (1991) Behçet's disease associated with HIV infection. J Rheumatol 18:1427–1428
16. Mercie P, Viallard JF, Cipriano C et al (2002) Aphthous stomatitis in a patient with Behçet's disease and HIV was associated with an increased HIV load. Clin Exp Rheumatol 20(Suppl. 26):S54
17. Buskila D, Gladman DD, Gilmore J, Saliut IE (1991) Behçet's disease in a patient with immunodeficiency virus infection. Ann Rheum Dis 50:115–116
18. Cooper LM, Patterson JA (1989) Allergic granulomatosis and angiitis of Churg-Strauss: case report in a patient with antibodies to human immunodeficiency virus and hepatitis B virus. Int J Der-

matol 28:597–599

19. Hall TN, Brennan B, Leahy MF, Woodroffe AJ (1998) Henoch-Schönlein purpura associated with human immunodeficiency virus infection. Nephrol Dial Transplant 13:988–990

20. Gherardi R, Belec L, Mhiri C et al (1993) The spectrum of vasculitis in human immunodeficiency virus-infected patients: a clinicopathologic evaluation. Arthritis Rheum 36:1164–1174

21. Font C, Miro O, Pedrol E et al (1996) Polyarteritis nodosa in human immunodeficiency virus infection: report of four cases and review of the literature. Br J Rheumatol 35:796–799

22. Calabrese LH (1991) Vasculitis and infection with the human immunodeficiency virus. Rheum Dis Clin North Am 17:131–147

23. Libman BS, Quismorio FP, Jr, Stimmler MM (1995) Polyarteritis nodosa-like vasculitis in human immunodeficiency virus infection. J Rheumatol 22:351–355

24. Gisselbrecht M, Cohen P, Lortholary O et al (1997) HIV-related vasculitis: clinical presentation and therapeutic approach on six patients. AIDS 11:121–123

25. O'Grady NP, Sears CL (1996) Therapeutic dilemmas in the care of a human immunodeficiency virus-infected patient with vasculitis: case re-port. Clin Infect Dis 23:559–561

26. Porwancher RSS (1992) Adult Kawasaki disease in HIV-infected patients. 8th International Conference on AIDS, Amsterdam, 1992

27. Martinez-Escibano JA, Redondo C, Galera S et al (1998) Recurrent Kawasaki syndrome in an adult with HIV-1 infection. Dermatology 197:96–97

28. Wolf CV 2nd, Wolf JR, Parker JS (1995) Kawasaki's syndrome in a man with the human immunodeficiency virus. Am J Ophthalmol 120:117–118

29. Porneuf M, Sotto A, Barbuat C, Ribou G, Jourdan J (1996) Kawasaki syndrome in an adult AIDS patient. Int J Dermatol 35:292–294

30. Viraben R, Dupre A (1987) Kawasaki disease associated with HIV infection. Lancet 1:1430–1431

31. Bayrou O, Philippoteau C, Artigou C et al (1993) Adult Kawasaki syndrome associated with HIV infection and anticardiolipin antibodies. J Am Acad Dermatol 29:663–664

32. Yoganathan K, Goodman F, Pozniak A (1995) Kawasaki-like syndrome in an HIV-positive adult. J Infect 30:165–166

33. Johnson RM, Little JR, Storch GA (2001) Kawasaki-like syndromes associated with human immunodeficiency virus infection. Clin Infect Dis 32:1628–1634

Chapter 12

HIV-Associated Pulmonary Hypertension

G. Barbaro

About 14 years ago, Kim and Factor reported the first case of HIV-associated pulmonary hypertension [1]. Since then more than 131 cases have been described in the literature [2]. For this reason, HIV-associated pulmonary hypertension has been included as a definite cause of precapillary pulmonary hypertension according to the executive summary of the World Health Organization (WHO) [3]. The incidence of HIV-associated pulmonary hypertension is 1 in 200, much higher than the 1 in 200,000 found in the general population [3]. No differences have been found in the clinical, histologic, and hemodynamic features between patients with HIV-associated pulmonary hypertension and HIV-uninfected patients affected by primary pulmonary hypertension.

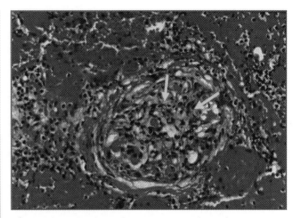

Fig. 1 Plexogenic pulmonary arteriopathy (*arrows*) in a patient with HIV-associated pulmonary hypertension (autopsy specimen). H&E, x20

Pathogenesis of HIV-Associated Pulmonary Hypertension

The histopathology of HIV-associated pulmonary hypertension is similar to that of primary pulmonary hypertension. The most common alteration in HIV-associated pulmonary hypertension is plexogenic pulmonary arteriopathy (Fig. 1), while thrombotic pulmonary arteriopathy and pulmonary veno-occlusive disease are more rare histologic findings. This observation may suggest that similar etiopathogenetic mechanisms are at the basis of both HIV-associated pulmonary hypertension and primary pulmonary hypertension.

The finding of an increased incidence of pulmonary hypertension in HIV-infected patients was at first related to viral infection. Although a direct role of HIV-1 in HIV-associated pulmonary hypertension has not been demonstrated [4, 5], several indirect mechanisms may link HIV infection to the pulmonary vascular changes. The principal pathogenetic hypotheses formulated for development of HIV-associated pulmonary hypertension with related clinical evidence are reported in Table 1.

Clinical Manifestations and Diagnosis of HIV-Associated Pulmonary Hypertension

In the largest clinical series of HIV-associated pulmonary hypertension, 47–54% of all

Table 1 Pathogenetic hypotheses of HIV-associated pulmonary hypertension

Pathogenetic hypothesis	Clinical evidence
Cytokines hypothesis (Fig. 2)	Several studies have found an increased production of cytokines–e.g., endothelin-1 (ET-1), interleukin-6 (IL-6), interleukin-1-beta (IL-1b), plateletderived growth factor (PDGF), and tumor necrosis-factor-alpha (TNF-α)–in patients affected by primary pulmonary hypertension, evoking a potential role of these substances in the pathogenesis of the disease [6–9].
α_1-Adrenergic hypothesis (Fig. 3)	In HIV-infected patients different factors can induce a chronic stimulation of α_1-adrenoreceptors of the pulmonary vasculature, including: chronic hypoxia, high circulating levels of norepinephrine, appetite suppressant agents, or cocaine use. The chronic stimulation of pulmonary vascular α_1-adrenoreceptors can induce the local production of a large amount of cytokines, particularly ET-1, IL-1b, IL-6, and PDGF, which in turn stimulate the growth of new pulmonary capillaries, induce vasoconstriction of resistance-sized pulmonary arteries, and have an anti-apoptosis effect [10].
Toxic substances	Patients with a history of chronic intravenous drug use may develop pulmonary hypertension. Pulmonary artery thrombosis is the main pathological finding in such conditions, and is believed to be due to foreign particle pulmonary emboli, following injections of solutions derived from heroin or from crushed oral medications in which talc was a frequent component [11, 12]. The use of appetite suppressant agents and/or cocaine has been associated with pulmonary hypertension, even in HIV-infected patients, possibly as a consequence of an increased α_1-adrenoreceptor stimulation [12, 13].
Liver disease and HIV-associated pulmonary hypertension	Porto-pulmonary hypertension is now a well-described disease characterized by a clinical and hemodynamic picture substantially identical to primary pulmonary hypertension. In liver cirrhosis, an increased production and a decreased metabolism of some cytokines (e.g., ET-1) have been reported. Kuddus et al. demonstrated that an enhanced synthesis and a reduced metabolism of ET-1 in hepatocytes can be an important mechanism of elevated endogenous and circulating ET-1 in patients affected by liver cirrhosis [14, 15]. Pellicelli et al. reported higher values of systolic pulmonary arterial pressure in HIV-infected patients with HCV/HBV-associated liver cirrhosis compared to other HIV-infected patients without cirrhosis [12].
Genetic factors (HLA antigens)	In a study conducted by Morse and co-workers, it was found that in ten racially mixed HIV-infected patients with HIV-associated pulmonary hypertension, there was a significant increase in the frequency of human leukocyte antigen (HLA) class II DR52 and DR6, and of the linked alleles HLA-DRB1-1301/2, -DRB3-0301, -DQB1 0603/4, compared to the frequencies of the same alleles in normal Caucasian control subjects [16]. HLA-DR6 and its DRB1-1301/2 subtypes were also significantly increased in HIV-associated pulmonary hypertension patients compared to the respective frequencies of racially diverse HIV-positive control subjects. Furthermore, HLA-DR6 and the DRB1-1301 subtype have also been reported to increase in HIV-positive patients who develop diffuse infiltrative lymphocytosis syndrome [17, 18]. It is possible that both entities represent different spectra of a common HLA-DR-determined host response to HIV-1.

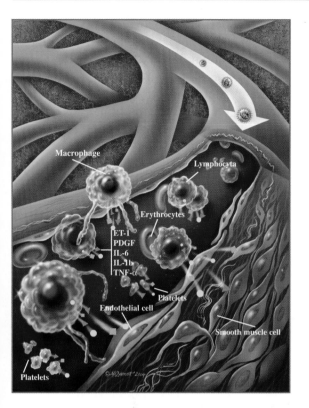

Fig. 2 The possible pathogenetic mechanisms involved in the development of HIV-associated pulmonary hypertension. HIV-infected macrophages, platelets, and lymphocytes may release multifunctional cytokines–endothelin-1 (ET-1), platelet-derived growth factor (PDGF), interleukin-6 (IL-6), interleukin-1 beta (IL-1b), tumor necrosis factor alfa (TNF-α)–which may affect the endothelial cells of the pulmonary vessels, inducing their proliferation and vasoconstriction by a reduction of nitric oxide (NO) production. Moreover, ET-1 produced by endothelial cells may affect the smooth muscle cells of the pulmonary vessels inducing their migration and proliferation. (From [20], with permission from Teri McDermott. ©2004 Teri McDermott CMI)

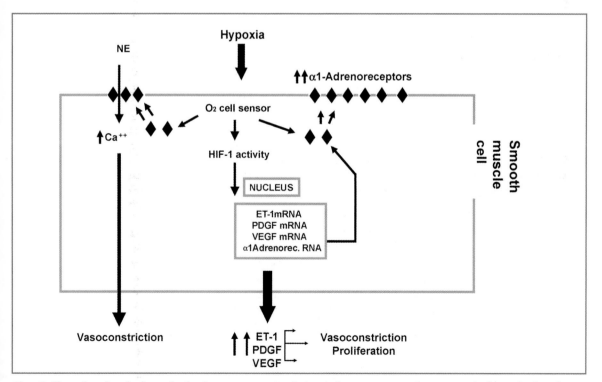

Fig. 3 Chronic stimulation of α1-adrenoreceptors of the pulmonary vasculature can induce the local production of a large amount of cytokines and particularly of ET-1, IL-1b, IL-6, and PDGF, which in turn stimulate the growth of new pulmonary capillaries, induce vasoconstriction of resistance-sized pulmonary arteries, and have an anti-apoptosis effect. (From [21], with permission from Wiley-Blackwell)

the patients were male, and the age at the time of diagnosis ranged from 2 to 56 years (mean 33 years). Intravenous drug use was the most common risk factor and ranged from 50 to 58%, while homosexual behavior was present in 20% of the patients, hemophilia in 9%, heterosexual contacts in 9%, and other risk factors in 6% of the patients [2, 11, 12], reflecting the epidemiology of HIV infection in the general population. The mean CD4+ count was 300 mm^3 (range 0–937/mm^3). Currently, no correlation has been found between the CD4+ count and the presence of opportunistic infections and the development of pulmonary hypertension.

The most common presenting symptom was dyspnea (from 49 to 85%), while pedal edema ranged from 11 to 30% of the patients, nonproductive cough from 7 to 19%, syncope from 8 to 12%, and chest pain was present in 7% of the patients. Raynaud's syndrome, which is more frequently found in patients affected by pulmonary hypertension associated to connective tissue disease, was present in only one patient (1%) [2, 12].

Signs of pulmonary hypertension on physical examination are subtle and often overlooked. An accentuated pulmonary component of the second heart sound, audible at the apex, may be noted in more than 90% of patients, reflecting an increased force of pulmonary valve closure due to elevated pulmonary artery pressure [19]. Other signs of increased pulmonary artery pressure may include the following [19]:

a. An early systolic ejection click due to sudden interruption of pulmonary valve opening
b. A midsystolic ejection murmur caused by turbulent transvalvular pulmonary flow
c. A palpable left parasternal lift produced by the impulse of the hypertrophied high-pressure right ventricle
d. A right ventricular S4 gallop
e. A prominent jugular "a" wave suggesting high right ventricular filling pressure

Physical signs of more advanced disease include the diastolic murmur of pulmonary regurgitation and the holosystolic murmur of tricuspid valve regurgitation, which is audible at the lower left sternal border and augmented with inspiration. A right ventricular S3 gallop, marked distension of the jugular veins, pulsatile hepatomegaly, peripheral edema, and ascites are indicative of right ventricular failure [19]. The principal diagnostic tests used for diagnosis of HIV-associated pulmonary hypertension with related clinical verification are reported in Table 2.

Table 2 Principal diagnostic tests for diagnosis of HIV-associated pulmonary hypertension

Diagnostic test	Clinical verification
Laboratory tests	A comprehensive laboratory evaluation which includes complete blood count, prothrombin time, partial thromboplastin time, hepatic profile, autoimmune panel, HIV viral load, HCV antibodies, and HBsAg may be helpful in excluding pulmonary hypertension secondary to systemic diseases. Serum D-dimer, produced during fibrinolysis, if higher than 500 ng/ml may be suggestive of pulmonary thromboembolism.
Electrocardiogram (ECG) (Fig. 4)	The ECG most often (15–50%) shows right-axis deviation (S1Q3T3 aspect or McGinn-White sign) along with R>7 mm in V1-V2. Other findings on the ECG include tall, prominent P waves (>3 mm) in leads II, III, aVF (secondary to right atrial enlargement), complete or incomplete right bundle branch block, or sinus tachycardia.
Chest radiogram (Fig. 5)	The chest radiograph frequently has a prominent main pulmonary artery (71–90%) along with enlarged hilar vessels (80%), "pruning," or a decrease in peripheral vessels (51%) and cardiomegaly (72%).

cont. →

Table 2 *cont.*

Diagnostic test	Clinical verification
Transthoracic echocardiography (TTE) (Figs. 6–9)	The most frequent findings on TTE are: systolic flattening of the interventricular septum, right atrial and right ventricular enlargement, and tricuspid regurgitation. Additionally, TTE can estimate pulmonary arterial systolic pressure by measuring the Doppler flow through the tricuspid valve according to the modified Bernulli formula: $P=4V2$ (where P is pressure gradient and V is peak retrograde velocity). The right atrial pressure is nominally estimated at 10 mmHg. The grade of pulmonary hypertension is categorized as grade I (36–45 mmHg), grade II (46–55 mmHg), and grade III (> 56 mmHg). Finally, the TTE can evaluate secondary causes of pulmonary hypertension such as congenital heart disease or valvular disease.
Pulmonary function tests (PFTs)	The most frequent abnormality seen on PFTs in patients with pulmonary and arterial blood gases (ABG) hypertension is a decrease in the diffusing capacity for carbon monoxide (DLco; mean, 69% of predicted). A mild restrictive pattern (mild decrease in total lung capacity) may also be seen. ABG are frequently obtained along with the PFTs and most commonly demonstrate hypoxemia and a respiratory alkalosis (hypocapnea).
Ventilation-perfusion (V/Q) scan	An abnormal V/Q scan should not necessarily be interpreted as evidence of thromboembolic disease; patients with non-thromboembolic pulmonary hypertension often have abnormal V/Q scans, most commonly displaying a diffuse patchy pattern. In HIV-associated pulmonary hypertension the most common findings observed in V/Q scans is a patchy distribution of the tracer or normal lung scan.
Spiral computerized tomography (CT)	It is a fast, safe, minimally invasive procedure which shows the thrombus in segmental and subsegmental arteries and gives further information suggesting or confirming alternative clinical diagnoses frequently observed in HIV-infected patients (pneumonia, pulmonary fibrosis, cardiovascular diseases, pulmonary neoplasms, pleural diseases).
Pulmonary angiography and right heart cardiac catheterization (Fig. 10)	Pulmonary angiography is restricted to cases with unclear or negative spiral CT scans but with a strong clinical suspicion of pulmonary hypertension. Right heart cardiac catheterization is the standard for diagnosis and measurement of hemodynamic values.

Treatment of HIV Pulmonary Hypertension

The treatment of HIV-associated pulmonary hypertension is complex and controversial. To date, no controlled clinical trial has evaluated the agent of choice for the treatment of this disease. The principal drugs currently used in the treatment of HIV-associated pulmonary hypertension with related clinical evidence are reported in Table 3.

Conclusion

Pulmonary hypertension associated with HIV infection is a cardiovascular complication that has been recognized with increasing frequency in the last few years. The etiology of HIV-associated pulmonary hypertension is unknown. At present, a multifactorial pathogenesis of HIV-associated pulmonary hypertension has been hypothesized. In this clinical condition, the endothelial

Table 3 Treatment of HIV-associated pulmonary hypertension

Therapy	Clinical evidence
Highly active antiretroviral therapy (HAART)	Opravil et al. [22] reported a reduction of right systolic ventricular pressure — right atrial pressure gradient in six patients who received antiretroviral treatment compared to seven patients not receiving antiretroviral therapy. Zuber et al. retrospectively analyzed 47 patients with HIV-associated pulmonary hypertension in the Swiss HIV Cohort Study [23]. According to the data reported by these authors, HAART significantly decreased mortality caused by HIV-associated pulmonary hypertension as well as other causes, suggesting a beneficial effect of HAART in this condition [23]. In an open-label prospective study, Barbaro et al. reported that HAART alone did not significantly influence the cardiopulmonary haemodynamic parameters in HIV-infected patients with pulmonary hypertension, especially in those with a more advanced stage of the disease (mPAP> 50 mm Hg and exercise capacity < 200 m at baseline) [24].
Epoprostenol	In a study by Petiprez et al., a short-term treatment with i.v. administered epoprostenol was evaluated in 19 HIV-infected patients with pulmonary hypertension compared to 86 control patients. The proportion of responders to epoprostenol was equal in both groups, and the level of acute pulmonary vasodilatation (percent fall in total pulmonary resistance) achieved with epoprostenol in HIV-infected and non-HIV-infected patients was similar [25]. Aguilar et al. treated six patients with HIV-associated pulmonary hypertension with continuous i.v. infusion of epoprostenol. At 1 year, the mean pulmonary artery pressure and the pulmonary vascular resistance decreased by 21 and 54% with respect to baseline values. They concluded that epoprostenol infusion is effective in improving hemodynamic and functional status acutely as well as in the long term in patients with HIV-associated hypertension [26]. Currently, it is not clear whether early administration of epoprostenol could substantially improve the prognosis of HIV-infected patients with pulmonary hypertension. Epoprostenol therapy is generally limited to seriously ill patients because of its cost and the need for continuous i.v. infusion with associated risk of infection.
Beraprost	Beraprost can improve the adherence to a long-lasting antiretroviral therapy. Beraprost can be absorbed easily and can be administered in a t.i.d. or q.i.d. fashion. In different studies in non-HIV-associated pulmonary hypertension, the oral administration of beraprost seemed to have beneficial effects on the survival and on the hemodynamic parameters of the patients [12]. Indeed, controlled clinical studies are needed to establish the efficacy of this treatment in HIV-associated pulmonary hypertension.
Bosentan	Bosentan is a dual endothelin-1 receptor antagonist and may be an effective approach to therapy for pulmonary arterial hypertension. Bosentan increased exercise capacity and improved hemodynamics in HIV-infected patients with pulmonary hypertension without any negative impact on control of HIV infection if administered in combination with HAART [24, 27]. Bosentan in combination with HAART appears to be a suitable option in the management of patients with symptomatic HIV-associated pulmonary hypertension, especially those with a baseline mPAP >50 mm Hg and a 6 min walk test <200 m, because in this subset of patients the combination treatment appears to be more effective than HAART alone [24]. However, the therapeutic efficacy of bosentan in patients with HIV-associated pulmonary hypertension needs to be tested in further controlled prospective studies.

cont. →

Table 3 *cont.*

Therapy	Clinical evidence
Calcium channel blockers	Treatment with calcium channel blockers seems to be another alternative in the therapy of HIV-associated pulmonary hypertension. However, reports regarding a small sample of patients with HIV-associated pulmonary hypertension treated with this kind of therapy have shown contrasting response rates [12]. Moreover, calcium channel blockers should be used with caution in patients receiving HAART, since they interact with protease inhibitors.
Sildenafil	Oral sildenafil seems to be beneficial as a selective pulmonary vasodilator in patients with primary pulmonary hypertension. Sildenafil may preferentially inhibit cGMP-specific phosphodiesterase, which is abundant in lung tissue [12, 25]. Therefore, the possibility of treatment needs to be evaluated prospectively in patients with HIV-associated pulmonary hypertension.

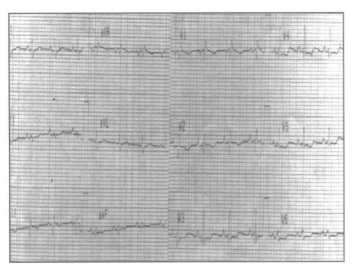

Fig. 4 ECG recording in a patient with HIV-associated pulmonary hypertension. A right-axis deviation (S1Q3T3 aspect or McGinn-White sign) along with tall, prominent P waves in leads II, III, aVF (secondary to right atrial enlargement) and complete right bundle branch block is evident

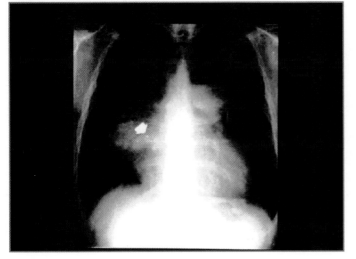

Fig. 5 Chest radiogram in a patient with HIV-associated pulmonary hypertension. A prominent main pulmonary artery along with enlarged hilar vessels (*arrow*) accompanied by a decrease in peripheral vessels and cardiomegaly is evident. (From [28], with permission from Wiley-Blackwell)

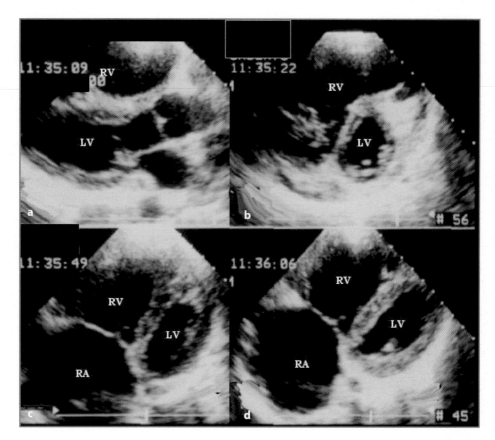

Fig. 6 a-d Transthoracic echocardiographic findings in HIV-associated pulmonary hypertension. It is possible to observe a systolic flattening of the interventricular septum and right atrial (*RA*) and right ventricular enlargement (*RV*). *LV*, left ventricle. (From [28], with permission from Wiley-Blackwell)

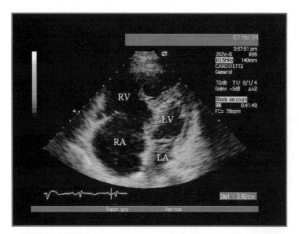

Fig. 7 Transthoracic echocardiographic findings in HIV-associated pulmonary hypertension. A systolic flattening of the interventricular septum and right atrial (*RA*) and right ventricular enlargement can be observed (*RV*). *LV*, left ventricle; *LA*, left atrial

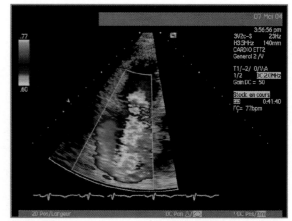

Fig. 8 Transthoracic echocardiographic findings in HIV-associated pulmonary hypertension. A significant tricuspid regurgitation is observed

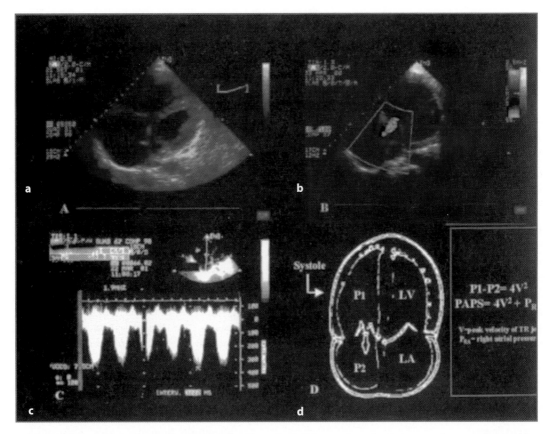

Fig. 9 a–d Transthoracic echocardiographic findings in HIV-associated pulmonary hypertension. The pulmonary arterial systolic pressure can be estimated by measuring the Doppler flow through the tricuspid valve according to Bernulli's modified formula: P=4V2 (where P is pressure gradient and V is peak retrograde velocity). The right atrial pressure (PRA) is nominally estimated at 10 mmHg. LV, left ventricle; LA, left atrium

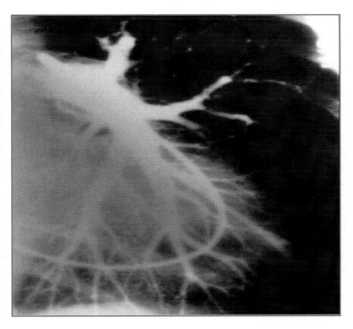

Fig. 10 Pulmonary angiography in a patient with HIV-associated pulmonary hypertension. It is possible to observe a "pruning" aspect with enlargement of the left pulmonary artery and decrease in peripheral vessels

dysfunction, the deregulation of circulating cytokines, and genetic factors seem to be implicated in the pathogenesis of this disease. In particular, as in primary pulmonary hypertension, an increase in the plasma concentrations of ET-1, IL-6, and TNF-α has been found in patients with HIV-associated pulmonary hypertension. The role of antiretroviral therapy is still being debated. Vasodilator agents such as prostaglandin I2 analog (beraprost), and ET-1 receptor antagonists such as bosentan, seem to be interesting therapeutic alternatives in the treatment of HIV-associated pulmonary hypertension compared to continuous intravenous infusion of epoprostenol. The use of cGMP-specific phosphodiesterase inhibitors such as sildenafil, is promising, but long-term controlled clinical trials are needed in this specific subset of patients.

References

1. Kim KK, Factor SM (1987) Membrano-proliferative glomerulonephritis and plexogenic pulmonary arteriopathy in a homosexual man with acquired immunodeficiency syndrome. Hum Pathol 18:1293–1296
2. Mehta NJ, Khan IA, Mehta RN et al (2000) HIV-related pulmonary hypertension: analytic review of 131 cases. Chest 118:1133–1141
3. Rich S (2000) Executive summary from the World Symposium on Primary Pulmonary Hypertension. Evian, France, 6–10 September 1998, cosponsored by World Health Organization. http://www.who.int/ncd/cvd/pph.html. Cited 14 April 2000
4. Mette SA, Palevsky HI, Pietra GG et al (1992) Primary pulmonary hypertension in association with human immunodeficiency virus infection: a possible viral etiology for some forms of hypertensive pulmonary arteriopathy. Am Rev Respir Dis 145:1196–1200
5. Humbert M, Monti G, Fartouk M et al (1998) Platelet-derived growth factor expression in primary pulmonary hypertension: comparison of HIV seropositive and HIV seronegative patients. Eur Respir J 11:554–559
6. Giaid A, Yanagisawa M, Langleben D (1993) Expression of endothelin-1 in the lungs of patients with pulmonary hypertension. N Engl J Med 328:1732–1739
7. Giaid A (1998) Nitric oxide and endothelin-1 in pulmonary hypertension. Chest 114:208S–212S
8. Cacoub P, Dorent R, Nataf P et al (1997) Endothelin-1 in the lungs of patients with pulmonary hypertension. Cardiovasc Res 33:196–200
9. Pellicelli AM, Palmieri F, D'Ambrosio C et al (1998) Role of human immunodeficiency virus in primary pulmonary hypertension: case reports. Angiology 49:1005–1011
10. Salvi SS (1999) Alfa1-adrenergic hypothesis for pulmonary hypertension. Chest 115:1708–1719
11. Tomashefski JF, Hirsch CS (1980) The pulmonary vascular lesions of intravenous drug abuse. Hum Pathol 11:133–145
12. Pellicelli AM, Barbaro G, Palmieri F et al (2001) Primary pulmonary hypertension in HIV patients: a systematic review. Angiology 52:31–41
13. Branch CA, Knuepfer MM (1992) Adrenergic mechanisms underlying cardiac and vascular responses to cocaine in conscious rats. J Pharmacol Exp Ther 263:742–751
14. Hadengue A, Benhayoun MK, Lebrec D et al (1991) Pulmonary hypertension complicating portal hypertension: prevalence and relation to splanchnic hemodynamics. Gastroenterology 100:520–528
15. Kuddus RH, Nalesnik MA, Subbotin VM et al (2000) Enhanced synthesis and reduced metabolism of endothelin-1 (ET-1) by hepatocytes: an important mechanism of increased endogenous levels of ET-1 in liver cirrhosis. J Hepatol 33:725–732
16. Morse JH, Barst RJ, Itescu S et al (1996) Primary pulmonary hypertension in HIV infection: an outcome determined by particular HLA class II alleles. Am J Respir Crit Care Med 153:1299–1301
17. Itescu S, Dalton J, Zhang HZ, Winchester R (1993) Tissue infiltration in a CD8 lymphocytosis syndrome associated with human immunodeficiency virus-1 infection has the phenotypic appearance of an antigenically driven response. J Clin Invest 91:2216–2225
18. Itescu S, Brancato LJ, Winchester W (1989) A sicca syndrome in HIV infection: association with HLA-DR5 and CD8 lymphocytosis. Lancet 2:466–468
19. McGoon M, Gutterman D, Steen V et al (2004) Screening, early detection and diagnosis of pulmonary arterial hypertension: ACCP Evidence-Based Clinical Practice Guidelines. Chest 126:14S–34S
20. Barbaro G (2004). Reviewing the clinical

aspects of HIV-associated pulmonary hypertension. J Respir Dis 25: 289–293

21. Pellicelli A, Palmieri F, Cicalini S et al (2001) Pathogenesis of HIV-related pulmonary hypertension. Ann NY Acad Sci 946:82–94

22. Opravil M, Pechère M, Speich R et al (1997) HIV-associated primary pulmonary hypertension. Am J Respir Crit Care Med 155:990–995

23. Zuber JP, Calmy A, Evison JM et al (2004) Pulmonary arterial hypertension related to HIV infection: improved hemodynamics and survival associated with antiretroviral therapy. Clin Infect Dis 38:1178–1185

24. Barbaro G, Lucchini A, Pellicelli AM et al (2006) Highly active antiretroviral therapy compared with HAART and bosentan in combination in patients with HIV-associated pulmonary hypertension. Heart 92:11641166

25. Petiprez P, Brenot F, Azarian R et al (1994) Pulmonary hypertension in patients with human immunodeficiency virus infection: comparison with primary pulmonary hypertension. Circulation 89:2722–2727

26. Aguilar RV, Farber HW (2000) Epoprostenol (prostacyclin) therapy in HIV-associated pulmonary hypertension. Am J Respir Crit Care Med 162:1846–1850

27. Sitbon O, Gressin V, Speich R et al (2004) Bosentan for the treatment of human immunodeficiency virus-associated pulmonary arterial hypertension. Am J Respir Crit Care Med 170:1212–1217

28. Petrosillo N, Pellicelli AM, Boumis F et al (2001) Clinical manifestations of HIV-related pulmonary hypertension. Ann NY Acad Sci 946:223–235

Chapter 13

Coagulative Disorders in HIV-Infected Patients

L. Drouet

Coagulative disorders in human immunodeficiency virus (HIV)-infected patients can lead to two opposite conditions:
1. Thrombotic conditions;
2. Hemorrhagic conditions.

Coagulative Disorders in HIV-Infected Patients Leading to Thrombotic Conditions

Coagulative Disorders in HIV Patients Undergoing HAART and Arterial Risk of Thrombosis

Emphasis has been placed on the deleterious associations/consequences of coagulative disorders and the two main high cardiovascular risk conditions of HIV patients undergoing highly active antiretroviral therapy (HAART): the metabolic and lipodystrophic syndromes. These conditions are associated with an overwhelming risk of cardiovascular events among the numerous metabolic and hemostatic pathways that are modified in these conditions: the coagulative systems and mostly the fibrinolytic systems are affected. The best-documented coagulative abnormalities associated with these conditions are an increase of plasminogen activator inhibitor-1 (PAI-1) and a decrease of fibrinolytic potential.

Coagulative Disorders in HIV Patients Undergoing HAART Linked to the Increased Risk of Cardiovascular Disorders

Hypofibrinolysis is associated with insulin resistance in HIV-infected patients receiving HAART, especially in those with metabolic syndrome.

The levels of PAI-1 and fibrinogen are significantly increased in patients receiving protease inhibitors (PIs) compared with control subjects, independently of HAART-associated metabolic syndrome. PAI-1 — and tissue plasminogen activator (tPA) — levels have been shown to be independently correlated to the use of PIs, triglyceride and insulin levels, body mass index, and gender in several studies (Fig. 1) [1]. Metformin treatment induces an improvement in PAI-1 levels. Changes in insulin AUC correlate significantly with changes in tPA antigen concentration. By reducing PAI-1 and tPA antigen concentrations, metformin may ultimately reduce the cardiovascular risk in patients with fat redistribution and insulin resistance [2].

Plasma PAI-1 concentrations are increased in direct proportion to liver fat content in HIV patients with lipodystrophy receiving HAART. Rosiglitazone decreases liver fat content, serum insulin, and plasma PAI-1 without changing the size of other fat

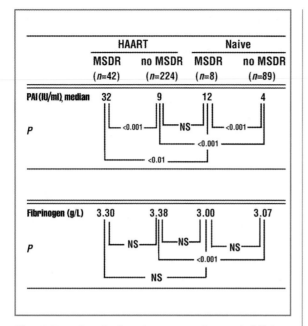

Fig. 1 Levels of plasminogen activator inhibitor type 1 (*PAI-1*) and fibrinogen in HIV-1-infected patients receiving protease inhibitor-containing higly active antiretroviral therapy (*HAART*) and treatment-naive HIV-1-infected patients with and without metabolic syndrome (*MSDR*) at the time of the cross-sectional study. *NS*, not significant. (From [1], with permission)

depots or PAI-1 mRNA in subcutaneous fat. These observations suggest that liver fat contributes to plasma PAI-1 concentrations in these patients (Fig. 2) [3].

HAART Reduces Markers of Endothelial and Coagulation Activation in HIV-1-Infected Patients

Endothelial-derived proteins — soluble vascular cell adhesion molecule-1 (sVCAM-1), soluble intercellular adhesion molecule-1 (sICAM-1), and von Willebrand's factor (VWF) — are markers of endothelial lesion and/or activation. These markers are increased in HIV-infected patients and they are usually considered as markers and/or agents of the accelerated atherosclerosis which characterizes HIV-infected patients independently of HAART and HAART-asso-

ciated metabolic syndrome. The increased plasma level of VWF [4] could be related to the inflammatory status, to antiretroviral treatment, but also to the direct lesion of

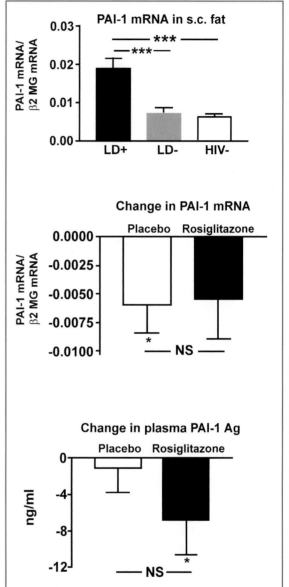

Fig. 2 PAI-1 mRNA expression in subcutaneous (*s.c.*) adipose tissue (*top*) and the change by rosiglitazone versus placebo treatment in PAI-1 mRNA (*middle*) and plasma PAI-1 antigen concentration (*bottom*). *LD+* indicates HIV+ patients with HAART-associated lipodystrophy; *LD–*, HIV+ patients using HAART but without LD; *HIV–*, HIV-normal subjects; *b2 MG*, b2-microglobulin. *NS*, not significant. *p<0.05, ***p<0.005. (From [3], with permission)

endothelium by HIV-1, and levels of sVCAM-1 and VWF factor are significantly correlated with HIV-1 viral load.

Great attention has been focused on VWF. In longitudinal testing, a persistent rise in VWF was associated with progression of HIV disease. The persistent elevation of functionally normal VWF during HIV infection, possibly reflecting a persistent endothelial cell activation, may have an important role in the pathogenesis of HIV infection. This elevated VWF is functionally normal as evaluated by plasma factor VIII (FVIII), ristocetin cofactor assay, and VWF multimer analyses. While HIV-infected patients showed enhanced platelet activation, platelets did not contribute substantially to the increased plasma VWF levels [5].

VWF plasma levels are correlated with HIV-1 viral load. Plasma levels of sVCAM-1, sICAM-1, and VWF decrease significantly after 5–13 months of HAART (Fig. 3). The pronounced decline in HIV RNA levels is associated with a corresponding decrease in VWF levels. D-dimer concentrations also decrease significantly after initiation of treatment. PI- and non-nucleoside reverse transcriptase inhibitor (NNRTI)-containing regimens have similar effects. However, contrary to markers of endothelial lesion/activation, HAART does not reduce the levels of the soluble markers of platelet activation (sP-selectin and CD40 ligand) (Table 1) [6]. The inhibition of markers of endothelial activation may be of benefit by counterbalancing the consequences of HAART-associated metabolic syndrome and potentially preventing the development of atherosclerosis in HIV-infected patients.

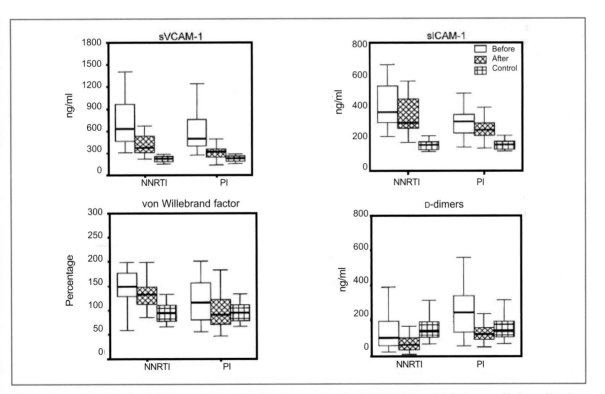

Fig. 3 Plasma levels of soluble vascular cell adhesion molecule (*sVCAM*)-1, soluble intercellular adhesion molecule (*sICAM*)-1, von Willebrand's factor, and D-dimers in HIV-infected patients who received treatment with protease inhibitors (*PIs*; *n*=21) or a non-nucleoside reverse transcriptase inhibitor (*NNRTI*; *n*=20), before and after initiation of treatment, compared to levels in healthy, HIV-negative control subjects (*n*=21). (From [6], with permission from the University of Chicago Press)

Table 1 Levels of endothelial, coagulation, and platelet activation markers in HIV-infected patients receiving protease inhibitors (PIs) or non-nucleoside reverse transcriptase inhibitors (NNRTIs) compared with levels in HIV-negative control subjects. (From [6], with permission from the University of Chicago Press)

Activation marker	Patients receiving PIs (n=21)		Patients receiving NNRTIs (n=20)		Control subjects (n=21)
	Before initiation of treatment	After initiation of treatment	Before initiation of treatment	After initiation of treatment	
Endothelial, mean (±SD)					
sVCAM-1, ng/ml	595 (266)[a]	381 (98)[a,b]	790 (442)[a]	515 (324)[a,b]	223 (42)
sICAM-1, ng/ml	313 (125)[a]	267 (86)[a,b]	444 (218)[a]	401 (249)[a,b]	168 (30)
von Willebrand factor, %	120 (45)	99 (39)[b]	149 (35)[a]	129 (33)[a,b]	98 (28)
Thrombomodulin, ng/ml	78 (16)[a]	77 (14)	46 (16)[a]	47 (17)[a]	67 (11)
Coagulation, mean (±SD)					
D-dimers, ng/ml	311 (248)	224 (320)b	141 (118)	74 (57)[b]	153 (68)
Thrombinantithrombin III complex, g/l	4.9 (7.7)	3.5 (2.6)	5.5 (5.7)	13 (18.3)[a]	3.2 (0.6)
Platelet, mean (±SD)					
sP-selectin, ng/ml	79 (84)[a]	67 (16)	49 (32)	58 (44)	34 (9)
Soluble CD40 ligand, ng/ml	2.3 (2.3)[a]	1.9 (0.7)[a]	2.3 (3.0)	3.1 (3.4)[a]	0.7 (0.3)

sICAM, soluble intercellular adhesion molecule; *sP*, soluble platelet; *sVCAM*, soluble vascular cell adhesion molecule.
[a] Statistically significantly higher than that of the control group (calculated using 1-way analysis of variance, Scheffé test, and Bonferroni correction; $p<0.05$).
[b] Statistically significantly lower than values before initiation of treatment (calculated using paired Wilcoxon rank sum test; $p< 0.01$)

HAART May Induce Thrombocytosis

Thrombocytosis has been reported in 9% of patients receiving HAART, with vascular complications being reported in up to 25% of the cases [7]. This side effect could contribute to the increased risk of arterial thrombosis among these patients.

Coagulative Disorders in HIV-Infected Patients Undergoing HAART Leading to the Risk of Venous Thrombosis

In recent years, several case reports [8] and a first epidemiological study [9] have focused attention on HIV-infected patients developing venous thromboembolic events under HAART [10, 11].

Thromboembolic Events and HIV Infection

Deep venous thrombosis of the lower arms [12, 13], pulmonary embolism [12], as well as thrombosis involving jugular and subclavian veins [14, 15], upper arm veins (apparently independent of intravenous drug abuse) [16], and cerebral [17], portal [18, 19], and retinal veins [20–23] have been described in HIV-infected patients, especially in those receiving HAART.

The risk factors of venous thromboembolic events (VTEE) identified in the general population (venous stasis, vascular lesions, hypercoagulability, and deficiency in the fibrinolytic system) are often found in HIV-infected patients, but additional factors may be present such as:

1. Acquired deficiency in coagulation inhibitors (protein S [23, 24], heparin cofactor II [25]);
2. Endothelial lesions;
3. Infection by HIV-1 itself [26, 27] or opportunistic infections (e.g., cytomegalovirus [28], chlamydia [29]);
4. Treatments (endothelial toxicity due to PIs and more specifically to indinavir [18] and ritonavir [30]);
5. Inflammatory and/or dysmetabolic states associated with HIV infection and HAART inducing hypofibrinolysis [increase in fibrinolysis inhibitors (mainly PAI-1) and a hypercoagulability state with increased coagulation factors (fibrinogen, VWF]. This results in an increase in global markers (D-dimers), due to inflammatory cytokines which induce a prothrombotic endothelial phenotype (decreased expression by endothelial cells of membrane thrombomodulin, of protein C receptor, hyperexpression by endothelial cells of tissue factor, increased synthesis of PAI-1 and of VWF) and the acquisition by leukocytes of a prothrombotic phenotype (mainly shedding of membrane microvesicles expressing tissue factor, complexes between leukocytes and platelets), and indirectly platelet activation;
6. Autoimmune state with a high frequency of auto-antibodies which act on coagulation such as those with specificity against phospholipids, cardiolipids, and prothrombinase (also called lupus anticoagulant) [31–34];
7. Potentially prothrombotic therapeutic molecules (as reported for indinavir [18], ritonavir [30], or megestrol acetate [18, 35, 36]), or invasive procedures (such as permanent indwelling catheters and implantable chambers);
8. HIV-associated malignancies (e.g., Kaposi's sarcoma [37]);
9. Vascular lesions related to intravenous drug administration [16].

Few studies have tried to quantify the incidence of VTEE in large cohorts of HIV patients. The Adult/Adolescent Spectrum of HIV Disease Project [9] reported the incidence of clinical VTEE and the associated risk factors in a population of HIV patients. This large epidemiological study had the advantage of being based on high numbers of patients (42,935 patients) with a long follow-up (2.4 years) and of being representative of a large spectrum of patients aged 13 years and over from more than 100 specialized medical centers in the United States. The calculated incidence of VTEE was 2.6/1,000 patient-years compared to 1/1,000 in the general population [38]. However, in this study, the incidence of VTEE was not the main endpoint, thus the real incidence may be underestimated.

The risk factors associated to VTEE were [9]:
- Age: above 45 years, the adjusted odds ratio (AOR) was 1.9 (CI 95%: 1.4–2.7);
- Cytomegalovirus infection or retinitis: AOR 1.9 (CI 95%: 1.2–2.9);
- Other opportunistic infection: AOR 1.5 (CI 95%: 1.1–2.2);
- Hospitalization: AOR 3.3 (CI 95%: 2.5–4.4);
- Use of megestrol acetate: AOR 2.0 (CI 95%: 1.3–3.9);
- Use of indinavir: AOR 2.4 (CI 95%: 1.4–4.3).

The occlusion of the retinal veins is mostly related to ocular infection such as that by the herpes virus [39], but can be of other origin [22], especially when they are bilateral [40] (it could be related to the endothelial affinity of HIV). Cerebral venous thrombosis can be associated to a deficiency of inhibitors such as protein S [41] or to local infections (meningitis or cerebral localization of cytomegalovirus [42], coccidioidomycosis [43]) or malignancy (e.g., non-Hodgkin's immunoblastic lymphoma) [44].

The increased plasma level of VWF and fibrinogen is more frequently associated with arterial thrombosis than venous thrombosis.

In HIV-infected patients, a high incidence of antiphospholipid antibodies has been reported. In a French study involving 342 HIV-infected patients, 64% had positive anticardiolipin antibodies, 50% had positive antiphosphatidyl choline antibodies, and 39% had antibodies with double specificity [45]. However, the specificity of the antiphospholipid antibodies usually associated with lupus and lupus-like syndromes was exceptional (anti-b2GP-1, lupus anticoagulant with antiprothrombinase specificity). Alteration of the immune system associated with HIV infection is different from that of lupus, probably explaining the differences in the specificity of antiphospholipid antibodies in the two diseases, but without explaining the pathogeny of their occurrence. One of theses differences is that, although antiphospholipid antibodies are commonly detected in patients with HIV disease, the clinical manifestations of antiphospholipid syndrome are uncommon and are still reported as case reports [46]. In HIV-infected patients, the main features of the antiphospholipid antibodies are not thrombotic but avascular (bone and cutaneous necrosis) [47].

Protein S has been studied in HIV-infected children (characterized by a minimal association of confounding risk factors), showing that the deficiency was mostly due to a deficit in free protein S antigen with a global functional deficiency in protein S [48]. This deficiency was correlated with the clinical evolution of the disease. The incidence was 33% in asymptomatic HIV-infected children and 75% in symptomatic HIV-infected children. The occurrence of protein S deficiency appears linked to the duration of the disease but not to the degree of immunodeficiency, since it is not correlated to the CD4+ lymphocytes count. Cell membrane phospholipids are usually not accessible, but if they are exposed in large amounts they could form a complex with and absorb protein S (in a process similar to that observed during the hemolytic crisis of sickle cell anemia). Similar exposure of cell membrane phospholipids (e.g., from endothelial origin during HIV contamination) could induce occurrence of antiphospholipid antibodies.

Most of these factors are correlated with each other [34] and with the markers of activation of the coagulation/fibrinolysis reaction (such as the D-dimers), with the status of immunodeficiency, with opportunistic infections, with cancer complications, and with the inflammatory status.

Three different types of mechanisms of VTEE linked to treatments can be differentiated:

- Those due to the central catheters required in patients with severe undernourishment [49]. It seems that among HIV-infected patients requiring total intravenous nutrition, a low-dose oral anticoagulant regimen does not have the efficacy encountered in other types of patients treated with a central catheter [50].
- Those related to the administration of megestrol acetate [35].
- Those related to PIs [18, 51]. This observation is in apparent opposition with two other types of observations on PI-related effects in HIV-infected patients:
- Effective antiretroviral treatment in HIV-infected patients decreases markers of endothelial activation/lesion [5] and markers of coagulation activation [6].
- Antiretroviral treatment exerts a prohemorrhagic effect in hemophilic patients infected by HIV-1 [52].

Treatment-Related VTEE in HIV-infected Patients

PIs are large lipophilic molecules metabolized by P450 cytochromes. The same P450 cytochrome system also metabolizes oral anticoagulants (warfarin) [53]. HIV-infected patients often have complex clinical signs such as thrombocytopenia or other clinical manifestations or treatment which often represents a contraindication to warfarin treatment so that other types of therapy may be required such as the use of low-molecular-weight heparin for long periods.

Coagulative Disorders in HIV-Infected Patients Leading to Microvascular Risk of Thrombosis

Microthrombotic Disease in HIV Patients

Thrombotic thrombocytopenic purpura (TTP) is a microthrombotic disease of rare occurrence. The most clinically sensitive microcirculations to TTP are those of the brain, kidney, and liver, explaining the most frequent clinical manifestations of the disease. One of the main pathogenic mechanism of TTP is a deficiency (hereditary or acquired) of an endogenous metalloprotease (ADAMS 13) which physiologically degrades the highest-molecular-weight forms of VWF into lower-molecular-weight fragments. The increased concentration of higher-molecular-weight forms of VWF trig-

gers in vivo platelet aggregation and formation of platelet microthrombi, which plug the microcirculations of the most sensitive organs. The treatment is based on plasma exchange and infusion of fresh frozen plasma to remove the highest-molecular-weight forms of VWF, to remove the inhibitors of ADAMS 13, and to replenish ADAMS 13. From an epidemiologic point of view, TTP in HIV infection is associated with opportunistic infections (cryptosporidiosis, cytomegalovirus infection) [54], with HIV-associated malignancies, or with HIV-associated wasting syndrome. The incidence of TTP is significantly reduced after the introduction of HAART (Fig. 4) [55, 56].

Coagulative Disorders in HIV-Infected Patients Leading to Hemorrhagic Condition

Thrombocytopenia

The most frequent hemorrhagic condition associated with HIV infection is thrombocytopenia [57]. Although often asymptomatic, thrombocytopenia may be linked to a variety of bleeding abnormalities. The underly-

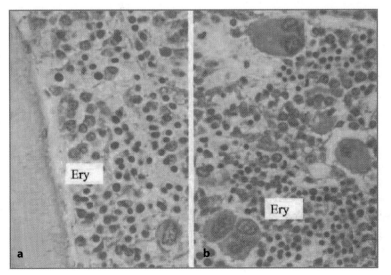

Fig. 4a, b Photomicrographs of bone marrow core biopsy. a Paratrabecular aggregates of erythroid precursor cells as seen in myelodysplasia. H&E, × 400. b Hypercellularity with erythroid and megakaryocytes hyperplasia. PAS, × 400. (From [56], with permission of Wiley-Liss, Inc., a subsidiary of John Wiley & Sons, Inc.)

ing pathophysiology includes accelerated peripheral platelet destruction and decreased ("ineffective") production of platelets from the infected megakaryocytes. In drug users, the disease appears to be of more rapid progression and more frequently complicated. HIV-associated thrombocytopenia responds to antiretroviral therapy, but this is less effective in drug users [58]. Some studies have evaluated the use of zidovudine (AZT) and have shown increased platelet production. HAART induces a sustained platelet response in HIV-associated thrombocytopenia, even in antiretroviral-experienced subjects and in those with AZT-resistant thrombocytopenia (Table 2) [59]. If antiretroviral agents fail to improve the platelet count or if antiretroviral agents cannot be used, other treatments, similar to those used in "classic" immune thrombocytopenia (ITP), can be employed, including steroids and intravenous immunoglobulins (intravenous anti-D). Splenectomy has been used to treat HIV-infected patients with refractory thrombocytopenia. Although it is an effective treatment, there are concerns about infections and selection of appropriate candidates. Other treatment modalities, such as interferon, vincristine, danazol, low-dose splenic irradiation, and staphylococcal protein A immunoadsorption have shown limited success in HIV-associated thrombocytopenia. Alternatively, thrombocytopenia in HIV-infected patients may be treated with pharmacological hyperstimulation of megakaryocytopoiesis (administration of PEG-rHuMGDF or TPO). The latest evidence indicates that the chemokine receptor CXCR4 (co-receptor for the cellular entry of lymphotropic HIV strains) is expressed on megakaryocytes; as a result, the development of chemokine receptor antagonists may modify the course of the disease.

Table 2 Platelet and CD4+ response to antiretroviral therapy in 34 HIV-infected patients with severe thrombocytopenia. (From [59], with permission from the British Infection Society)

Variable	No. of patients	Baseline[a]	Treatment[a]		Overall[b]		0–3rd month[c]	3rd-6th month[c]
			3rd month	6th month	c^2	p	p	p
HAART treatment	15							
PLT count (PLT x 10 9 /1)		32 (6 –49)	87 (34 –259)	108 (20 –195)	10.53	0.01	0.01	NS
CD4+(cells/µl)		58 (1 –392)	127 (10 –503)	142 (4 –387)	8.1	0.02	0.05	NS
AZT treatment	19							
PLT count (PLT x 10 9 /1)		29 (6 –47)	49 (12 –429)	79 (9 –253)	20.63	0.001	0.01	NS
CD4+(cells/µl)		96 (9 –177)	144 (16 –528)	99 (15 –378)	6.63	0.03	0.01	NS

[a]Values of each variable are median (range); [b]Friedmann test; [c]Wilcoxon-Wilcox test

Increased Hemorrhagic Tendency and Hemophiliac HIV Patients

One concerning side effect of HAART is the increased hemorrhagic tendency of hemophiliac patients contaminated and treated for HIV. Shortly after the introduction of PIs for the treatment of HIV infection, an association between these drugs and an increased bleeding tendency in patients with hereditary bleeding disorders was observed. The patients experience not only an increased bleeding frequency in usual sites, but bleeding can also occur in unusual sites such as the finger joints. Mucus membrane bleeding and hematuria are also common. Ritonavir appears to be associated with the highest risk of bleeding followed by indinavir. PI-associated bleeds tend to be more resistant to factor VIII concentrate treatment, and periods of prophylaxis may be required in individuals with frequent persistent bleeding. Patients continuing PI therapy tend to develop a tolerance to this adverse effect over time. The mechanism of the bleeding tendency has not been elucidated. There is no consistent evidence of a disturbance of coagulation, fibrinolysis, or platelet function, which raises the possibility that PIs may exert a direct local effect on blood vessels. It is very important that this class-specific side effect is recognized and understood by both the physicians and the patients [52].

References

1. Koppel K, Bratt G, Schulman S, Bylund H, Sandstrom E (2002) Hypofibrinolytic state in HIV-1-infected patients treated with protease inhibitor-containing highly active antiretroviral therapy. J Acquir Immune Defic Syndr 29:441–449
2. Hadigan C, Meigs JB, Rabe J et al (2001) Increased PAI-1 and tPA antigen levels are reduced with metformin therapy in HIV-infected patients with fat redistribution and insulin resistance. J Clin Endocrinol Metab 86:939–943
3. Yki-Jarvinen H, Sutinen J, Silveira A et al (2003) Regulation of plasma PAI-1 concentrations in HAART-associated lipodystrophy during rosiglitazone therapy. Arterioscler Thromb Vasc Biol 23:688–694
4. Drouet L, Scrobohaci ML, Janier M, Baudin B (1990) Endothelial cells: target for the HIV1 virus? Nouv Rev Fr Hematol 32:103–106
5. Aukrust P, Bjornsen S, Lunden B et al (2000) Persistently elevated levels of von Willebrand factor antigen in HIV infection. Downregulation during highly active antiretroviral therapy. Thromb Haemost 84:183–187
6. Wolf K, Tsakiris DA, Weber R, Erb P, Battegay M (2002) Antiretroviral therapy reduces markers of endothelial and coagulation activation in patients infected with human immunodeficiency virus type 1. J Infect Dis 185:456–462
7. Miguez-Burbano MJ, Burbano X, Rodriguez A, Lecusay R, Rodriguez N, Shor-Posner G (2002) Development of thrombocytosis in HIV+ drug users: impact of antiretroviral therapy. Platelets 13:183–185
8. Saif MW, Greenberg B (2001) HIV and thrombosis: a review. AIDS Patient Care STDS 15:15–24
9. Sullivan PS, Dworkin MS, Jones JL, Hooper WC (2000) Epidemiology of thrombosis in HIV-infected individuals: The Adult/Adolescent Spectrum of HIV Disease Project. AIDS 14:321–324
10. Majluf-Cruz A, Silva-Estrada M, Sanchez-Barboza R et al (2004) Venous thrombosis among patients with AIDS. Clin Appl Thromb Hemost 10:19–25
11. Callens S, Florence E, Philippe M, Van Der PM, Colebunders R (2003) Mixed arterial and venous thromboembolism in a person with HIV infection. Scand J Infect Dis 35:907–908
12. Becker DM, Saunders TJ, Wispelwey B, Schain DC (1992) Case report: venous thromboembolism in AIDS. Am J Med Sci 303:395–397
13. Tanimowo M (1996) Deep vein thrombosis as a manifestation of the acquired immunodeficiency syndrome? A case report. Cent Afr J Med 42:327–328
14. Vielhauer V, Schewe CK, Schlondorff D (1998) Bilateral thrombosis of the internal jugular veins with spasmodic torticollis in a patient with acquired immunodeficiency syndrome and disseminated cytomegalovirus infection. J Infect 37:90–91
15. Bayer DD, Sorbello AF, Condoluci DV (1995) Bilateral subclavian vein thrombosis in a patient with acquired immunodeficiency syndrome. J Am Osteopath Assoc 95:276–277
16. Laing RB, Brettle RP, Leen CL (1996) Venous

thrombosis in HIV infection. Int J STD AIDS 7:82–85

17. Meyohas MC, Roullet E, Rouzioux C et al (1989) Cerebral venous thrombosis and dual primary infection with human immunodeficiency virus and cytomegalovirus. J Neurol Neurosurg Psychiatry 52:1010–1011

18. Carr A, Brown D, Cooper DA (1997) Portal vein thrombosis in patients receiving indinavir, an HIV protease inhibitor. AIDS 11:1657–1658

19. Narayanan TS, Narawane NM, Phadke AY, Abraham P (1998) Multiple abdominal venous thrombosis in HIV-seropositive patients. Indian J Gastroenterol 17:105–106

20. Roberts SP, Haefs TM (1992) Central retinal vein occlusion in a middle-aged adult with HIV infection. Optom Vis Sci 69:567–569

21. Mansour AM, Li H, Segal EI (1996) Picture resembling hemicentral retinal vein occlusion in the acquired immunodeficiency syndrome: is it related to cytomegalovirus? Ophthalmologica 210:108–111

22. Park KL, Marx JL, Lopez PF, Rao NA (1997) Noninfectious branch retinal vein occlusion in HIV-positive patients. Retina 17:162–164

23. Stahl CP, Wideman CS, Spira TJ, Haff EC, Hixon GJ, Evatt BL (1993) Protein S deficiency in men with long-term human immunodeficiency virus infection. Blood 81:1801–1807

24. Bissuel F, Berruyer M, Causse X, Dechavanne M, Trepo C (1992) Acquired protein S deficiency: correlation with advanced disease in HIV-1-infected patients. J Acquir Immune Defic Syndr 5:484–489

25. Toulon P, Lamine M, Ledjev I et al (1993) Heparin cofactor II deficiency in patients infected with the human immunodeficiency virus. Thromb Haemost 70:730–735

26. Muller MM, Griesmacher A (2000) Markers of endothelial dysfunction. Clin Chem Lab Med 38:77–85

27. Gujuluva C, Burns AR, Pushkarsky T et al (2001) HIV-1 penetrates coronary artery endothelial cells by transcytosis. Mol Med 7:169–176

28. Madalosso C, de SN Jr, Ilstrup DM et al (1998) Cytomegalovirus and its association with hepatic artery thrombosis after liver transplantation. Transplantation 66:294–297

29. Kaukoranta-Tolvanen SS, Ronni T, Leinonen M et al (1996) Expression of adhesion molecules on endothelial cells stimulated by Chlamydia pneumoniae. Microb Pathog 21:407–411

30. Zhong DS, Lu XH, Conklin BS et al (2002) HIV protease inhibitor ritonavir induces cytotoxicity of human endothelial cells. Arterioscler Thromb Vasc Biol 22:1560–1566

31. Stimmler MM, Quismorio FP Jr, McGehee WG et al (1989) Anticardiolipin antibodies in acquired immunodeficiency syndrome. Arch Intern Med 149:1833–1835

32. Karmochkine M, Raguin G (1998) Severe coronary artery disease in a young HIV-infected man with no cardiovascular risk factor who was treated with indinavir. AIDS 12:2499

33. Ankri A, Bonmarchand M, Coutellier A, Herson S, Karmochkine M (1999) Antiphospholipid antibodies are an epiphenomenon in HIV-infected patients. AIDS 13:1282–1283

34. Feffer SE, Fox RL, Orsen MM et al (1995) Thrombotic tendencies and correlation with clinical status in patients infected with HIV. South Med J 88:1126–1130

35. Force L, Barrufet P, Herreras Z, Bolibar I (1999) Deep venous thrombosis and megestrol in patients with HIV infection. AIDS 13:1425–1426

36. Hirsh J, Hull RD, Raskob GE (1986) Epidemiology and pathogenesis of venous thrombosis. J Am Coll Cardiol 8(6 Suppl B):104B–113B

37. Kaufmann T, Nisce LZ, Metroka C (1991) Thromboembolism in AIDS-related Kaposi's sarcoma. JAMA 266:2834

38. Heit JA (2002) Venous thromboembolism epidemiology: implications for prevention and management. Semin Thromb Hemost 28(Suppl 2):3–13

39. Biswas J, Roy CB, Krishna KS et al (2001) Detection of Mycobacterium tuberculosis by polymerase chain reaction in a case of orbital tuberculosis. Orbit 20:69–74

40. Friedman SM, Margo CE (1995) Bilateral central retinal vein occlusions in a patient with acquired immunodeficiency syndrome. Clinicopathologic correlation. Arch Ophthalmol 113:1184–1188

41. Iranzo A, Domingo P, Cadafalch J, Sambeat MA (1998) Intracranial venous and dural sinus thrombosis due to protein S deficiency in a patient with AIDS. J Neurol Neurosurg Psychiatry 64:688

42. Biswas J, Kumar AA, George AE et al (2000) Ocular and systemic lesions in children with HIV. Indian J Pediatr 67:721–724

43. Kleinschmidt-DeMasters BK, Mazowiecki M, Bonds LA et al (2000) Coccidioidomycosis meningitis with massive dural and cerebral venous thrombosis and tissue arthroconidia. Arch Pathol Lab Med 124:310–314

44. Doberson MJ, Kleinschmidt-DeMasters BK (1994) Superior sagittal sinus thrombosis in a patient with acquired immunodeficiency syndrome. Arch Pathol Lab Med 118:844–846

45. Abuaf N, Laperche S, Rajoely B et al (1997) Autoantibodies to phospholipids and to the coagulation proteins in AIDS. Thromb Haemost 77:856–861

46. Shahnaz S, Parikh G, Opran A (2004) Antiphospholipid antibody syndrome manifesting as a deep venous thrombosis and pulmonary embolism in a patient with HIV. Am J Med Sci 327:231–232

47. Ramos-Casals M, Cervera R, Lagrutta M et al (2004) Clinical features related to antiphospholipid syndrome in patients with chronic viral infections (hepatitis C virus/HIV infection): description of 82 cases. Clin Infect Dis 38:1009–1016

48. Sugerman RW, Church JA, Goldsmith JC, Ens GE (1996) Acquired protein S deficiency in children infected with human immunodeficiency virus. Pediatr Infect Dis J 15:106–111

49. Melchior JC, Messing B (1999) Home parenteral nutrition in acquired immunodeficiency syndrome patients. Nutrition 15:68–69

50. Duerksen DR, Ahmad A, Doweiko J et al (1996) Risk of symptomatic central venous thrombotic complications in AIDS patients receiving home parenteral nutrition. JPEN J Parenter Enteral Nutr 20:302–305

51. George SL, Swindells S, Knudson R, Stapleton JT (1999) Unexplained thrombosis in HIV-infected patients receiving protease inhibitors: report of seven cases. Am J Med 107:624–630

52. Wilde JT, Lee CA, Collins P et al (1999) Increased bleeding associated with protease inhibitor therapy in HIV-positive patients with bleeding disorders. Br J Haematol 107:556–559

53. Llibre JM, Romeu J, Lopez E, Sirera G (2002) Severe interaction between ritonavir and acenocoumarol. Ann Pharmacother 36:621–623

54. Rerolle JP, Canaud G, Fakhouri F et al (2004) Thrombotic microangiopathy and hypothermia in an HIV-positive patient: importance of cytomegalovirus infection. Scand J Infect Dis 36:234–237

55. Gervasoni C, Ridolfo AL, Vaccarezza M et al (2002) Thrombotic microangiopathy in patients with acquired immunodeficiency syndrome before and during the era of introduction of highly active antiretroviral therapy. Clin Infect Dis 35:1534–1540

56. Gruszecki AC, Wehrli G, Ragland BD et al (2002) Management of a patient with HIV infection-induced anemia and thrombocytopenia who presented with thrombotic thrombocytopenic purpura. Am J Hematol 69:228–231

57. Scaradavou A (2002) HIV-related thrombocytopenia. Blood Rev 16:73–76

58. Burbano X, Miguez MJ, Lecusay R et al (2001) Thrombocytopenia in HIV-infected drug users in the HAART era. Platelets 12:456–461

59. Carbonara S, Fiorentino G, Serio G et al (2001) Response of severe HIV-associated thrombocytopenia to highly active antiretroviral therapy including protease inhibitors. J Infect 42:251–256

Chapter 14

Cardiovascular Complications in HIV-Infected Children

D. Bonnet

Longitudinal cardiovascular follow-up of HIV-infected children has shown that all components of the cardiovascular system might be affected during the course of the disease. The most frequent feature observed in the pediatric population is left ventricular dysfunction [1–12]. In developed countries, antiviral therapy has dramatically improved morbidity and mortality in HIV-infected children. Consequently, the spectrum of HIV-related concerns has shifted from reduction of mortality towards longer-term complications of HIV infection and adverse effects associated with the use of antiretroviral therapy. With regards to the cardiovascular system, efforts have been made to describe the long-term outcome in children. In this chapter, we review the different cardiac diseases that occur in HIV-infected children. HIV-related cardiac complications are very similar to the spectrum of disease described in adults, with a few exceptions. There have been descriptions of fetal and neonatal complications due to the common vertical transmission of the virus in most cases and the possible adverse intrauterine effects of maternal HIV infection with or without fetal HIV infection [12, 13]. The pathogenesis of some cardiac manifestations remains uncertain. Although in some cases the myocardial [14], endocardial [15], or pericardial disease [16, 17] may be attributed to an opportunistic infection, it is likely that HIV-related cardiac disease has a multifactorial origin due to HIV, secondary infections, other concurrent disease states, side effects of therapy, nutritional deficiencies, or yet-unknown mechanisms. However, it is recommended that children with active HIV infection should be monitored for cardiac disease because symptoms of cardiac failure are delayed and interventions might be required to reduce cardiac morbidity and mortality. Finally, the long-term "vascular" outcome might be impaired either by the HIV infection or by the metabolic effects of the antiretroviral therapy or their synergistic effect on endothelium. Early atherosclerosis may be a new emerging disease in HIV-infected children, and this raises concern on the prevention of vascular damage.

Myocardial Involvement

Dilated cardiomyopathy is the most common cardiac complication of HIV infection in children and is an adverse prognostic indicator in patients with HIV infection. The Prospective Pediatric Pulmonary and Cardiac Complications Study of HIV (P2C2) showed a 5-year cumulative incidence of dilated cardiomyopathy as high as 28% in vertically HIV-infected children [12]. Further, the mortality rate in children who exhibited congestive heart failure was 52.5% (95% CI, 30.5–74.5) in this study. In addition, the authors suggest that the incidence of left ventricular dysfunction in HIV-infected children is underestimated in this population because of the low sensitivity of the commonly used noninvasive echocardiographic techniques to examine left ventricular performance [18].

The reported incidence of cardiac involvement in HIV-infected children varies from 0.9% of congestive heart failure in a study using hospital diagnosis codes [19] to 14% in later studies using the shortening fraction of the left ventricle as an indicator of systolic function [20]. Lipshultz et al. reported that cardiac abnormalities were seen in up to 93% of patients who had undergone more extensive cardiac testing at a referral center [16]. Two patterns of left ventricular function abnormalities were described when using load-independent indexes of contractility: (1) hyperdynamic left ventricular performance with enhanced contractility and reduced afterload, and (2) diminished contractility associated with symptomatic cardiomyopathy. Serial evaluations revealed that 89% of the patients had progressive left ventricular dysfunction.

The most important study designed to assess the incidence of cardiac dysfunction in HIV-infected children is the P2C2 HIV study [10, 12, 21–23]. This study began in 1990 and data collection continued through January 1997. Left ventricular function was evaluated every 4–6 months for up to 5 years in a birth cohort of 805 infants born to women infected with HIV-1. In total, 205 vertically HIV-infected children (group I) and 600 subjects enrolled during fetal life (group II, neonatal inception cohort; n=432) or before 28 days of age (n=168) were included in the study. Their final HIV status was unknown at the time of enrolment in the study. Of these, 93 were finally HIV-infected and 463 HIV-uninfected. In addition, a cross-sectionally measured comparison group of 195 healthy children born to mothers who were not infected with HIV was also recruited as external controls. Main outcome measures were the cumulative incidence of an initial episode of left ventricular dysfunction, cardiac enlargement, and congestive heart failure. Because cardiac abnormalities tended to cluster in the same patients, the number of children who had cardiac impairment defined as hav-ing left ventricular fractional shortening (LV FS) <25% after 6 months of age, congestive heart failure, or treatment with cardiac medications was also determined. In group I, the cumulative incidence of left ventricular dysfunction after 5 years in the study was 28%. In group II, the 5-year cumulative incidence of left ventricular dysfunction was 9.3% in the HIV-infected neonatal group compared with 2.9% in the uninfected children (p=0.02). During the follow-up period, 21 children in group I had congestive heart failure (cumulative incidence rate 14%). The use of cardiac medication after a diagnosis of cardiomyopathy was 25%. In the group II-infected children, four cases of congestive heart failure occurred and the 5-year cumulative incidence rate was 5.1%, with four additional patients receiving medications for a cardiomyopathy. This study and the previous reports show that cardiac dysfunction occurs frequently in HIV-infected children with a wide range of abnormalities. The relative risk of death in infected children is 8.5–14.6 times higher than in children without these complications. This risk is even higher in rapid progressors defined as infants having an AIDS-defining condition, severe immunodepression (CDC immunologic category 3), or both [12]. This worrisome study has led to controversies regarding the fact that cardiomyopathy is a major cause of or contributor to mortality in HIV-infected children, since several groups in Europe did not have this experience. However, it suggests strongly that a routine echocardiographic follow-up should be proposed in this population.

When analyzing more precisely the echocardiographic parameters of left ventricular function and mass, additional prognostic factors appear [24]. Indeed, an abnormal thickness-to-dimension ratio from progressive left ventricular dilatation and inadequate hypertrophy and an increased ventricular mass are related with patient morbidity and mortality. Diastolic function estimated by isovolumic relaxation time was also found to be impaired in HIV-infected children and to decline further with time. These markers may be a harbinger of congestive heart failure.

The pathogenesis of left ventricular dysfunction in HIV-infected children remains unclear and its specific origin might be difficult to address as the prevalence of this complication is thought to be rare today. HIV cardiomyopathy is probably not due to any one single mechanism. In the majority of cases of AIDS-related cardiomyopathy in both pediatric and adult age groups, no precise etiology is found. A few autopsy studies described the pathologic findings of cardiomyopathy in pediatric patients with HIV. In one of the earlier series of five fatal pediatric cases, the heart showed biventricular dilatation with an increased diameter of myocardial fibers, nuclear enlargement, myocyte vacuolation, interstitial edema with or without foci of myxoid change, small foci of myocardial fibrosis, and endocardial thickening [25]. Mononuclear inflammatory infiltrates with small foci of myocyte necrosis were not found in any patient in this study or in later ones. The pathologic findings of lymphocytic myocarditis, which is common in adults with AIDS, are similar to those found in pediatric age groups [26]. Electron microscopy, done in very few cases, showed mitochondrial and sarcoplasmic reticulum changes. The specificity of these anomalies and the fact that these structures may be related to the development of cardiomyopathy in AIDS patients have not been demonstrated [27].

In a minority of cases of lymphocytic myocarditis in adults, an associated pathogen is found. In one pediatric case, cytomegalovirus inclusions were noted in the endocardium and endothelial cells without myocardial involvement [25]. The other microorganisms reported to involve the heart in cases of AIDS (cryptococcus, *Candida*, *Toxoplasma gondii*, *Sarcocystis*, bacterial infection during tuberculosis, Coxsackie virus, and *Aspergillus*) are only rarely reported or have not been described yet.

HIV has been detected within myocardial cells by different methods, suggesting that the virus itself may be a cause of cardiomyopathy and lymphocytic myocarditis in some patients. The role of dendritic cells in the pathogenesis has been suggested because PCR detected HIV more frequently in these cells [28]. The mechanism leading to cardiac dysfunction remains unclear. It may involve cytokines, a susceptibility to myocarditis in HIV-infected patients, and/or auto-immunity [29].

The toxicity of antiretroviral therapy may also contribute to the pathogenesis of cardiomyopathy. The introduction of highly active antiretroviral therapy regimens has significantly modified the course of HIV disease particularly in children, with longer survival rates and improvement of life quality in HIV-infected subjects. However, adverse cardiovascular effects of different drugs have been proposed. In a retrospective study of 137 HIV-infected children, Domanski et al. found that a cardiomyopathy was 8.4 times more likely to occur in children who had been previously given zidovudine than in those who had never taken this drug [30]. Although the cause of this difference is uncertain, it may be due to an inhibition of cardiac mitochondrial DNA replication by zidovudine. In our experience, we had only one case with proven mitochondrial respiratory chain deficiency on endomyocardial biopsy in a child receiving zidovudine. In a more recent study [31], 382 infants without HIV infection born to HIV-infected women (36 with zidovudine exposure) and 58 HIV-infected infants (12 with zidovudine exposure) underwent serial echocardiography from birth to 5 years of age. Zidovudine exposure was not associated with significant abnormalities in mean left ventricular fractional shortening, end-diastolic dimension, contractility, or mass in both the non-HIV-infected and the HIV-infected infants. The authors concluded that zidovudine was not associated with acute or chronic abnormalities in left ventricular structure or function in infants exposed to the drug in the perinatal period. While controversial, these results suggest that careful follow-up is necessary in an HIV-infected child with cardiomyopathy receiving zidovudine. Finally, nutritional deficiencies such as selenium deficiency and prolonged immunosuppression have also been proposed to be causal or deleterious additional factors [32].

The treatment of congestive heart failure in children with HIV should begin with routine anticongestive measures. Although not formally studied in HIV-infected children, angiotensin-converting inhibitors can be used judiciously. Recent nonrandomized studies using chronic β-blockers in children yielded encouraging preliminary results [33]. Lipshultz et al. reported normalization of the left ventricular dilatation and diminished wall thickness of HIV-infected children with monthly intravenous immunoglobulin infusion, possibly because of an improvement in immunologically mediated left ventricular dysfunction [34]. The question of whether asymptomatic HIV-infected children with left ventricular dilatation should be treated with angiotensin-converting inhibitors is unresolved.

Pericardial Involvement

Pericardial effusion has been reported in pediatric patients infected with HIV and even in fetuses. The prevalence of this cardiac complication may increase as the incidence of HIV infection rises in the pediatric age group. In children, pericardial effusion has been reported in up to 26% of cases [16]. These pericardial effusions are usually small and asymptomatic. Kovacs et al. reported three cases of sudden death of infants with HIV who had symptomatic pericardial effusions, two with tamponade

and one with large pericardial effusion and cardiac compromise [35]. In most cases of pericardial effusion, no established cause is found. In the published studies, there was no evidence of cardiac infection by pathogens other than HIV. Noninfectious causes such as lymphoma, Kaposi's sarcoma, or myocardial infarction have not been reported in children.

Endocardial Involvement

Infective endocarditis, either acute or subacute, has been rarely reported in pediatric AIDS patients [1]. Nonbacterial thrombotic endocarditis, usually an incidental finding in adults, has not yet been described in children.

Vascular Involvement

Although rare, coronary artery abnormalities have been described in the earliest case reports of cardiac complications in children [35–38]. Joshi et al. found macroscopic lesions in small and medium-sized arteries in six children with AIDS. The pathologic findings in the coronary artery wall were characterized by intimal fibrosis, fragmentation of the elastic lamellae, and calcification of the media. In one out of six cases, this arterial remodeling involved the coronary arteries and had led to a fatal myocardial infarction by aneurysms and thrombosis of the right coronary artery. The pathophysiology of these arterial anomalies is unknown. It may be related to the viral infection, given the absence of other cardiovascular risk factors. Whether HIV itself is the causal agent or other viruses such as herpes or cytomegalovirus has to be elucidated. The adverse effects of antiretroviral drugs, including dyslipidemia, lipodystrophy, and insulin resistance, are problems in the long-term management of HIV infection. This is of particular importance in children because HIV infection has become a chronic disease in this population. HIV-infected children may live two decades longer than HIV-infected adults. As in the adult population, metabolic toxicity of antiretroviral therapy has been observed in children [39–41], but the long-term cardiovascular consequences in children are unknown. Atherogenic lipoprotein changes in adults treated with protease inhibitors (PIs) have been found and are associated with endothelial dysfunction and increased intima-media thickness [42–44]. However, the relative contributions of antiretroviral therapy, chronic inflammation due to the viral infection, classic cardiovascular risk factors, and their interactions are very difficult to identify. Bozzette et al. showed that the benefit in terms of mortality associated with the extensive use of therapies for HIV was not diminished by any increase in the rate of cardiovascular or cerebrovascular events or related mortality [45]. The pediatric population offers a unique opportunity to study vascular function during HIV infection in the absence of classic cardiovascular risk factors. Symptomatic atherosclerosis is evidently absent at this age, but endothelial function and arterial stiffness can be investigated by noninvasive echo-tracking techniques. We have recently shown that HIV-infected children have a vascular dysfunction that may be an early step in the development of atherosclerosis. We did not find any difference between children receiving antiretroviral therapy and patients who had never been treated [46]. Differences with the control subjects indicate that the HIV infection itself may have a deleterious effect on vascular function. However, others found a contribution of antiretroviral therapy to the vascular impairment in children [47]. This is consistent with autopsy studies during the pre-antiretroviral era, reporting eccentric atherosclerosis lesions in the absence of traditional risk factors [36]. The

HIV envelope protein, gp120, activates human arterial smooth muscle cells to express tissue factor, the initiator of the coagulation cascade [48]. In addition, inflammatory cytokines and viral proteins synergistically promote endothelial activation, apoptosis, or cell proliferation [49]. Consequently, the arterial remodeling observed in patients who had never been treated could be a result of direct viral infection, or of the activation of bystander cells (smooth muscle cells and endothelial cells), by HIV viral proteins. Hsue et al. recently proposed that in adults, immunodeficiency and traditional coronary risk factors might contribute to atherosclerosis rather than the deleterious effects of PI treatment [50]. In children, it is possible that antiretroviral therapy counterbalances, at least transiently, HIV-induced injury to the developing vascular bed by reversing or stabilizing the HIV-induced vascular dysfunction.

Mild and nonprogressive aortic root dilation was also seen in children with vertically transmitted HIV infection from 2 to 9 years of age. Aortic root size was not significantly associated with markers for stress-modulated growth; however, aortic root dilation was associated with left ventricular dilation, increased viral load, and lower CD4 cell count in HIV-infected children. The aortic root dilation could also be a consequence of increased arterial stiffness affecting the aorta. As prolonged survival of HIV-infected patients becomes more prevalent, some patients may require long-term follow-up of aortic root size [51–52].

Conduction System Involvement

Various atrial and ventricular arrhythmias as well as atrioventricular blocks have been described in patients with HIV. Bharati et al. studied histologically the conduction system in six children who died of AIDS [53].

Vasculitis, myocarditis, and fragmentation with lobulation and fibrosis of the conduction system were found. In a prospective series of 31 pediatric patients with AIDS, Lipshultz et al. found frequent conduction defects and dysrrhythmias [16]. Brady et al. reported the case of an infant with AIDS who died suddenly of probable cardiac arrhythmia due to involvement of the conduction system by myocarditis [14].

Fetal Heart Involvement

A recent study by Hornberger sought to determine whether vertically transmitted HIV infection and maternal infection with HIV are associated with altered cardiovascular structure and function in utero. Fetal echocardiography was performed in 173 fetuses of 169 HIV-infected mothers (mean gestational age, 33.0 weeks; SD=3.7 weeks) at five centers. Fetuses determined after birth to be HIV-infected had similar echocardiographic findings as fetuses determined to be HIV-uninfected later, except for slightly smaller left ventricular diastolic dimensions (p=0.01). Differences in cardiovascular dimensions and Doppler velocities were identified between fetuses of HIV-infected women and previously published normal fetal data. The reason for the differences may be a result of maternal HIV infection, maternal risk factors, or selection bias in the external control data [54]. The P2C2 study describing the cardiovascular status of infants and children of HIV-infected women shows that children infected with HIV-1 had significantly more cardiac abnormalities than external control subjects [13]. Study analysis showed that HIV-1-infected children had a statistically significant higher heart rate at all ages. In addition, all children born to HIV-1-infected women had a low left ventricular fractional shortening at birth, which improved in the uninfected children by 8 months of age but not quite up to the normal level as seen in children in the external control group. The left ventricular fractional shortening remained persistently lower in the HIV-infected children for up to 20 months. Similarly, left ventricular mass was the same at birth for both HIV-infected and uninfected children but became significantly higher in HIV-infected children aged between 4 and 30 months. The study results extend previous reports from the P2C2 study showing that fetal echocardiograms indicated fetal cardiovascular abnormalities in pregnant HIV-1-infected women, irrespective of whether the children turned out to be HIV-1 infected after birth. Based on the results of the current cohort study, the authors conclude that irrespective of their HIV-1 status, infants born to HIV-1-infected women have significantly worse cardiac function than other infants, suggesting that the uterine environment has an important role in postnatal cardiovascular abnormalities. The authors also suggest that appropriate treatment strategies should be considered for all children born to HIV-1-infected women, as even mild left ventricular dysfunction has shown to effect mortality over time. The P2C2 study led to many commentaries dealing particularly with the reliability of the methods used to assess ventricular function. Indeed, in another P2C2 report, there was unacceptable variability of many M-mode cardiac measurements, including fractional shortening, between the local and central institutions [18]. A less variable method of measuring cardiac function should be identified and used in future studies that attempt to evaluate early treatment of HIV-associated cardiac depression with novel therapeutic approaches. Other groups have not confirmed the results of this study [10], which do no reflect the experience of European countries.

The effects of maternal HIV infection and mother–infant HIV transmission on the prevalence and distribution of congenital cardiovascular malformations in the children of HIV-infected mothers have been investigated in a few studies. The Italian Multicenter Study demonstrated a trend toward a higher prevalence of congenital cardiovascular malformations in HIV-infected children as compared to general population-based data, but the number of cases was small (5/165, 2.4%) [55]. There was no difference between HIV-infected and HIV-uninfected children. Vogel et al. reported a series of five patients with congenital heart disease from a population of 175 children exposed prenatally to maternal HIV infection (2.8%) [56]. The P2C2 HIV study indicates a congenital cardiovascular malformation prevalence of 12.3% in children of HIV-infected mothers [57]. Again, this proportion is very surprising and has not been confirmed. It is of note that in the first study [54], the methodology pertaining to the identification of cardiac defects was not provided and that in the P2C2 study, most of the lesions were clinically unapparent and were detected by routine echocardiography as part of the study protocol. Our personal experience shows that the prevalence of symptomatic heart defects in children born to HIV-infected mothers is comparable to the general population. The pathophysiologic factors leading to a higher prevalence of cardiac malformations in fetuses of HIV-infected mothers may include alterations of fetal flow patterns related to increased placental vascular resistances. Additional maternal risk factors that may significantly affect fetal organogenesis such as increased alcohol use, cocaine addiction, and poor nutritional status also have to be considered. There are no reports on cardiac teratogenicity related to zidovudine.

Cardiac complications of AIDS or vertically transmitted HIV in children appear to be frequent. However, the actual prevalence of severe cardiac compromise remains difficult to assess and very few groups have reported their own experience. The P2C2 HIV study is the most important study sharing its data with the medical community in charge of these infants and children. This study presents very disquieting results regarding cardiac involvement in infants from HIV-infected mothers, but the numbers of commentaries published after these results were evidence of a rising controversy. The evolving antiviral therapy may change the profile of cardiac manifestations of HIV in the pediatric age group, as fewer children are infected in developed countries. The emerging concern is the vascular dysfunction that may lead to early atherosclerosis. Longitudinal studies are needed to address this worrisome issue in the pediatric population.

References

1. Stewart JM, Kaul A, Gromisch DS, Reyes E et al (1989) Symptomatic cardiac dysfunction in children with human immunodeficiency virus infection. Am Heart J 117:140–144
2. Bierman FZ (1991) Guidelines for diagnosis and management of cardiac disease in children with HIV infection. J Pediatr 119(Pt 2):S53–56
3. Lewis W, Dorn GW 2nd (1993) Cardiac structure and function in HIV-infected children. N Engl J Med 328:513–514
4. Croft NM, Jacob AJ, Godman MJ et al (1993) Cardiac dysfunction in paediatric HIV infection. J Infect 26:191–194
5. Luginbuhl LM, Orav EJ, McIntosh K, Lipshultz SE (1993) Cardiac morbidity and related mortality in children with HIV infection. JAMA 269:2869–2875
6. Levin BW, Krantz DH, Driscoll JM Jr, Fleischman AR (1995) The treatment of non-HIV-related conditions in newborns at risk for HIV: a survey of neonatologists. Am J Public Health 85:1507–1513
7. Johann-Liang R, Cervia JS, Noel GJ (1997) Characteristics of human immunodeficiency virus-infected children at the time of death: an experience in the 1990s. Pediatr Infect Dis J 16:1145–1150
8. Plein D, Van Camp G, Cosyns B et al (1999) Cardiac and autonomic evaluation in a pediatric population with human immunodeficiency virus. Clin Cardiol 22:33–36
9. Bowles NE, Kearney DL, Ni J et al (1999) The detection of viral genomes by polymerase chain

reaction in the myocardium of pediatric patients with advanced HIV disease. J Am Coll Cardiol 34:857–865

10. Lipshultz SE, Easley KA, Orav EJ et al (2000) Cardiac dysfunction and mortality in HIV-infected children: The Prospective P2C2 HIV Multicenter Study. Pediatric Pulmonary and Cardiac Complications of Vertically Transmitted HIV Infection (P2C2 HIV) Study Group. Circulation 102:1542–1548

11. Keesler MJ, Fisher SD, Lipshultz SE (2001) Cardiac manifestations of HIV infection in infants and children. Ann N Y Acad Sci 946:169–178

12. Starc TJ, Lipshultz SE, Easley KA et al (2002) Incidence of cardiac abnormalities in children with human immunodeficiency virus infection: The Prospective P2C2 HIV Study. J Pediatr 141:327–334

13. Lipshultz SE, Easley KA, Orav EJ et al (2002) Cardiovascular status of infants and children of women infected with HIV-1 (P2C2 HIV): a cohort study. Lancet 360:368–373

14. Brady MT, Reiner CB, Singley C et al (1988) Unexpected death in an infant with AIDS: disseminated cytomegalovirus infection with pancarditis. Pediatr Pathol 8:205–214

15. Anderson DW, Virmani R (1990) Emerging patterns of heart disease in human immunodeficiency virus infection. Hum Pathol 21:253–259

16. Lipshultz SE, Chanock S, Sanders SP et al (1989) Cardiovascular manifestations of human immunodeficiency virus infection in infants and children. Am J Cardiol 63:1489–1497

17. Rudin C, Meier D, Pavic N et al (1993) Intrauterine onset of symptomatic human immunodeficiency virus disease. The Swiss Collaborative Study Group "HIV and Pregnancy". Pediatr Infect Dis J 12:411–414

18. Lipshultz SE, Orav EJ, Sanders SP et al (1994) Limitations of fractional shortening as an index of contractility in pediatric patients infected with human immunodeficiency virus. J Pediatr 125:563–570

19. Turner BJ, Denison M, Eppes SC et al (1993) Survival experience of 789 children with the acquired immunodeficiency syndrome. Pediatr Infect Dis J 12:310–320

20. Scott GB, Hutto C, Makuch RW et al (1989) Survival in children with perinatally acquired human immunodeficiency virus type 1 infection. N Engl J Med 321:1791–1796

21. Starc TJ, Langston C, Goldfarb J et al (1999) Unexpected non-HIV causes of death in children born to HIV-infected mothers. Pediatric Pulmonary and Cardiac Complications of Vertically Transmitted HIV Infection Study Group. Pediatrics 104:e6

22. Pitt J, Schluchter M, Jenson H et al (1998) Maternal and perinatal factors related to maternal–infant transmission of HIV-1 in the P2C2 HIV study: the role of EBV shedding. Pediatric Pulmonary and Cardiovascular Complications of Vertically Transmitted HIV-1 Infection (P2C2 HIV) Study Group. J Acquir Immune Defic Syndr Hum Retrovirol 19:462–470

23. Lipshultz SE, Easley KA, Orav EJ et al (1998) Left ventricular structure and function in children infected with human immunodeficiency virus: the prospective P2C2 HIV Multicenter Study. Pediatric Pulmonary and Cardiac Complications of Vertically Transmitted HIV Infection (P2C2 HIV) Study Group. Circulation 97:1246–1256

24. Lipshultz SE, Grenier MA (1997) Left ventricular dysfunction in infants and children infected with the human immunodeficiency virus. Prog Pediatr Cardiol 7:33–43

25. Joshi VV, Gadol C, Connor E et al (1988) Dilated cardiomyopathy in children with acquired immunodeficiency syndrome: a pathologic study of five cases. Hum Pathol 19:69–73

26. Anderson DW, Virmani R, Reilly JM (1988) Prevalent myocarditis at necropsy in the acquired immunodeficiency syndrome. J Am Coll Cardiol 11:792–799

27. Flomenbaum M, Soeiro R, Udem SA et al (1989) Proliferative membranopathy and human immunodeficiency virus in AIDS hearts. J Acquir Immune Defic Syndr 2:129–135

28. Rodriguez ER, Nasim S, Hsia J et al (1991) Cardiac myocytes and dendritic cells harbor human immunodeficiency virus in infected patients with and without cardiac dysfunction: detection by multiplex, nested, polymerase chain reaction in individually microdissected cells from right ventricular endomyocardial biopsy tissue. Am J Cardiol 68:1511–1520

29. Beschorner WE, Baughman K, Turnicky RP et al (1990) HIV-associated myocarditis. Pathology and immunopathology. Am J Pathol 137:1365–1371

30. Domanski MJ, Sloas MM, Follmann DA et al (1995) Effect of zidovudine and didanosine treatment on heart function in children infected with human immunodeficiency virus. J Pediatr 127:137–146

31. Lipshultz SE, Easley KA, Orav EJ et al (2000) Absence of cardiac toxicity of zidovudine in infants. Pediatric Pulmonary and Cardiac Complications of Vertically Transmitted HIV Infection Study Group. N Engl J Med 343:759–766

32. Dworkin BM, Antonecchia PP, Smith F et al (1989) Reduced cardiac selenium content in the acquired immunodeficiency syndrome. JPEN J Parenter Enteral Nutr 13:644–647

33. Shaddy RE, Curtin EL, Sower B et al (2002) The Pediatric Randomized Carvedilol Trial in Children with Heart Failure: rationale and design. Am Heart J 144:383–389

34. Lipshultz SE, Orav EJ, Sanders SP, Colan SD (1995) Immunoglobulins and left ventricular structure and function in pediatric HIV infection. Circulation 92:2220–2225

35. Kovacs A, Hinton DR, Wright D et al (1996) Human immunodeficiency virus type 1 infection of the heart in three infants with acquired immunodeficiency syndrome and sudden death. Pediatr Infect Dis J 15:819–824

36. Joshi VV, Pawel B, Connor E et al (1987) Arteriopathy in children with acquired immune deficiency syndrome. Pediatr Pathol 7:261–275

37. Bharati S, Lev M (1989) Pathology of the heart in AIDS. Prog Cardiol 2:261–272

38. Lipshultz SE (1994) Cardiovascular problems. In: Pizzo PA, Wilfert CM (eds) Pediatric AIDS, the challenge of HIV infection in infants, children and adolescents, 2nd edn. Williams and Wilkins, Baltimore, pp 122–148

39. Melvin AJ, Lennon S, Mohan KM, Purnell JQ (2001) Metabolic abnormalities in HIV type 1-infected children treated and not treated with protease inhibitors. AIDS Res Hum Retroviruses 17:1117–1123

40. Lainka E, Oezbek S, Falck M et al (2002) Marked dyslipidemia in human immunodeficiency virus-infected children on protease inhibitor-containing antiretroviral therapy. Pediatrics 110:e56

41. Jaquet D, Levine M, Ortega-Rodriguez E et al (2000) Clinical and metabolic presentation of the lipodystrophic syndrome in HIV-infected children. AIDS 14:2123–2128

42. Seminari E, Pan A, Voltini G et al (2002) Assessment of atherosclerosis using carotid ultrasonography in a cohort of HIV-positive patients treated with protease inhibitors. Atherosclerosis 162:433–438

43. Mercie P, Thiebaut R, Lavignolle V et al (2002) Evaluation of cardiovascular risk factors in HIV-1 infected patients using carotid intima-media thickness measurement. Ann Med 34:55–63

44. Chironi G, Escaut L, Gariepy J et al (2003) Brief report: carotid intima-media thickness in heavily pretreated HIV-infected patients. J Acquir Immune Defic Syndr 32:490–493

45. Bozzette SA, Ake CF, Tam HK et al (2003) Cardiovascular and cerebrovascular events in patients treated for human immunodeficiency virus infection. N Engl J Med 348:702–710

46. Bonnet D, Aggoun Y, Szezepanski I et al (2004) Arterial stiffness and endothelial dysfunction in HIV-infected children. AIDS 18:1037–1041

47. Charakida M, Donald AE, Green H, et al (2005) Early structural and functional changes of the vasculature in HIV-infected children: impact of disease and antiretroviral therapy. Circulation 112:103–109

48. Schecter AD, Berman AB, Yi L et al (2001) HIV envelope gp120 activates human arterial smooth muscle cells. Proc Natl Acad Sci USA 98:10142–10147

49. Chi D, Henry J, Kelley J et al (2000) The effects of HIV infection on endothelial function. Endothelium 7:223–242

50. Hsue PY, Lo JC, Franklin A et al (2004) Progression of atherosclerosis as assessed by carotid intima-media thickness in patients with HIV infection. Circulation 109:1603–1608

51. Lai WW, Colan SD, Easley KA et al (2001) Dilation of the aortic root in children infected with human immunodeficiency virus type 1: The Prospective P2C2 HIV Multicenter Study. Am Heart J 141:661–670

52. Zareba KM, Lavigne JE, Lipshultz SE (2004) Cardiovascular effects of HAART in infants and children of HIV-infected mothers. Cardiovasc Toxicol 4:271–279

53. Bharati S, Joshi VV, Connor EM et al (1989) Conduction system in children with acquired immunodeficiency syndrome. Chest 96:406–413

54. Hornberger LK, Lipshultz SE, Easley KA et al (2000) Cardiac structure and function in fetuses of mothers infected with HIV: The Prospective PCHIV Multicenter Study. Am Heart J 140:575–584

55. Italian Register for HIV Infection in Children (1994) Features of children perinatally infected with HIV-1 surviving longer than 5 years. Lancet 22(343):191–195

56. Vogel RL, Alboliras ET, McSherry GD et al (1988) Congenital heart defects in children of human immunodeficiency virus positive mothers. Circulation 78:II–17

57. Lai WW, Lipshultz SE, Easley KA et al (1998) Prevalence of congenital cardiovascular malformations in children of human immunodeficiency virus-infected women: The Prospective P2C2 HIV Multicenter Study. P2C2 HIV Study Group, National Heart, Lung, and Blood Institute, Bethesda, Maryland. J Am Coll Cardiol 32:1749–1755

Chapter 15

Cardiac Surgery and the Human Immunodeficiency Virus

N. Bonnet, P. Leprince, S. Varnous, I. Gandjbakhch

Twenty years after the first antibody test for the human immunodeficiency virus (HIV), highly active antiretroviral therapy (HAART) became available in Western countries. Although cardiac surgery in HIV-infected patients remains rare — 0.2% of interventions with extracorporeal circulation (ECC) in La Pitié Institute — and has some particularities, the majority of cardiac surgeons believe that the surgical strategies and techniques should be the same for HIV-infected patients as for other patients.

Although some standard cardiac operations have been performed on asymptomatic and unknown HIV-infected patients, the first deliberate open-heart operation on a patient known to be infected with HIV was performed by Frater et al. in December 1984 for tricuspid endocarditis in a bisexual heroin addict [1–3]. During the 1980s, the indications for cardiac surgery in AIDS patients were limited to urgent life-threatening conditions: severe infectious endocarditis and tamponade [4]. These urgent indications are still frequent in patients with advanced AIDS, but standard elective cardiac surgery in asymptomatic HIV-infected patients is increasing proportionally.

From the beginning of the AIDS pandemic, surgical teams were faced with unusual questions in this new and very peculiar population of patients, whose main characteristic was that they were young. The first questions were about the feasibility of surgery in patients with severe immunodeficiency and the benefit of surgery in patients with poor short-term prognosis. Other questions concerned the risk of HIV transmission from the patient to the surgical staff and vice versa during surgery. The risk of blood-borne virus transmission between the patient and the surgical team is now well known and fortunately low after the adoption of universal precautions.

We can now briefly answer the first and second questions: surgery, even complex cardiac surgery with ECC, is feasible in patients with severe immunodeficiency with higher but tolerable mortality; however, the benefit is low a fortiori in patients with uncontrolled HIV and opportunistic infections. Every surgeon agrees that a life-threatening lesion, despite poor conditions in HIV-infected patients, should be operated on, but thanks to HAART, this situation is now less frequently encountered, and a new question arises: how to operate on a patient with HIV-controlled infection and good long-term prognosis?

Today, this disease is considered to be a chronic illness. For this reason, it is reasonable to expect an increasing number of HIV-infected patients who will require heart surgery. Cardiac surgeons should be prepared to manage these patients.

HIV-Infected Patients Referred for Cardiac Surgery and Indications for Surgery

In most cardiac centers, 0.2–0.4% of cardiac surgeries are performed on HIV-infected patients, a relatively rare but increasing situation [4, 5] (La Pitié experience). The routine use of antiretroviral therapies has led directly to dramatic declines in morbidity and mortality among HIV-1-infected patients with advanced immunodeficiency [6]. Mortality declined from 29.4 per 100 person-years in 1995 to 8.8 per 100 person-years in mid-1997. A number of patients infected with HIV-1 may develop cardiovascular diseases or complications and require cardiac surgery.

During the last 10 years, the profile of HIV-infected patients referred for cardiac surgery in Western countries has changed. These patients are still young—41 years old for Trachiotis et al. [7], 36 years old for Mestres et al. [8], 44 for Abad et al. [4]—the majority are men (100% for Abad et al. [4]), frequently drug addicts or homosexual, but there is also an increasing proportion of women and older patients. At La Pitié, only 1 of 22 patients (4.5%) operated on during the 1990s was a woman; since the beginning of 2000, 5 of 27 patients (14.8%) operated on have been women.

The indications for cardiac surgery in HIV-infected patients have increased and changed for three reasons. First, the survival is greater and HIV-infected patients are exposed for longer periods to specific and classic cardiac lesions requiring surgery. Second, HAART itself is suspected to induce specific cardiac lesions, particularly coronary artery disease. Third, because the HIV infection is controlled with a long survival, we can consider complex therapeutic strategies in these patients such as heart transplantation and soon artificial hearts. Figure 1 reports the increasing number of coronary artery bypass grafting in HIV-infected patients during the last 6 years at La Pitié Institute. Because of the epidemiological profile of the HIV-infected population in Western countries in the HAART era, the major indications for cardiac surgery are coronary artery disease and cardiomyopathy.

Pericardial Effusion and Tamponade

Before the introduction of HAART, the prevalence of pericardial effusion in asymptomatic AIDS patients was estimated at 11% [9], and was particularly high in those with end-stage disease. HAART has significantly reduced the overall incidence of pericardial effusion in HIV patients. Pericardial effusion in HIV disease may be related to opportunistic infections (tuberculosis and nontubercu-

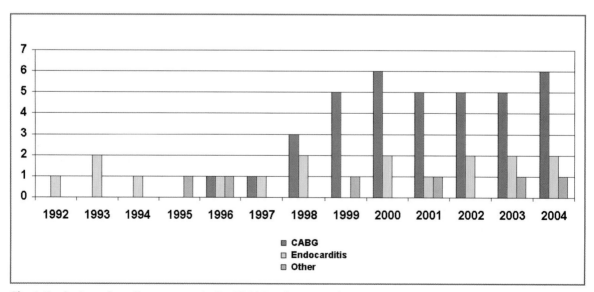

Fig. 1 Evolution of cardiac surgery in La Pitié Institute, Paris. *CABG*, coronary artery bypass grafting

losis mycobacteria [10], *Nocardia* [11], *Cryptococcus* [12], and cytomegalovirus), malignancy (Kaposi's sarcoma [13], non-Hodgkin's lymphoma [14]), and valve endocarditis or bacterial pericarditis [15] (*Streptococcus pneumoniae*), but most often a clear etiology is not found. Hypoalbuminemia, which is associated with ascites and pleural effusions, is a potential cause of pericardial effusion in end-stage HIV infection. Pericardial effusion may be part of capillary leak syndrome. A pericardial effusion is a marker of shortened survival.

The majority of pericardial effusions are small and asymptomatic, but sometimes there is a cardiac tamponade which requires urgent pericardial drainage (only 1 case among 231 patients over a 5-year period for Heidenreich) [9]. An HIV test is required for each patient with pericardial effusion. In young patients with cardiac tamponade, the coexistence of fever and pulmonary infiltrates is suggestive of underlying HIV infection [16]. The indications of pericardiocentesis or pericardial window are not different between HIV-infected and other patients in cases of cardiac tamponade. Because the effusions are frequently small and rarely progressive, an exhaustive search for a diagnosis with pericardiocentesis is not indicated. The surgical techniques are the same as those used on non-HIV patients, with a preference for percutaneous or videoscopic techniques limiting the risk of viral transmission to the surgical team.

Valvular Surgery

Valvular surgery is the most common cardiac surgery performed on HIV patients, particularly in the pre-HAART era when severe infectious endocarditis was frequent in patients with significant immunodeficiency. In these patients, two factors which increase the incidence of infective endocarditis are frequently associated: intravenous drug abuse and immunodeficiency [17–19]; this association was found in 85% of 40 patients reported by Aris et al. in 1993 [20] and in all 11 patients for Frater et al. in 1989 [1]. The indications for cardiac surgery (replacement or valve repair) are classic (heart failure, valve destruction, emboli, annular abscess) with a higher number of interventions for persistent infection despite proper antibiotic treatment. In cases of tricuspid endocarditis, the indication for cardiac surgery is rare except for infections with yeasts.

The prevalence of infective endocarditis in HIV-infected patients is similar to that of patients in other risk groups such as intravenous drug users. Estimates of endocarditis prevalence vary from 6.3 to 34% in HIV-infected patients who use intravenous drugs independently of HAART regimens. Right-sided valves are predominantly affected and the most frequent agents are *Staphylococcus aureus, Streptococcus pneumoniae, Haemophilus influenzae, Candida albicans, Aspergillus fumigatus*, and *Cryptococcus neoformans* [21, 22]. Infective organisms are common; nevertheless, yeasts (*Candida albicans*) and rare bacteria such as corynebacteria should be suspected particularly in right-sided endocarditis in intravenous drug abusers.

Good results have been achieved with the use of mechanical heart valves, bioprosthetic valves, and homografts (Fig. 2) in patients who have endocarditis [23]. Most surgeons use the following standards for heart-valve replacement: (1) a mechanical heart valve in adults, young patients, and pediatric patients when there is no contraindication to long-term anticoagulation; (2) a bioprosthetic valve in most patients over 65 or 70 years, patients with a proven short life expectancy, those requiring right-heart valve replacement, those in whom anticoagulation poses a high risk, and those with contraindication to long-term anticoagulation. Because survival is longer in HIV-controlled infection, at La Pitié, similar to Abad et al. [4], the same policies are applied to all patients who are HIV-

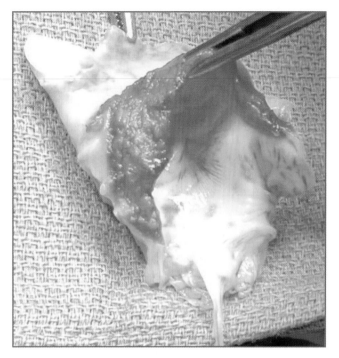

Fig. 2 Aortic homograft

positive, whether they are drug addicts or not. Using a homograft in an aortic position is supported when the lesions are very destructive with a large annular abscess [4]. In summary, the policy for choosing a valve substitute is identical in HIV-positive and HIV-negative patients (Figs. 2–4).

Valvular endocarditis is still the most common finding in HIV-positive patients (Figs. 3, 4). However, it is possible that in the future, with the aging of this population due to longer survival as a result of HAART, valvular surgery will be performed for noninfective lesions like aortic stenosis.

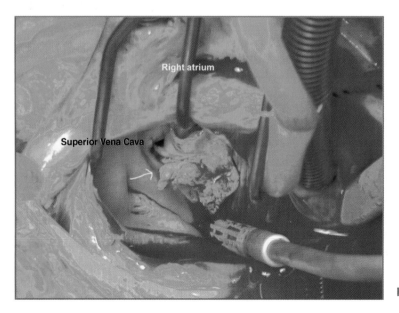

Fig. 3 Mitral vegetations

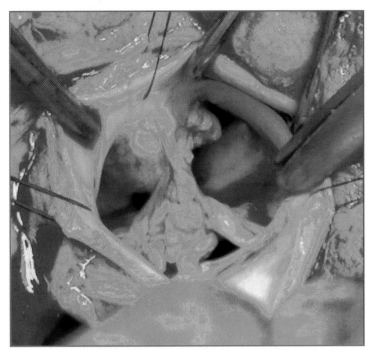

Fig. 4 Aortic vegetations

Coronary Artery Bypass Grafting

An increased rate of acute coronary syndromes has been reported in HIV-infected patients after the introduction of protease inhibitors. However, the substantial benefits of combination antiretroviral therapy clearly continue to outweigh the increased risk of myocardial infarction associated with this therapy [24]. Although valvular surgery was and is still the most common cardiac intervention in HIV-infected patients (70% of the HIV-infected patients for Mestre et al. [8], 65% at La Pitié), coronary artery bypass grafting (CABG) is more and more frequent in HIV-infected patients (30 CABG among 37 interventions for Trachiotis et al. [7]). According to the limited experience reported by different surgical centers (Table 1), the perioperative course of these patients is unremarkable [25, 26]. Surgical revascularization is sometimes performed in an urgent or emergent condition involving the lesions of coronary arteries but never in patients with end-stage HIV disease. These patients are younger than other patients referred for CABG, with the majority being men. The surgical strategy and technique are unremarkable. Full arterial revascularization is a good option because of the age of these patients. The incidence of mediastinitis despite bilateral mammary harvesting, frequent diabetes mellitus, and immunodeficiency is not higher than in comparable patients (2.7%) [7]. Due to the lack of controlled trials and large patient reviews, no firm recommendations about the strategy and technique of surgical revascularization can be provided [25].

Aneurysm or false aneurysm of the coronary artery is a rare lesion in HIV-positive patients; it can require cardiac surgery under ECC (exclusion of the aneurysm and CABG). After CABG, lipid-lowering therapy should be prescribed cautiously in HIV-infected patients because of the potential of a lethal interaction between statin (except pravastatin, fluvastatin and rosuvastatin) and protease inhibitors.

Table 1 Cardiac surgery excluding transplantation in HIV-infected patients

Author	Year of publication	Number of patients	Valvular surgery	CABG	Pericardium
Frater [1]	1989	11	11		
Sousa Uva [27]	1992	10	10		
Carrel [17]	1993	6	6 Endocarditis		
Aris [20]	1993	40	38		
Flum [25]	1997	4	4	0.13% of CABG	
Abad [4]	2000	5	4 Endocarditis		1 Tamponade
Trachiotis [7]	2001	37	9–3 with CABG	27	
Mestres [8]	2003	31	26–21 Endocarditis	5	
La Pitié (personal data)	2004	60	21–16 Endocarditis	37	2

CABG, coronary artery bypass grafting

Heart Transplantation

HIV disease is recognized as an important cause of dilated cardiomyopathy with a reported prevalence of 3.6% among patients with cardiomyopathy, a proportion that is increasing as patients with HIV infection live longer. The pathogenesis of HIV-related cardiomyopathy is very likely to be multifactorial. HIV-associated symptomatic heart failure may become one of the leading causes of heart failure worldwide [21]. It explains why, despite a complex pharmacological and immunological status in these patients, several heart transplantations following other solid-organ transplantations [28–30] have been reported in HIV-positive recipients (Table 2) [31]. Although Calabrese et al. [32] reported a successful cardiac transplantation in 2003 in an HIV-infected patient with advanced disease, we reserve this therapeutic strategy to well-controlled HIV-positive patients (undetectable viral load, CD4 count >400/mm3)

Table 2 Cardiac transplantations

Author	Year of publication	Number
Tzakis [34]	1990	1
Calabrese [31]	2003	1
Bisleri [30]	2003	1
La Pitié (personal data)	2004	2

without opportunistic infection and without a history of Kaposi's sarcoma. Two cardiac transplantations with a simple postoperative course and no specific complications during follow-up have been performed at La Pitié during the last 2 years. A multidisciplinary team is required for this therapeutic technique because numerous complex and unpredictable pharmacological and immunological adverse events can occur (Fig. 5) [33].

There is no report of a cardiac assist device

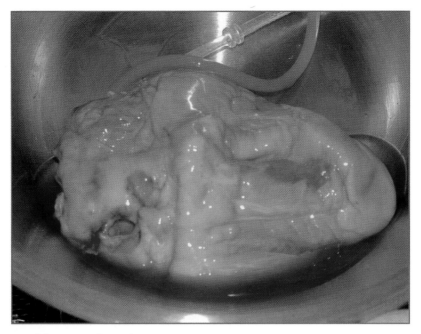

Fig. 5 Heart prepared for transplantation

in HIV-infected patients, but it is only a matter of time before these devices are used in HIV patients. When the patient is on the waiting list for cardiac transplantation, he or she is eligible for a mechanical bridge. Nevertheless, this therapy will be a challenge because the major complication of ventricular assist devices is sepsis. If the number of HIV-infected patients on waiting lists for cardiac transplantation increases in a high proportion, we should ask the controversial question concerning the harvesting of a heart in HIV-infected donors.

Cardiac Malignancy

Malignant cardiac tumor is rare in HIV- and non-HIV-infected patients. Cardiac Kaposi's sarcoma and non-Hodgkin's lymphoma have been described in HIV-infected patients, but there is no specific surgery for these tumors except pericardial drainage and biopsy for diagnosis or tamponade.

Risk of HIV Transmission to Operating Room Personnel

From the beginning of the HIV pandemic, the risk of HIV transmission by contact with infected blood, a fortiori, in case of injuries was put forward. This fear was so high that some surgeons asked if it was possible to refuse an intervention in HIV-infected patients under the pretext that the risk to themselves was too high. In France and in the majority of European countries, the law does not permit routine testing for HIV infection in all surgical candidates. At La Pitié Institute, we performed this test after the patient's consent in more than 80% of cases; this test is always done before transplantation.

Accidents involving exposure to blood are not rare during surgery and particularly cardiac surgery. For example, Trachiotis [7] reported six injuries with a solid needle during 37 cardiac operations, and three injuries occurred (one with a hollow needle, two with sternal wire) at La Pitié during 49 interventions. These accidents needed prophylactic antiretroviral therapy. It is now standard practice to prescribe a course of anti-HIV agents in the event of a percutaneous injury based on the evidence that early use after exposure to the virus reduces the chance of infection [35]. No cases of seroconversion were observed. Moreover, there continues to be no known case of transmission of HIV to personnel as a result of a solid needle injury.

According to Beekman et al. [36] and Klatt et al. [37], the risk of accidental infection to operating-room personnel through blood contact during surgical procedures is low and can be avoided by adherence to universal precautions with proper training of personnel.

The universal precautions are:

- Impermeable gowns.
- Two pairs of surgical gloves [38].
- Protective glasses.
- Reinforced masks.
- Needles and other sharp instruments should be handled cautiously (one operator, count of sharp tools, solid box for infected sharps tools).
- Knowledge of the serology of the patient. This point is questionable because the universal precautions should be precisely universal and thus followed independently of the serological status of the patient. Moreover, knowledge of the serological status can generate fear and stress and could be a risk factor for percutaneous injuries. Nevertheless, when a patient is known to be HIV-infected in our institution, this fact is clearly mentioned in the medical file. HIV testing is not systematic before cardiac surgery in our institution and this practice is very different from one center to another [39]. HIV testing in patients and personnel is systematic and urgently done in case of percutaneous injury with bleeding.

- Continuous training of the entire staff about these universal precautions.
- Continuous training of the entire staff about the procedure in case of percutaneous injury with blood from the patient.
- Antiretroviral therapy should be continued until the day of surgery and restarted as soon as possible.
- The patient should have a viral load as low as possible; the intervention can be reported in case of excessive viral load, nonurgent surgery, and high probability of reducing the viral load with antiretroviral therapy adaptation.

Because the risk of contact with the patient's blood is higher during cardiac surgery, particularly in cases of extracorporeal bypass, special precautions have to be taken and if possible generalized to all patients:

- The kit for ECC is preconnected.
- The ECC machine is handled with gloves.
- Suturing and reparation of the sternum with steel wire should be done very cautiously and with only one operator (no tandem surgery) [40].

Videoscopic surgery, even robotically assisted surgery (Fig. 6), reduces the risk of percutaneous injuries compared to open surgery (0.01 vs. 1% for Kjaegard et al. [40] in thoracic surgery). The fear of HIV transmission should not divert the surgeon's attention from the higher risk of acquiring other fatal infections such as HBV and HCV. This is why precautions against blood-borne infection have to be universal.

Risk of HIV Transmission to Patients

The risk of HIV transmission through blood transfusion is well known in France, and is higher during cardiac surgery because blood transfusion is very common during cardiac surgery with ECC (in our institution, 41% of patients who underwent cardiac surgery with ECC were transfused with heterologous blood). This risk has been

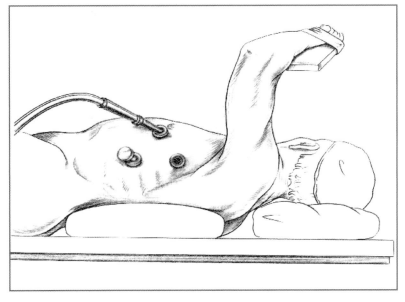

Fig. 6 Videoscopic surgery

reduced by screening blood donors and blood units. Serologic screening of donors for antibodies to HIV-1 and HTLV-I coupled with exclusion of donors from groups having a relatively high risk for infection has led to a low incidence of transfusion-transmitted HIV-1 and HTLV-I/II infection. A small risk remains, however, despite these measures. The residual risk for HIV-1 and HTLV-II infection from transfusion of screened blood was about 1 in 60,000 units [41], 1 in 100,000 per unit for Cohen et al. [42], and is now 1 in 32,5000 for Pillonel et al. [43].

Pooling of plasma donations increases the risk for blood-borne infections. In solvent- or detergent-treated plasma, lipid-enveloped viruses are efficiently inactivated; transfusion of solvent-/detergent-treated plasma was found to be safe with regard to lipid-enveloped viruses [44].

The risk of infection has been further reduced by limitation of blood transfusion itself. After the discovery in the 1980s that HIV can be transmitted via blood transfusion, there has been increased interest in technologies that reduce the amount of allogeneic blood used during and after surgery. These technologies include various drugs (aprotinin, tranexamic acid, epsilon-aminocaproic acid, erythropoietin), devices (cell salvage; Fig. 7), and techniques (acute hemodilution, predeposited autologous donation). Enhancement of comprehension

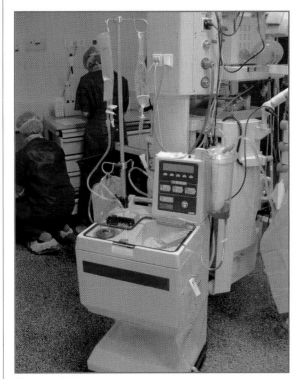

Fig. 7 Cell saver

and assumption of hemostasis before, during, and after cardiac surgery has resulted in a major reduction in the incidence of reoperation for bleeding and heterologous blood transfusion. Other new therapeutics such as the recombinant factor VIIa (Novo-Seven) should be of interest for reduction of blood transfusions [45].

Information about transfused patients is legal in France. Thus, in the HIV Information Project, six previously unsuspected HIV-seropositive cases were diagnosed after studying 1,793 patients who underwent cardiac surgery between 1980–1985 [46].

Transmission of HIV from healthcare workers to patients has been documented in one report. A retrospective review was conducted of 612 patients of an HIV-positive cardiothoracic surgeon, in an attempt to identify any instance of viral transmission. A total of 189 patients received HIV testing and counseling and no positive test results were obtained [47]. Pathogens can be transferred through contact between patients undergoing surgery and the surgical team, resulting in postoperative or blood-borne infections in patients or blood-borne infections in the surgical team. Both the patient and the surgical team need to be protected from this risk. Implementing protective barriers such as wearing surgical gloves can reduce this risk. Wearing two pairs of surgical gloves instead of one pair is considered as providing an additional barrier, further reducing the risk of contamination. Wearing two pairs of latex gloves significantly reduces the number of perforations to the innermost glove.

Results

Data available to date show no conclusive evidence of acceleration of HIV infection into AIDS associated with cardiac surgery [5]. Five of 25 investigators (20%) saw HIV infection progress to AIDS within a maxi-

mum period of 74 months [5]. In a short report of six patients, Lemma et al. [46] could not demonstrate any deleterious effect of ECC in HIV-infected patients. Preoperative and postoperative absolute lymphocyte T-helper (CD4) and T-suppressor (CD8) counts did not show a close association between the temporary lymphopenia induced by cardiopulmonary bypass and progression to AIDS [48]. The fear that cardiopulmonary bypass might cause acceleration of the disease has not been borne out [3].

Cardiac surgery in HIV-infected patients is complicated by higher mortality and morbidity rates than in other patients (20% hospital death for Aris et al. [20] with the majority occurring in valvular surgery [27]), but this fact has tended to decrease substantially (2.7% of hospital death for Trachiotis et al. [7] with the majority involving a CABG). This group of high-risk patients has the following characteristics: immunodepression, poor general condition, associated diseases, infections, intravenous drug abuse, homosexual/bisexual behavior, high rate of infectious valve endocarditis, frequent recurrence of postoperative infection, and increased risk of transmission to clinical staff. The long-term survival is difficult to describe because there is still a high mortality in patients operated on for severe endocarditis; however, the mid-term results of CABG are unremarkable.

Risk of Lactic Acidosis

Open-heart surgery may be a risk factor for nonischemic (type B) lactic acidosis in patients taking nucleoside-analog reverse-transcriptase inhibitors [49]. This rare complication should be weighed against the benefit of antiretroviral therapy and particularly the interest of reducing the viral load in order to lower the risk of HIV transmission to the surgical staff.

Conclusion

HIV-infected patients are eligible for classic cardiac surgery, even for cardiac transplantation. The surgical strategy and technique should be the same for HIV-infected and other patients.

References

1. Frater RW, Sisto D, Condit D (1989) Cardiac surgery in human immunodeficiency virus (HIV) carriers. Eur J Cardiothorac Surg 3:146–150
2. Frater RW (1999) As originally published in 1989: human immunodeficiency virus and the cardiac surgeon: a survey of attitudes. Updated in 1999. Ann Thorac Surg 67:1203–1204
3. Frater RW (2000) Cardiac surgery and the human immunodeficiency virus. Semin Thorac Cardiovasc Surg 12:145–147
4. Abad C, Cardenes MA, Jimenez PC et al (2000) Cardiac surgery in patients infected with human immunodeficiency virus. Tex Heart Inst J 27:356–360
5. Everson D, Zeigler R, Sabbaga AM et al (1999) Significance of the human immunodeficiency infection in patients submitted to cardiac surgery. J Cardiovasc Surg 40:477–479
6. Palella FJ Jr, Delaney KM, Moorman AC et al (1998) Declining morbidity and mortality among patients with advanced human immunodeficiency virus infection. HIV Outpatient Study Investigators. N Engl J Med 338:853–860
7. Trachiotis GD, Alexander EP, Benator D, Gharagozloo F (2003) Cardiac surgery in patients infected with the human immunodeficiency virus. Ann Thorac Surg 76(4):1114–1118
8. Mestres CA, Chuquire JE, Claramonte X et al (2003) Long-term results after cardiac surgery in patients infected with the human immunodeficiency virus type-1 (HIV-1). Eur J Cardiothorac Surg 23:1007–1016
9. Heidenreich PA, Eisenberg MJ, Kee LL et al (1995) Pericardial effusion in AIDS, incidence and survival. Circulation 92:3229–3234
10. Cegielski JP, Ramiya K, Lallinger GJ et al (1990) Pericardial disease and human immunodeficiency virus in Dar es Salaam, Tanzania. Lancet 335:209–212
11. Holtz H, Lavery D, Kapila R (1985) Actinomycetales infection in AIDS. Ann Intern Med 102:203–205
12. Schuster M, Valentine F, Holzman R (1985) Cryptococcal pericarditis in an intravenous drug abuser. J Infect Dis 152:842
13. Stotka JL, Good CB, Downer WR, Kapoor WN (1989) Pericardial effusion and tamponade due to Kaposi's sarcoma in acquired immunodeficiency syndrome. Chest 95:1359–1361
14. Holladay AO, Siegel RJ, Schwartz DA (1992) Cardiac malignant lymphoma in acquired immune deficiency syndrome. Cancer 70:2203–2207
15. Karve MM, Murali MR, Shah HM, Phelps KR (1992) Rapid evolution of cardiac tamponade due to bacterial pericarditis in two patients with HIV-1 infection. Chest 101:1461–1463
16. Kwan T, MM, Emerole O (1993) Cardiac tamponade in patients infected with HIV: a report from an inner-city hospital. Chest 104:1059–1062
17. Carrel T, Schaffner A, Vogt P et al (1993) Endocarditis in intravenous drug addicts and HIV infected patients: possibilities and limitations of surgical treatment. J Heart Valve Dis 2:140–147
18. De Rosa FG, Cicalini S, Canta F et al (2007) Infective endocarditis in intravenous drug users from Italy: the increasing importance in HIV-infected patients. Infection 35:154–160
19. Gebo KA, Burkey MD, Lucas GM et al (2006) Incidence of, risk factors for, clinical presentation, and 1-year outcomes of infective endocarditis in an urban HIV cohort. J Acquir Immune Defic Syndr 43:426–432
20. Aris A, Pomar JL, Saura E (1993) Cardiopulmonary bypass in HIV-positive patients. Ann Thorac Surg 55:1104–1107
21. Barbarini G, Barbaro G (2003) Incidence of the involvement of the cardiovascular system in HIV infection. AIDS 17(Suppl 1):S46–S50
22. Nahass RG, Weinstein MP, Bartels J, Gocke DJ (1990) Infective endocarditis in intravenous drug users: a comparison of human immunodeficiency virus type 1-negative and -positive patients. J Infect Dis 162:967–970
23. Mestres CA, Castella M, Moreno A et al; Hospital Clinico Endocarditis Study Group (2006) Cryopreserved mitral homograft in the tricuspid position for infective endocarditis: a valve that can be repaired in the long-term (13 years). J Heart Valve Dis. 15:389–391
24. Friis-Moller N, Reiss P, Sabin CA et al; the DAD Study Group (2007). Class of antiretroviral drugs and the risk of myocardial infarction. N Engl J Med 356:1723–1735
25. Flum DR, Tyras DH, Wallack MK (1997) Coronary artery bypass grafting in patients with human immunodeficiency virus. J Card Surg 12:98–101

26. Filsoufi F, Salzberg SP, Harbou KT et al (2006). Excellent outcomes of cardiac surgery in patients infected with HIV in the current era. Clin InfectDis 43:532–536

27. Sousa Uva M, Jebara VA, Fabiani JN et al (1992) Cardiac surgery in patients with human immunodeficiency virus infection: indication and results. J Card Surg 7:204–204

28. Ragni MV, Dodson SF, Hunt SC et al (1999) Liver transplantation in a hemophilia patient with acquired immunodeficiency syndrome. Blood 93:113–114

29. Roland ME, Stock PG (2003) Review of solid-organ transplantation in HIV-infected patients. Transplantation 75:425–429

30. Halpern SD, Ubel PA, Caplan AL (2002) Solid-organ transplantation in HIV-infected patients. N Engl J Med 347:284–287

31. Bisleri G, Morgan J, Deng M et al (2003) Should HIV-positive recipients undergo heart transplantation? J Thorac Cardiovasc Surg 126:1639–1640

32. Calabrese LH, Albrecht M, Young Y et al (2003) Successful cardiac transplantation in an HIV-1-infected patient with advanced disease. N Engl J Med 348:2323–2328

33. Jahangiri B, Haddad H (2007) Cardiac transplantation in HIV-positive patients: Are we there yet? J Heart Lung Transplant 26:103–107

34. Tzakis AG, Cooper MH, Dummer JS et al (1990) Transplantation in HIV(+) patients. Transplantation 49:354–358

35. Henderson DK (1997) Postexposure antiretroviral chemoprophylaxis: embracing risk for safety's sake. N Engl J Med 337:1542–1543

36. Beekman SE, Vlahov D, Koziol DE et al (1994) Implementation of universal precautions was temporally associated with a sustained progressive decrease in percutaneous exposures to blood or body fluids. Clin Infect Dis 18:562–569

37. Klatt EC (1994) Surgery and human immunodeficiency virus infection: indications, pathologic findings, risks, and risk prevention. Int Surg 79:1–5

38. Tanner J, Parkinson H (2004) Double gloving to reduce surgical cross-infection (Cochrane Review). In: The Cochrane Library, issue 3. Wiley, Chichester, NY

39. Kendall JB, Hart CA, Pennefather SH, Russel GN (2003) Infection control measures for adult cardiac surgery in the UK: a survey of current practice. J Hosp Infect 54:174–178

40. Kjaegard HK, Thiis J, Wiinberg N (1992) Accidental injuries and blood exposure to cardiothoracic surgical teams. Eur J Cardiothorac Surg 6:215–217

41. Nelson KE, Donahue JG, Munoz A et al (1992) Transmission of retroviruses from seronegative donors by transfusion during cardiac surgery: a multicenter study of HIV-1 and HTLV-I/II infections. Ann Intern Med 117:612–614

42. Cohen ND, Munoz A, Reitz BA et al (1989) Transmission of retroviruses by transfusion of screened blood in patients undergoing cardiac surgery. N Engl J Med 320:1172–1176

43. Pillonel J, Laperche S, Groupe "Agents Transmissibles par Transfusion" de la Societe francaise de transfusion sanguine, Etablissement francais du sang, Centre de transfusion sanguine des armees (2004) Risque résiduel de transmission du VIH, du VHC et du VHB par transfusion sanguine entre 1992 et 2002 en France et impact du dépistage génomique viral. Transfus Clin Biol 11:81–86

44. Solheim BG, Rollag H, Svennevig JL et al (2000) Viral safety of solvent/detergent-treated plasma. Transfusion 40:1149–1150

45. Tanaka K, Waly A, Cooper W, Levy J (2003) Treatment of excessive bleeding in Jehovah's Witness patients after cardiac surgery with recombinant factor VIIa (NovoSeven). Anesthesiology 98:1513–1515

46. King SM, Murphy T, Corey M et al (1995) The HIV information project: transfusion recipients a decade after transfusion. Arch Pediatr Adolesc Med 149:680–685

47. Babinchak TJ, Renner C (1994) Patients treated by thoracic surgeon with HIV: a review. Chest 106:681–683

48. Lemma M, Vanelli P, Beretta L et al (1992) Cardiac surgery in HIV-positive intravenous drug addicts: influence of cardiopulmonary bypass on the progression to AIDS. Thorac Cardiovasc Surg 40:279–282

49. Vasseur BG, Kawanishi H, Shah N, Anderson ML (2002) Type B lactic acidosis: a rare complication of antiretroviral therapy after cardiac surgery. Ann Thorac Surg 74:1251–1252

Chapter 16

Cardiological Emergencies in HIV-Infected Patients

G. Barbaro

Many cardiac complications in acquired immunodeficiency syndrome (AIDS) that may be faced by emergency department (ED) physicians are due to opportunistic infections or malignancy, but they may also be associated with other aspects of human immunodeficiency virus (HIV) disease and its treatment (Table 1) [1]. The clinical expression of cardiac involvement is variable and is affected by the stage of HIV dis-

Table 1 Frequent cardiac abnormalities in HIV disease and related emergencies. Modified from [1] with permission from Elsevier

HIV-associated cardiac disease	Cardiac emergencies
Myocardial	
Dilated cardiomyopathy Lymphocytic myocarditis	Congestive heart failure (CHF), cardiogenic pulmonary edema, arrhythmias
Noninflammatory myocardial necrosis (microvascular spasm, catecholamine excess, opportunistic infections, toxic drug reaction)	CHF
Right ventricular hypertrophy due to HIV-associated pulmonary hypertension Right ventricular hypertrophy with secondary pulmonary hypertension (pulmonary infections, pulmonary emboli)	CHF, pulmonary embolism, pulmonary infarction
Coronary artery disease (atherogenic effects of protease inhibitors, coronary arteritis, aortitis)	Unstable angina, myocardial infarction
Neoplastic (Kaposi's sarcoma, non-Hodgkin's lymphoma)	Arrhythmias, pericardial tamponade
Endocardial	
Infective endocarditis	Septic shock, acute valvular regurgitation (cardiogenic pulmonary edema, CHF), septic embolization (pulmonary and cerebral infarction)
A. Autoimmune response to infection B. Bacterial (*Staphylococcus aureus, Salmonella* species, *Streptococcus* species, *Enterococcus, Haemophilus parainfluenza, S.epidermidis, Pseudallescheria boydii*)	

cont. →

Table 1 *cont.*

HIV-associated cardiac disease	Cardiac emergencies
C. Fungal/yeast (*Candida albicans, Aspergillus fumigatus, Cryptococcus neoformans*)	
Nonbacterial thrombotic endocarditis	Systemic embolization (lung, brain, kidney, spleen) disseminated intravascular coagulopathy

Pericardial
Pericardial effusion/pericarditis
A. Infectious
   1. Bacterial (*Mycobacterium tuberculosis, M. avium intracellulare, Nocardia asteroides*)
   2. Viral (Coxsackievirus, Epstein-Barr virus, cytomegalovirus, adenovirus, herpes virus)
   3. Fungal (*Histoplasma capsulatum, Cryptococcus neoformans*)
	Cardiac tamponade, arrhythmias, CHF (for chronic pericardial effusions)

B. Idiopathic (HIV, autoimmune)	
C. Uremic	
D. Neoplastic (Kaposi's sarcoma, non-Hodgkin's lymphoma)	

ease, the degree of immunodeficiency, and the drugs used to treat HIV disease–i.e., zidovudine and protease inhibitors (PIs) in the era of highly active antiretroviral therapy (HAART) regimens–or to treat or prevent opportunistic infections and neoplasms (e.g., pentamidine, cotrimoxazole, interferon α) [2].

Myocarditis

In the ED, suspecting acute myocarditis in HIV-infected patients is important as this condition may evolve to include life-threatening congestive heart failure and arrhythmias. Fever and infection of the upper respiratory tract or flu-like symptoms may precede exertional dyspnea by as little as hours or days. Signs and symptoms may occur at rest and include palpitations, atypical chest pain, and electrocardiographic alterations (ST-segment elevation followed by T-wave inversion in different leads). Laboratory alterations may include elevated cardiac troponin I (cTnI) and myoglobin levels with or without increased levels of myocardial fraction of creatine kinase (CK-MB). A clinical diagnosis of myocarditis or congestive heart failure in an HIV-infected patient may be difficult to make due to the masking of symptoms by concomitant bronchopulmonary disease and/or wasting syndromes. Differentiating myocarditis from myocardial infarction may also be difficult. A careful clinical history and physical examination, electrocardiogram (ECG) review, and analysis of traditional risk factors expanded to include HIV-specific therapies (i.e., PIs in the context of HAART regimens) may direct the diagnosis.

Myocardial enzyme testing will help to detect myocardial injury rapidly with high sensitivity and specificity. Markers of cardiac injury should be interpreted in relation to the timing of the onset of the patient's symptoms. An elevation of myoglobin in the absence of an elevated cTnI level in subsequent samples may be related to an inflammatory muscle disease. Myositis is more likely to occur in HIV-infected patients, making myoglobin a much less specific marker for cardiac injury.

An isolated positivity of cTnI suggests a minimal myocardial damage of small areas of the myocardium (micronecrosis). In HIV-positive patients, micronecrosis may be caused by an inflammatory process secondary to myocarditis or pericarditis with extended epicarditis (perimyocarditis) or secondary to autoimmune mechanisms induced by infections or antiviral drugs. In case of a positive CK-MB and/or cTnI in patients with a nondiagnostic ECG (e.g., presence of left bundle-branch block, chronic ischemic alterations), clinical skills and echocardiography should help guide the differential diagnosis of myocarditis (absence or reversible hypokinesia) or acute myocardial infarction (with or without ST-segment elevation). However, endomyocardial biopsy represents the gold standard in the diagnosis of myocarditis. According to the Dallas criteria, myocarditis is defined as "a process characterized by a lymphocytic infiltrate of the myocardium with necrosis and/or degeneration of adjacent myocytes not typical of the ischemic damage associated with coronary artery disease" [3].

Intravenously administered immunoglobulins may be useful in improving the clinical outcome and the echocardiographic measurements of cardiac mass and function. The apparent efficacy of immunoglobulin therapy may be the result of immunoglobulins inhibiting cardiac autoantibodies (i.e., anti-a-myosin autoantibodies) by competing for Fc receptors or dampening the secretion or effects of cytokines and cellular growth factors [4]. Serial therapy in children has been shown to improve fractional shortening and left ventricular mass and to stabilize the disease process. Immunomodulatory therapy may be helpful in HIV-infected adults and children with declining left ventricular function, but further study is needed to evaluate the efficacy of this therapy and its impact on mortality.

Infective Endocarditis

The diagnosis of infective endocarditis is based on clinical, echocardiographic, and bacterial culture data. HIV-infected patients usually present with fever, sweats, weight loss, coexisting pneumonia, and/or meningitis. Among intravenous drug addicts, the tricuspid valve is most frequently affected (Fig. 1). Vegetations may

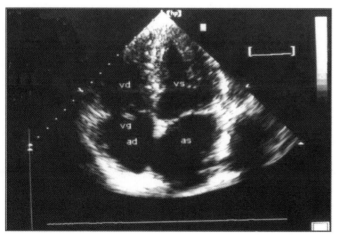

Fig. 1. Echocardiographic finding of Candida endocarditis in an intravenous heroin user suffering from AIDS. A vegetation (*vg*) is attached to the anterior leaflet of the tricuspid valve (apical four-chamber view). *ad*, right atrium; *as*, left atrium; *vd*, right ventricle; *vs*, left ventricle. (From [1], with permission from Elsevier)

form on the tricuspid or pulmonic valves with resultant pulmonary embolism and consequent septic pulmonary infarcts that appear as multiple opacities on chest radiograms. Systemic emboli may involve the coronary arteries, spleen, bowel, extremities, and central nervous system. Cardiac rhythm alterations (i.e., atrioventricular block) may suggest the presence of an abscess in proximity to the atrioventricular node. Peripheral pulses must be examined for signs of embolic occlusion or pulsating mass suggesting mycotic aneurysm. Mycotic aneurysms may occur in the intracranial arteries potentially leading to intracranial hemorrhage.

Echocardiographic findings in endocarditis include mobile echodense masses attached to the inflow side of the valvular leaflets or mural endocardium; pericardial effusion is frequently associated with this. Transthoracic echocardiography (TTE) is useful for detecting relatively large valvular mass(es); however, perivalvular abscess, leaflet perforation, or rupture of the valvular chordae are better assessed by transesophageal echocardiography (TEE). Both TTE and TEE, which may be performed in the ED, are also useful in guiding the duration of antibiotic therapy and evaluating the timing for surgery when necessary.

Assessment of infective endocarditis in an HIV-infected patient should include at least four sets of blood cultures separated by 30 min. Empiric broad-spectrum antibiotic therapy should be started within a maximum of 2–3 h from admission of the patient to the ED (after blood culture sets are obtained). According to our clinical experience, combination regimens including vancomycin 15 mg/kg i.v. (maximum 1 g) every 12 h, ampicillin 2 g i.v. every 4 h, and gentamycin 1 mg/kg i.m. every 8 h have significant bactericidal activity and cover methicillin-resistant *Staphylococcus aureus* [1].

Nonbacterial thrombotic endocarditis, also known as marantic endocarditis, is most common in patients with HIV wasting syndrome [1]. The incidence of marantic endocarditis and systemic embolization from marantic endocarditis is a rare cause of death in AIDS patients receiving HAART, whereas its frequency is increasing in developing countries (about 10%), where HAART availability is scanty, with a high mortality rate for systemic embolization [5].

Pericardial Effusion

Pericardial effusion in HIV disease is generally related to opportunistic infections (*Mycobacterium tuberculosis, M. avium intracellulare, S. aureus, Nocardia asteroides, Rhodococcus equi, Listeria monocytogenes, Chlamydia trachomatis*, coxsackievirus, Epstein-Barr virus, cytomegalovirus, adenovirus, herpes virus, *Histoplasma capsulatum, Cryptococcus neoformans*, and *Toxoplasma gondii*), or to malignancy (Kaposi's sarcoma, non-Hodgkin's lymphoma), but most often a clear etiology is not found. Fever, chest pain radiating to the left shoulder (often dull), aggravated by a supine posture and often decreased by sitting up and leaning forward, and pericardial friction rub (over the left sternal border, usually accentuated by sitting up and leaning forward) should suggest acute pericarditis. Pericardial effusion is suggested by absence or weakness of the apical impulse with an apparent increase in the area of dullness to percussion over the left chest and over the hepatocardiac angle as well as by muffled heart sounds, diffuse low-voltage ECG, electrical alternans of QRS complexes, and increased cardiac opacity on chest radiographs. Echocardiography confirms clinical suspicion by showing the pericardial effusion (Fig. 2a–b). An M-mode technique may help to demonstrate characteristic signs of cardiac tamponade: right atrial compression and diastolic right ventricular collapse. These echocardiographic signs pre-

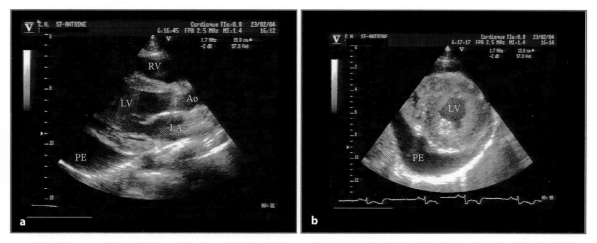

Fig. 2a, b Echocardiographic finding of posterior pericardial effusion in an AIDS patient. a Parasternal long-axis view; b Parasternal short-axis view; *LV*, left ventricle; *RV*, right ventricle; *Ao*, aorta; *LA*, left atrium; *PE*, pericardial effusion

cede pulsus paradox or severe dyspnea related to the hemodynamic effects of cardiac tamponade. CT scans can easily demonstrate pericardial effusion and help analyze the thickness of the pericardium and reveal signs of constrictive pericarditis (Fig. 3).

Pericardial effusion may resolve spontaneously in up to 42% of HIV-positive patients [1]. Pericardiocentesis is currently recommended only in large or poorly tolerated effusions, for diagnostic evaluation of systemic illness, or in the presence of cardiac tamponade [1].

Congestive Heart Failure

In HIV-infected patients, symptoms of heart failure may be masked by concomitant illness such as diarrhea or malnutrition, or may be disguised by bronchopulmonary

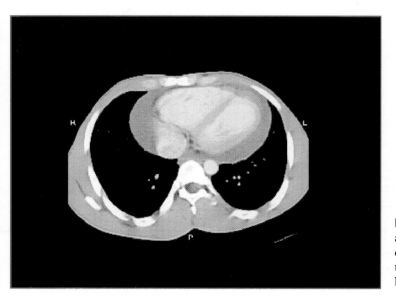

Fig. 3 CT scan finding of a large and circumferential pericardial effusion in an HIV-infected patient with *Mycobacterium M.* tuberculosis infection

infection. Left ventricular asynergy may develop due to regional differences in the distribution of cardiac sympathetic nerve endings, even in the context of acute myocarditis. In fact, an alteration of catecholamine dynamics (or autonomic function) has been associated with a transient extensive akinesis of the apical and mid portions of the left ventricle with hypercontraction of the basal segment (*takotsubo*-like dysfunction) in an HIV-infected patient with cytomegalovirus myocarditis leading to congestive heart failure [6]. Echocardiography is the only sensitive and specific method for the evaluation of ventricular function and pericardial effusion in this population and should be considered early in a patient with a change in clinical status (Fig. 4).

Standard heart failure treatment regimens are generally recommended for HIV-infected patients with dilated cardiomyopathy and congestive heart failure, even though these regimens have not been tested in this specific population. Patients with systolic dysfunction and symptoms of fluid retention should receive a loop diuretic and an aldosterone antagonist as well as an angiotensin-converting enzyme (ACE) inhibitor. ACE inhibitors are recommended on the basis of general heart failure studies, but may be poorly tolerated due to low systemic vascular resistance from diarrheal disease, infection, or dehydration. Digoxin may be added to the therapy regimen of patients with persistent symptoms or rapid atrial fibrillation. When the patient is euvolemic, a β-blocker (e.g., carvedilol, metoprolol, and bisoprolol) may be started because of its beneficial effects on circulating levels of inflammatory and anti-inflammatory cytokines.

Arrhythmias

Both tachy- and bradyarrhythmia may be observed in HIV-infected patients in relation to structural alterations of the endocardium (infective endocarditis), of the myocardium (myocarditis, dilated cardiomyopathy), and of the pericardium (infective and neoplastic pericarditis and myopericarditis). In HIV-infected patients with myocarditis, the most frequent arrhythmias are ventricular ectopic beats. Bradycardias (e.g., left bundle branch block and/or atrioventricular block) may be observed in patients with HIV-associated dilated cardiomyopathy resulting from fibrous degeneration of the conduction system [7].

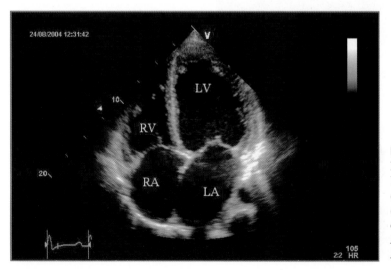

Fig. 4 Dilated cardiomyopathy in an HIV-infected patient (four-chamber apical view). Left ventriculalr ejection fraction: 25%. Note the dilatation of both left and right cardiac chambers. *RA*, right atrium; *RV*, right ventricle; *LA*, left atrium; *LV*, left ventricle

Side effects of both antiretroviral drugs or drugs used in the treatment and/or prophylaxis of opportunistic infections and neoplasms. Ganciclovir, amphotericin B, cotrimoxazole (trimethoprim-sulfamethoxazole), and pentamidine may cause Torsades de pointes (TdP) that can degenerate into ventricular fibrillation and sudden cardiac death (Fig. 5). Torsades de pointes (TdP) is related to prolongation of the ventricular action potential duration (QTc interval of the electrocardiogram >0.45 s) and it has also been described in relation to the administration of macrolide antibiotics (erythromycin, clarithromycin). Uncorrected electrolyte alterations (e.g., hypokalemia, hypomagnesemia, hypocalcemia) related to malnutrition and/or to chronic diarrhea or electrolyte imbalances induced by diuretics are also associated. These alterations, which should be evaluated and treated as early as possible, may further contribute to prolonging the QTc interval.

Use of central nervous system stimulant drugs (e.g., cocaine, amphetamines). Cocaine abuse has been associated with myocarditis, myocardial infarction, and dilated cardiomyopathy even in HIV-negative subjects, possibly because of intermittent microvas-cular spasm resulting from catecholamine surges associated with a high risk of ventricular arrhythmia.

Particularly in the ED, the first line of therapy for TdP is to stop medications suspected of prolonging the QT interval and to correct electrolyte imbalances. Intravenously administered magnesium sulfate is immediately indicated (loading dose of 1–2 g, mixed in 50–100 ml of saline, over 5–10 min followed by a continuous infusion of 1.0–2.0 g/h over 4–6 h), whereas i.v. infusion of isoproterenol (0.01–0.02 mcg/kg per minute) in the absence of known or suspected coronary artery disease may accelerate the heart rate and suppress ventricular arrhythmias while temporary ventricular pacing (overdrive pacing) is initiated [1].

In HIV-infected patients, hemodynamically stable sustained monomorphic wide-QRS complex tachycardia is another diagnostic challenge for the emergency physician, as ventricular tachycardia (VT) must be distinguished from supraventricular tachycardia (SVT). In particular, SVT with an accessory pathway, preexisting bundle-branch block, or rate-dependent bundle-branch block should be considered. SVT

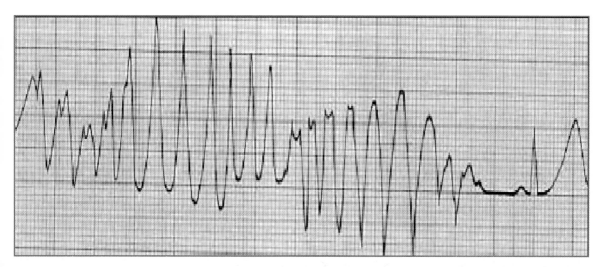

Fig. 5 Run of Torsade de pointes in an HIV-infected subject receiving pentamidine as prophylaxis for Pneumocystis carinii pneumonia during Holter electrocardiographic monitoring (lead CM5). Note the prolongation of the QT interval of the QRS complex following the arrhythmic run (0.50 s). (From [1], with permission from Elsevier)

with aberrant conduction is frequently observed in HIV-infected patients with dilated cardiomyopathy and histological diagnosis of myocarditis [1] (Fig. 6). In patients that are hemodynamically stable with no symptoms or clinical evidence of tissue hypoperfusion or shock, initial management should proceed under the presumption that the arrhythmia is VT, and electric cardioversion is the preferred therapy. If electrical cardioversion is not possible, empiric pharmacological therapy may be necessary with agents such as procainamide or amiodarone, which possess efficacy against VT and SVT and are also acceptable in patients with accessory pathway conduction [1].

Procainamide is administered in an infusion of 20 mg/min until the arrhythmia is suppressed or hypotension ensues, or when a total of 17 mg/kg of the drug has been given. Amiodarone is administered as 150 mg over 10 min, followed by 150 mg over the next 30 min, and then 1 mg/min infu-

sion for 6 h followed by 0.5 mg/min, to a maximum daily dose of 2 g. If the patient is in shock or in congestive heart failure (hemodynamically unstable), a wide-QRS complex tachycardia should be presumed to be VT, which requires immediate termination of synchronized cardioversion [1].

Coronary Heart Disease

Contraindications to thrombolytic therapy in HIV-infected patients with acute coronary syndrome include acute pericarditis, infective endocarditis, active cavitating pulmonary tuberculosis, and thrombocytopenia. Primary percutaneous transluminal coronary angioplasty, if feasible, seems the most appropriate treatment in some HIV-infected patients [8]. In patients presenting with unstable angina or non-Q-wave myocardial infarction without specific therapeutic contraindications, the best

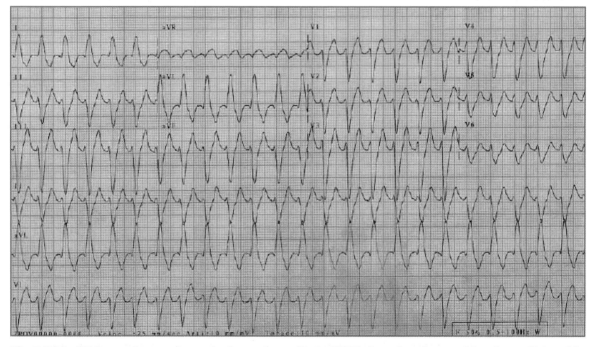

Fig. 6 Wide-QRS complex supraventricular tachycardia in HIV-infected patients with echocardiographic diagnosis of dilated cardiomyopathy (left ventricular ejection fraction: 30%) and diagnosis of myocarditis confirmed by histological examination of endomyocardial biopsy specimens

approach may be medical therapy (i.v. nitroglycerin, aspirin, low-molecular-weight heparin, IIb/IIIa platelet inhibitor, beta-blockers). Patients with unstable angina at high risk (recent severe angina, elevated cTnI, ischemic ECG changes, hypertension, elevated cholesterol, diabetes, active smokers) or with myocardial infarction without ST-segment elevation should undergo coronary angiography to define their anatomy and optimize treatment to prevent ischemic injury and sudden death. Cardiac revascularization has been shown to be beneficial in the treatment of HIV-infected patients with coronary artery disease [9]. Indeed, the extraordinary fruits of a massive research effort have made it reasonable to perform elective surgery and to offer major surgery to patients independent of their immunologic status; additionally, the concern that the surgical team would be exposed to a significant risk of acquiring HIV infection during surgery has proved to be unfounded. Cardiac surgeons should have a heightened awareness for the possibility of successful surgical treatment of HIV-infected patients with a definitive clinical diagnosis of coronary artery disease [9].

HIV-Associated Pulmonary Hypertension and Right Ventricular Dysfunction

Pulmonary embolism should be considered in HIV-positive patients with risk factors for pulmonary embolism (cancer, lower limb fractures, prolonged immobilization, recent surgery, infective endocarditis of the right-sided heart valves), the onset of acute paroxysmal dyspnea with jugular venous distension and normal physical examination of the chest with an ECG not suggestive of acute myocardial infarction as well as chest radiograms negative for acute pulmonary infiltrate. The onset of hemoptysis days after dyspnea, associated with fever,

stabbing chest pain (exacerbated by deep inspiration and coughing), and pleural friction rub, should suggest pulmonary infarction. Oxygen and steroids are generally used with conflicting results in the ED for HIV-infected patients with pulmonary hypertension. Calcium channel blockers (e.g., nifedipine and diltiazem), epoprostenol, and nitric oxide have been suggested in the treatment of HIV-associated pulmonary hypertension; however, controlled clinical trials have not been performed to confirm their efficacy. Studies on the effects of HAART therapy on pulmonary artery endothelial cells have shown contradictory results. Further information about the treatment of HIV-associated pulmonary hypertension is reported by G. Barbaro in a separate chapter in this volume.

Conclusion

Often, symptoms of congestive heart failure or pericardial effusion in HIV-infected patients are nonspecific and may be attributed to generalized illness or coinfection. Echocardiography noninvasively and accurately aids diagnosis during any change in clinical status and it also directs therapy. Patients will usually respond to early therapy for left ventricular dysfunction and increased left ventricular mass. Treatment based on these findings may prolong the quality and duration of life, and may also direct further patient evaluation.

The role of the ED cardiologist in the evaluation and treatment of patients with HIV infection should, therefore, be expanded to include patients who are being evaluated for or who are receiving HAART regimens, especially those with underlying risk factors, since the HAART-associated metabolic syndrome may increase the risk of acute coronary syndromes and stroke. Careful clinical and echocardiographic evaluation is also required for HIV-infected patients who receive drugs with a recognized cardiotoxic action (doxorubicin, interferon alpha, pentamidine), since they may worsen the clinical outcome of HIV-associated cardiomyopathy and increase the risk of potentially fatal arrhythmias [1].

References

1. Barbaro G, Fisher SD, Giancaspro G, Lipshultz SE (2001) HIV-associated cardiovascular complications: a new challenge for emergency physicians. Am J Emerg Med 19:566–574
2. Morris A, Huang L (2004) Intensive care of patients with HIV infection: HAART warming improvement but beware of future HAART (and heart) attacks. Chest 15:1602–1604
3. Aretz HT (1987) Myocarditis: the Dallas criteria. Hum Pathol 18:619–624
4. Lipshultz SE, Orav EJ, Sanders SP, Colan SD (1995) Immunoglobulins and left ventricular structure and function in pediatrics HIV infection. Circulation 92:2220–2225
5. Nzuobontane D, Blackett KN, Kuaban C (2002) Cardiac involvement in HIV-infected people in Yaounde, Cameroon. Postgrad Med J 78:678–681
6. Barbaro G, Pellicelli A, Barbarini G et al. (2006) Takotsubo-like left ventricular dysfunction in HIV-infected patient. Curr HIV Res; 4:239–241
7. Barbaro G, Di Lorenzo G, Grisorio B, Barbarini G (1996) Clinical meaning of ventricular ectopic beats in the diagnosis of HIV-related myocarditis: a retrospective analysis of Holter electrocardiographic recordings, echocardiographic parameters, histopathological and virologic findings. Cardiologia 41:1199–1207
8. Boccara F, Teiger E, Cohen A et al (2006) Percutaneous coronary intervention in HIV-infected patients: immediate results and long- term prognosis. Heart 92:543–544.
9. Frater RW, Sisto D, Condit D (1989) Cardiac surgery in human immunodeficiency virus (HIV) carriers. Eur J Cardiothorac Surg 3:146–150

Guidelines for the Prevention of Cardiovascular Risk in HIV-Infected Patients Treated with Antiretroviral Drugs

D. Scevola, L. Oberto, G. Barbarini, G. Barbaro

Introduction

Highly active antiretroviral therapy (HAART) has decreased by two-thirds [1] the lethality of AIDS and opportunistic infections. However, the improved survival of HIV patients receiving HAART has become associated with metabolic complications including insulin resistance, impaired glucose tolerance, loss of skeletal muscle mass (sarcopenia) and performance, osteopenia, lipid abnormalities such as dyslipidemia and body-fat distribution [2–19], which increase cardiovascular morbidity, compromising the patient's quality of life and the efficacy of HAART. As a consequence of prolonged survival and the direct effect of HAART [16], AIDS is changing from a "slim disease" to a "lipodystrophic disease" [20] and the care of the HIV-infected patients "has shifted from prevention and treatment of opportunistic infections and malignancies to management of the metabolic and related complications"[17]. The risk of cardiovascular disease (CVD) in HIV patients is increased two- to three-fold by disturbances in fat metabolism [15, 17]. New strategies addressed to prevent and manage such emerging disorders, including muscle and bone disorders (sarcopenia and osteopenia) [17, 21, 22], are needed. Moreover, coronary heart disease (CHD) is the leading cause of death and a common cause of morbidity in Western countries. Approximately 14 million Americans have CHD, according to NHANES III data [23]. Annually, about 1.1 million of them experience a heart attack and about 500,000 die from CHD (Fig. 1).

The objective proposed by various health authorities for the year 2010 is to reduce CHD deaths to no more than 51 in 100,000, "enhancing the cardiovascular health and quality of life of all Americans through improvement of medical management, prevention and control of risk factors, and promotion of healthy lifestyle behaviors" [24]. In light of this policy also adopted by the European Union, particular attention must be devoted to HIV-infected individuals who, in the near future, could represent an emerging population at a more elevated risk of CHD due to the prolonged life expectancy and/or metabolic disturbances induced by therapy [25–30]. Elevated triglycerides (TG), low-density lipoprotein (LDL) cholesterol, very low-density lipoprotein (VLDL) cholesterol, and reduced levels of high-density lipoprotein (HDL) cholesterol are associated with body-fat redistribution characterized by visceral fat accumulation, peripheral lipodystrophy/lipoatrophy, and CHD. It has been reported that 5–75% of HIV patients receiving HAART experience a worse lipid metabolism and body-fat distribution after 10–12 months of therapy [15, 17].

Our guidelines, based on our own and the experience of others [31–37], meet the intervention criteria defined by the American National Cholesterol Education Program (NCEP) [38], including evaluation criteria, diet prescription, drug and exercise treatment — preliminary discussion included in The Pavia Consensus Statement, Octo-

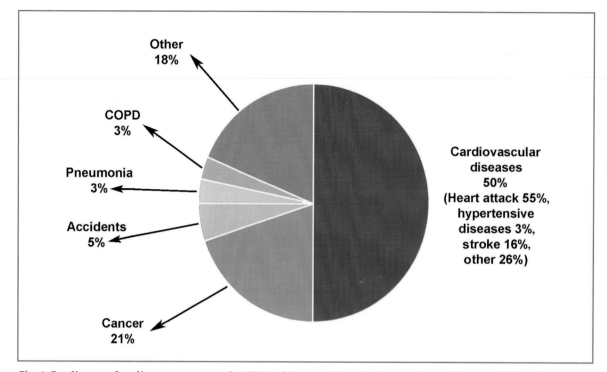

Fig. 1 Cardiovascular diseases account for 50% of the total deaths in the United States. *COPD*, chronic obstructive pulmonary disease

ber 2001 [39, 40], the recommendations of the HIV Medicine Association of the Infectious Disease Society of America and the Adult AIDS Clinical Trials Group (AACTG) [41], and the 2007 updated scientific statement from the American Heart Association Council on Clinical Cardiology and Council on Nutrition, Physical Activity and Metabolism [42]. Our study is also based on algorithms and approaches developed in classic physiology and sports Medicine for healthy people, the elderly, diseases such as diabetes and CVD [42–48].

Patient Evaluation Criteria

Patients at risk of CVD/CHD must be routinely evaluated for risk factors (Fig. 2) such as family history, smoking, hypertension, hormonal status, body-fat distribution and obesity, physical activity (Fig. 3), alcohol abuse, hypogonadism, hypothyroidism,

diabetes, and renal or hepatic disease. Guidelines include the measurement of total cholesterol, HDL, LDL, and VLDL cholesterol, TG, lactate [39–41, 49], the measure of body compartments, body circumferences and skinfolds [28], and resting metabolic rate (RMR) as a measure of the energy expended for maintenance of physiologic functions which generally represents the largest portion of daily energy expenditure (60–75%) [31–33]. We use the WHO equations for body weights and heights [34, 50] along with bioimpedance analysis (BIA) and indirect calorimetry to predict the RMRs and energy expenditure for different age and sex groups [35, 36, 51]. Energy production is estimated by measuring O_2 consumption and CO_2 production using a special calorimeter (e.g., Datex-Engstron Division Instrumentarium Corp. Helsinki, Finland; type MBM-200-23-01). RMR values normally range between 0.7 and 1.6 kcal/min according to the subject's body composition, gender, and level of training.

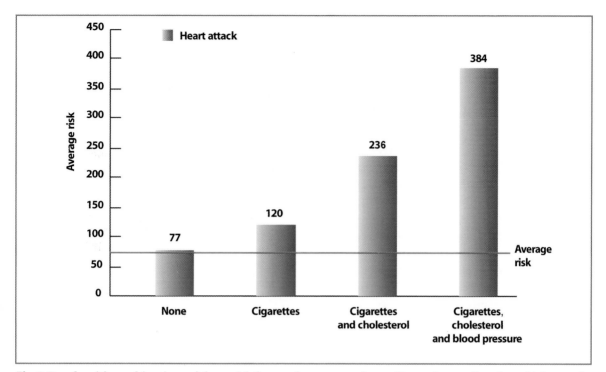

Fig. 2 People with combinations of three risk factors for coronary heart disease have a five times higher probability of heart attack than persons without risk factors. Physical inactivity is an additional risk factor

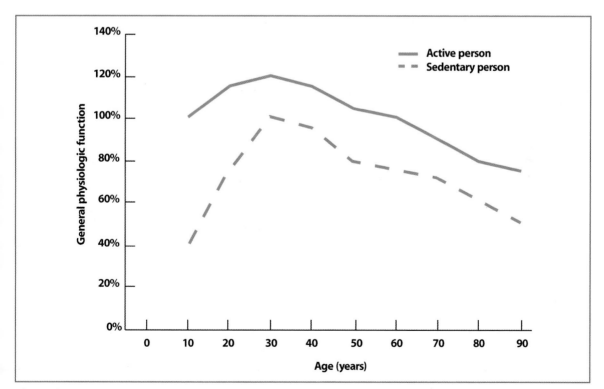

Fig. 3 Changes in physiologic functions with age and physical activity. The functional capacity of organs (e.g., cardiac index, breathing capacity, nerve conduction velocity, liver, kidneys, brain activity) declines with age and inactivity

Intervention Criteria

Nutritional and Pharmacological Approach

No universally accepted guidelines exist for the nutritional treatment of lipid metabolism disturbances in HIV patients, but according to NCEP [25, 38], our own studies as well as the studies of others [21, 28, 36, 39–41, 52] of patients with preexisting CHD, we advise dietary intervention when the LDL cholesterol level ranges between 100 mg/dl and 130 mg/dl, adding drug therapy if LDL cholesterol exceeds 130 mg/dl.

Among patients without CHD, but presenting two or more risk factors (Fig. 2), dietary intervention is strongly indicated when the LDL cholesterol is between 130 and 160 mg/dl. Drug therapy must be added when the LDL exceeds 160 mg/dl. With fewer than two risk factors, dietary modifications should be recommended when LDL levels range between 160 and 190 mg/dl. Drug therapy should be considered with LDL levels over 190 mg/dl. For patients with very high TG levels (>400 mg/dl), the AACTG [39] suggests a dietary intervention when total cholesterol is higher than 240 mg/dl or HDL cholesterol is lower than 35 mg/dl. Patients with isolated hypertriglyceridemia (fasting serum levels >200 mg/dl) should follow an adequate diet and physical exercise program. If levels exceed 1,000 mg/dl, pharmacological therapy should be strongly suggested because of the risk of pancreatitis. The same indication is mandatory for patients with a history of pancreatitis having TG levels over 500 mg/dl.

To reduce hypercholesterolemia, dietary and exercise treatments are recommended before pharmacological intervention. In patients suffering from wasting and lipid disturbances, it seems preferable to treat the wasting first [36, 53, 54].

For each patient, the guidelines for nutritional intervention must consider RMR, gut functions, concomitant diseases, hormonal status, appetite, and social conditions, as previously described [28, 39, 41]. At the first sign of malnutrition, suitable nutritional treatment is advised [36] because of the positive effect on the infection and on the quality of life. A balanced supply of n-6 and n-3 polyunsaturated fatty acids (PUFA) including eicosapentaenoic acid (EPA) and docosahexaenoic acid (DHA; the main components of fish oil) may modulate cytokine production. EPA, as a direct suppressant of lipid mobilization factor, counteracts weight loss, lipolysis, and protein catabolism [55]. Amino acids (1.5–2 g/kg per day) must be administered to block protein loss. A quota of them (<0.7 g/kg per day) should include essential amino acids. Branched chain amino acids are useful in hepatic encephalopathy. An early and aggressive nutritional treatment of wasting and lipid metabolism disturbances improves the general clinical status, reducing the length of hospital stay. Unfortunately, the National Health Services do not support nutritional therapy programs. Pharmacological intervention concerning appetite and metabolic pathways with drugs such as cyproheptadine [56], progestin derivatives [53, 57–59], insulin-like growth factor-1 [60], steroids, and growth hormone [28, 61, 62], contributes to the success of any nutritional program.

Drugs Lowering Lipids

Because only 40% of patients [25] treated via diet and physical exercise have reduced lipid levels, therapy with statins and/or fibrates for hypercholesterolemia and/or hypertriglyceridemia becomes necessary [39]. In the group of 3-hydroxy-3-methylglutaryl coenzyme A reductase inhibitors, pravastatin 10–40 mg PO q.i.d. is to be preferred because it is the least susceptible to interactions with protease inhibitors. Fluvastatin 20–80 mg PO b.i.d. is an alternative. In the group of fibrates, clofibrate 1 g

PO b.i.d., gemfibrozil 600 mg PO b.i.d. before meals, and fenofibrate 54–160 mg PO q.i.d. with meals are the first-line choice for isolated hypertriglyceridemia or mixed hypercholesterolemia plus hypertriglyceridemia. Because of the high risk of pancreatitis, an isolated increase of TG levels over 1,000 mg/dl, with normal HDL values, needs treatment with statin or fibrates and replacement of saturated fats with nonsaturated fats. In combined disorders (high cholesterol, high TG), statins and fibrates together may control lipid metabolism, but can also cause muscle damage (rhabdomyolysis). In some patients, gemfibrozil (600 mg b.i.d.), atorvastatin (10 mg q.i.d.), or their combination (G+A) reduces total cholesterol by 32, 19, and 30%, respectively, and TG by 59, 21, and 60%. The antilipidemic drugs pose a risk of toxicity because the majority of them (atorvastatin, lovastatin, simvastatin, bezafibrate, ciprofibrate, fenofibrate, gemfibrozil) are metabolized by the same CYP3A liver enzymes as protease inhibitors and other drugs taken by HIV-infected patients. Pravastatin and fluvastatin, on the contrary, have other mechanisms of excretion. Protease inhibitors, macrolides, and imidazole derivatives have an inhibitory effect on CYP3A and can raise statin levels by 10- to 20-fold, potentially leading to increased muscle and liver toxicity. CHD due to lipid metabolism alterations takes 5–10 years to develop, while heart attacks seen after a few weeks or months of HAART are attributed to thrombosis and not to arteriosclerosis. The use of metformin can reduce central fat and insulin resistance [63], but it also reduces general body fat and muscle mass. Troglitazone (Rezulin), which is active on glucose levels without effects on lipids and body fat [64], was removed from the market because of liver toxicity. Rosiglitazone (Avandia) and pioglitazone (Actos) are related compounds with a lower risk of hepatic toxicity. In spite of a confirmed improvement of insulin resistance, contrasting findings have been reported on the use of glitazones in the treatment of HIV-associated lipodystrophy/lipoatrophy [65]. Growth hormone [61, 62, 66] reduces abdominal fat without having an influence on peripheral fat loss and lipids. Androgenic anabolic steroids (oxandrolone, nandrolone decanoate) increase muscular body mass without changes in lipids and body fat [67]. Niacin 50–100 mg PO b.i.d./t.i.d. and bile acid sequestering agents may have side effects, while fish oil 3–5 g PO q.i.d. is well tolerated [68]. We usually administer fish oil and/or vegetable derivative PUFAs [28, 67, 69], associated with l-carnitine, in order to increase the beta-oxidative processes of long-chain fatty acids and we replace saturated fats with polyunsaturated fats. In patients without other risk factors such as smoking, preexisting cardiovascular diseases, or dyslipidemia, "wait and see" may be an appropriate strategy [14].

Physical Exercise

Loss of skeletal muscle mass (sarcopenia) and impairment of muscle performance are well documented during HIV infection [17–19, 29] and with the elderly [70]. Exercise has been extensively studied in patients with known coronary artery disease. It has been shown to induce a beneficial adaptation in the cardiovascular system as well as the peripheral musculature [36, 42, 71–75] (Fig. 4; Table 1). Aerobic exercise and resistance exercise are the most popular methods of preventing or treating sarcopenia and increasing muscular performance [45, 47, 76]. In our experience, both aerobic and anaerobic exercise associated with a personalized training diet improve muscular endurance and body composition in HIV patients, in accordance with results obtained by Stringer [77] and Smith [72].

For developing complete muscular strength, three exercise methods are commonly used: weight training, isometric (static) training, and isokinetic training.

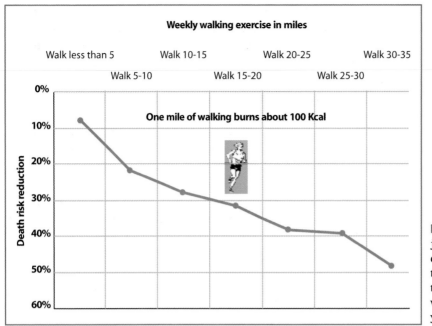

Weekly walking exercise in miles

Fig. 4 Regularly walking/ jogging more than 3 miles a day proportionally reduces the risk of death. No additional benefits are obtained with energy expenditure beyond 3,500 kcal per week

Table 1 Beneficial effects of muscular exercise

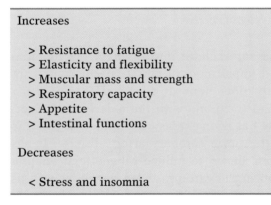

Increases

> Resistance to fatigue
> Elasticity and flexibility
> Muscular mass and strength
> Respiratory capacity
> Appetite
> Intestinal functions

Decreases

< Stress and insomnia

The neck, arms, and shoulders; the chest, abdomen, and back; and the buttocks and legs can be conditioned separately by specific exercises. All our exercise programs include progressive resistance training of the major muscle groups, according to the studies and indications of many authorities in the field of physical activity in health and disease[19, 42–44, 76, 78–84].

HDL levels may be favorably increased in sedentary people who engage in aerobic training. Concurrently, the LDL levels are lowered so that the net result is a considerably improved ratio of HDL to LDL or HDL to total cholesterol. This exercise effect appears to be independent of whether or not the diet is low in fat or whether or not the exerciser is overweight. The effect of regular endurance-type exercise on the blood lipid profile is certainly a strong argument for incorporating vigorous physical activity into a total program of health maintenance in HIV patients receiving HAART. It is well known that exercise improves myocardial circulation and metabolism and enhances vascularization, cardiac glycogen stores, and glycolitic capacity, which protects the heart from hypoxic stress [42, 75]. Mechanical and contractile properties of the myocardium are improved, enabling the conditioned heart to maintain or increase contractility during a specific challenge. Heart rate and blood pressure are favorably reduced so the work of the myocardium is significantly reduced at rest and during exercise.

Exercise reduces the symptoms and medication doses needed and it corrects the nutritional imbalances and side effects of drugs and altered diet. Many clinical signs and symptoms are responsive to exercise: atrophy of muscle and bone, postural hypotension, joint stiffness, reflexes, cardiovascular deconditioning, anorexia, gastrointestinal motility, insomnia, and depression. Exercise is the way to stimulate the muscles not only to move the body better but also to increase biochemical reactions devoted to energy production. The predominant energy pathways required in physical activities are the ATP-CP system, the lactic acid system, and the oxygen or aerobic system that are often operative simultaneously (Fig. 5). However, their relative con-

tributions to the total energy requirement during an exercise may differ markedly. This contribution is related directly to the length of time and intensity that a specific activity is performed.

Anaerobic Conditioning (Resistance Training or Dynamic-Anaerobic Strength Exercise)

During intense, maximal bursts of energy lasting no more than 6 s, the energy is provided anaerobically almost exclusively by the stored high-energy molecules of phos-

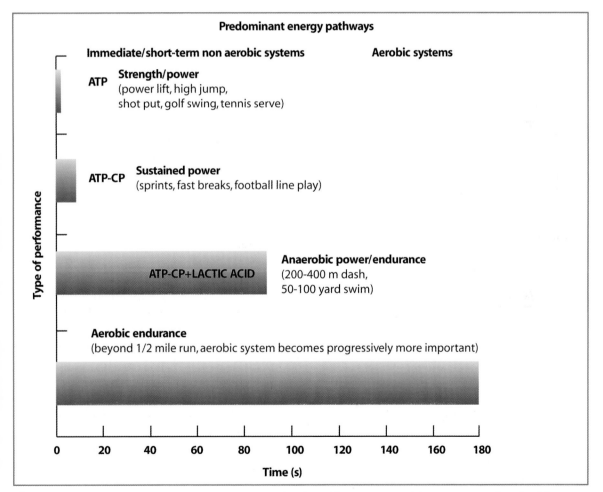

Fig. 5 The three energy systems (ATP-CP system, lactic acid system, aerobic system) are involved in some physical activities. In exercises with an intense, short burst of energy, the energy is provided anaerobically almost exclusively by the stored reserve of ATP and CP. In performances lasting between 10 and 90 s, the energy from lactic acid production becomes an important source. After 2–4 min of continuous activity, the energy is released almost exclusively from aerobic reactions

phates (ATP and CP). Overload of the ATP-CP pool can be achieved by engaging specific muscles in maximum bursts of effort for 5 or 10 s. In physical activities chosen to enhance the ATP-CP energy capacity of specific muscles, the subject must perform numerous bouts of intense, short-duration exercise. The energy for performances lasting between 10 and 90 s is still supplied predominantly by anaerobic reactions, but lactic acid becomes a more important source of energy. To improve the lactic acid energy system, the training program must be of sufficient intensity and duration to stimulate lactic-acid production as well as to overload the ATP-CP energy system. An effective way to increase near-maximum levels and overload the lactic acid system is repeat bouts of up to 1 min of extreme running, swimming, or cycling, stopped 30–40 s before exhaustion. The exercise bout should be repeated several times after 1–2 min of recovery. Recovery time from the exercise can be considerable when large amounts of lactic acid are produced (Fig. 5).

Aerobic Conditioning (Endurance Exercise or Dynamic-Aerobic Exercise)

After 2–4 min of continuous exercise, any physical activity becomes progressively more dependent on aerobic energy for the resynthesis of the phosphates. Under aerobic conditions, pyruvic acid from carbohydrate metabolism and molecules from fat and protein are transformed into various intermediate substances with the final formation of CO_2, H_2O, and large amounts of energy. If the O_2 supply and utilization are adequate, lactic acid does not accumulate and fatigue is absent. We can reach a condition of endurance or aerobic fitness in which the body's ability to generate ATP aerobically exceeds the energy produced from anaerobic reactions. To have a practical measure of cardiovascular capacity of the subject, we use the step-up test (Fig. 6), which provides the heart-rate response to aerobic exercise: a low heart rate during exercise and a small increment with more

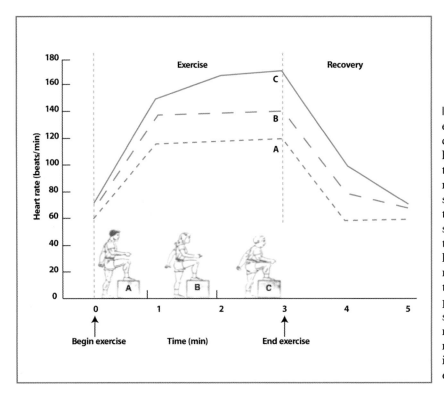

Fig. 6 Step-up exercise to evaluate the cardiovascular capacity: the different heart-rate responses of three individuals during 3 min of regular stepping. The subjects are basically conditioned differently: a professional football player, A, at the end of 3 min reaches a heart rate of 115 beats per minute; for B, a gym-trainer, the heart rate is 140 beats per minute, while C, a sedentary young person, reaches 170 beats per minute. Heart rate recovery is complete 2 min after the end of exercise

intense exercise reflect a high level of cardiovascular fitness. A simple method to recover heart rates for evaluation of relative fitness for aerobic exercise is the Tecumseh step test [72].

In the Tecumseh step test, the stepping cadence must be 22 steps per minute for women and 24 for men, with a stepping height of 20 cm. After 3 min of stepping and exactly 30 s after stopping, the subject must measure the pulse for 30 s in a standing position. The number of pulse beats, from the 30-s to the 1-min post-exercise period, is the heart rate score (Fig. 7). By means of special equations and the recovery heart rate, the maximal O_2 consumption can be calculated [73]. Because aerobic capacity declines with age and the population of old HIV infected patients is growing older [29], particular attention must be devoted to pre-

scribe adequate programs of physical activity in this group of patients.

Determination of Frequency, Duration, and Intensity of Training

The intensity of training is the most critical factor that influences successful aerobic conditioning and can be expressed in different ways: as calories consumed, as a percentage of maximal O_2 consumption, as heart rate or percentage of maximum heart rate, or as multiples of RMR required to perform the work. The exercise must be sufficient to produce an increase in heart rate to at least 130–140 beats per minute, equivalent to about 50–55% of the maximum aerobic capacity or about 70% of the maximum exercise heart rate (Fig. 8).

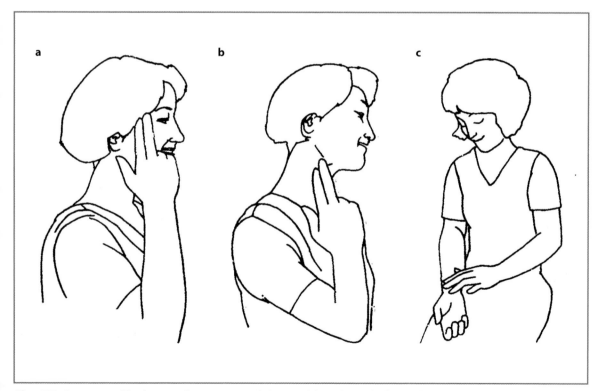

Fig. 7 Pulse rate self-taken at the **a** temporal, **b** carotid, and **c** radial arteries

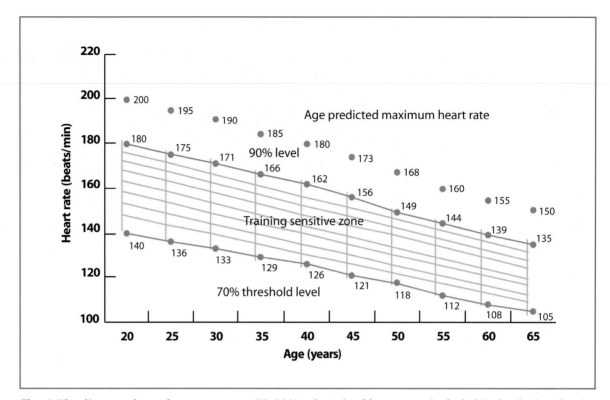

Fig. 8 The diagram shows the percentages (70–90%) of maximal heart rate (included in the depicted training zone) required to train aerobic systems of energy production in different age groups. The subject must exercise for 3–5 min in order to obtain a desired pulse rate, counting for 10 s after stopping. For example, a training heart rate equal to 70% of the age-related maximal value for a man of 40 years can be calculated using the formula (0.70¥180=126 beats per minute). Exercise must be performed at least for 20 min. A training response occurs if an exercise is performed two or preferably three times each week for at least 6 weeks. Both continuous as well as intermittent overload are effective in improving aerobic capacity. A single 3–5 min of vigorous exercise performed three times a week improves aerobic capacity as much as a less exhausting but steady-state exercise for 20 min. Our aerobic training program is conducted 3 days a week utilizing 20–30 min of continuous exercise of sufficient intensity to expend about 300 kcal. For example, subjects trained on a bicycle ergometer 20–30 min a day (~300 kcal), three times a week for 8 weeks, with a training intensity of 85% of maximum heart rate improved maximal O_2 uptake by 7.8%

Conclusion

In HIV patients like in people with and without CVD [42], both anaerobic and aerobic training induce some health benefits and improve physical fitness at different levels of body functions (Table 2), but the prescription and supervision of resistance training remain a medical task based on some limitations (Table 3).

Table 2 Physiological and biochemical effects of aerobic exercise (endurance) and anaerobic exercise (resistance training). Adapted [42, 43 and 84]

Parameters	Endurance	Resistance training
Body composition, metabolism and muscle strength		
Bone density	++	++
Body fat (%)	- -	-
Lean body mass	0	++
Basal metabolic rate	+/0	+
Muscle strength	0/+	+++
Biochemistry		
Cholesterol		
HDL	+/0	+/0
LDL	-/0	-/0
Triglycerides	—	-/0
Insulin (basal)	-	-
Insulin sensitivity	++	++
Insulin response to glucose	—	—
Cardiovascular system		
Resting heart rate	—	0
Systolic blood pressure	-/0	0
Diastolic blood pressure	-/0	0
Vo$_2$ max	+++	+/0
Resting cardiac output	0	0
Maximal cardiac output	++	0
Resting and maximal stroke volume	++	0
Submaximal and maximal endurance time	+++	++
Submaximal exercise rate-pressure product	—-	—

Table 3 Clinical conditions totally or partially contraindicating aerobic and resistance exercise

	Absolute contraindication	With caution
Cardiovascular diseases (CVD)		
Uncontrolled CVD	x	
Heart failure	x	
Aortic stenosis or dissection	x	
Myocarditis	x	
Endocarditis	x	
Pericarditis	x	
Pulmonary hypertension	x	
Arrhythmias	x	
Others		
Diabetes		x
Marfan syndrome	x	
Musculoskeletal (myopathies, osteoarthritis etc.)		x
Risks for CVD		x
Uncontrolled hypertension (180–110mm Hg)	x	
Uncontrolled hypertension (160–100mm Hg)		x
Pacemaker/defibrillator carriers		x

References

1. Palella FJ, Delaney KM, Mooreman AC et al (1998) Declining morbidity and mortality among patients with advanced human immunodeficiency virus infection. N Engl J Med 338:853–860
2. Dubè MP, Sattler FR (1998) Metabolic complications of antiretroviral therapies. AIDS Clinical Care 10:41–44
3. Sullivan AK, Nelson MR (1997) Marked hyperlipidaemia on ritonavir. AIDS 11:938–939
4. Hengel RL, Watts NB, Lennox JL (1997) Benign symmetric lipomatosis associated with protease inhibitors. Lancet 350:1596
5. Miller KD, Jones E, Yanovski JA et al (1998) Visceral abdominal-fat accumulation associated with use of indinavir. Lancet 351:871–875
6. Carr A, Samaras K, Burton S et al (1998) A syndrome of peripheral lipodystrophy, hyperlipidaemia and insulin resistance in patients receiving HIV protease inhibitors. AIDS 12:F51–F58
7. Lo JC, Mulligan K, Tai VW et al (1998) "Buffalo hump" in men with HIV-infection. Lancet 351:867–870
8. Carr A, Samaras K, Chisholm DJ, Cooper DA (1998) Pathogenesis of HIV-1-protease inhibitor-associated peripheral liopdystrophy, hyperlipidemia, and insulin resistance. Lancet 352:1881–1883
9. Rosenberg HE, Mulder J, Sepkowitz K et al (1998) "Protease-paunch" in HIV+ persons receiving protease inhibitor therapy: incidence, risks and endocrinologic evaluation. Fifth Conference on Retroviruses and Opportunistic Infections, Chicago, February 1998, abstract 408
10. Kotler DP, Rosenbaum KB, Wang J et al (1998) Alterations in body fat distribution in HIV-infected men and women. Twelfth World AIDS Conference, Geneva, Switzerland, June–July 1998, abstract 32173
11. Engelson ES, Kotler DP, Tan YX et al (1998) Altered body fat distribution in HIV infection: regional body composition measurements by whole body MRI and DXA scans. Twelfth World AIDS Conference, Geneva, Switzerland, June–July 1998, abstract 32181
12. Boyle BA (1999) Lipodystrophy: A new phenomenon? AIDS Reader 9:15–17
13. Gervasoni C, Ridolfo AL, Trifirò G et al (1999) Redistribution of body fat in HIV-infected women undergoing combined antiretroviral therapy. AIDS 13:465–471
14. Bernasconi E (1999) Metabolic effects of protease inhibitor therapy. AIDS Reader 9:254–269
15. Grinspoon S, Carr A(2005) Cardiovascular risk and body-fat abnormalities in HIV-infected adults. N Engl J Med 352:48–62
16. Mangili A, Murman DH, Zampini AM, Wanke CA (2006) Nutrition and HIV infection: review of weight loss and wasting in the era of highly active antiretroviral therapy from nutrition for healthy living cohort. Clin Infect Dis 42:836–842
17. Morse CG, Kovacs JA (2006) Metabolic and skeletal complications of HIV infection: the price of success. JAMA 296:844–854
18. Authier FJ, Chariot P, Gherardi RK (2005) Skeletal muscle involvement in human immunodeficiency virus (HIV)-infected patients in the era of highly active antiretroviral therapy (HAART). Muscle Nerve 32:247–260
19. Scott WB, Oursler KK, Katzel LI et al (2007) Central activation, muscle performance, and physical function in men infected with human immunodeficiency virus. Muscle Nerve 36(3) (published online: 6 June 2007). doi:10.1002/mus.20832
20. Scevola D, Di Matteo A, Giglio O, Uberti F (2006) HIV Infection-related cachexia and lipodystrophy In: Mantovani G (ed) Cachexia and wasting: a modern approach. Springer, Milan, pp 407–428
21. Scevola D, Di Matteo A, Uberti F et al (2000) Reversal of cachexia in patients treated with potent antiretroviral therapy. AIDS Reader 10:365–375
22. Henry K, Zackin R, Dube M et al (2001) Metabolic status and cardiovascular disease risk for a cohort of HIV-1-infected persons durably suppressed on an indinavir-containing regimen(ACTG 372A). Program and abstracts of the 8th Conference on Retroviruses and Opportunistic Infections, Chicago, ILL, 4–8 February 2001, abstract 656
23. Adams PF, Marano MA (1995) Current estimates from the National Health Interview Survey, 1994, National Center for Health Statistics. Vital Health Stat 10:193
24. Anonymous (1999) Healthy people 2010: draft for public comment. Department of Health and Human Services, Washington, DC
25. Henry K, Melroe H, Huebesh J et al (1999) Experience with the National Cholesterol Education Program (NCEP) guidelines for the identification and treatment of protease inhibitor related lipid abnormalities: results of a prospective study. 6th Conference on Retroviruses and Opportunistic Infections, Chicago, ILL, 31 Jan–4 Feb 1999, abstract 671
26. Grunfeld C, Feingold KR (1992) Metabolic disturbances and wasting in the acquired immunodeficiency syndrome. N Engl J Med 5:329–337

27. Lonergan JT, Havlir D, Barber E, Mathews WC (2001) Incidence and outcome of hyperlactatemia associated with clinical manifestations in HIV-infected adults receiving NRTI-containing regimens. Program and abstracts of the 8th Conference on Retroviruses and Opportunistic Infections, Chicago, ILL, 4–8 February 200,1 abstract 624

28. Scevola D, Bottari G, Oberto L, Faggi A (1996) AIDS cachexia: basics and treatment. In: Ruf B, Pohle HD, Goebel FD, L'age M (eds) HIV-Infektion, Pathogenese, Diagnostik und Therapie. Socio-medico Verlag, Wessobrunn, Germany, pp 281–327

29. Oursler KK, Sorkin JD, Smith B, Katzel LI (2006) Reduced aerobic capacity and physical functioning in older HIV-infected men. AIDS Res Hum Retroviruses 22:1113–1121

30. Watson RR (ed) (2004) AIDS and heart disease. Informa Healthcare, London, 496 pp

31. Melchior JC, Salmon D, Rigaud D et al (1991) Resting energy expenditure is increased in stable, malnourished HIV-infected patients. Am J Clin Nutr 53:437–441

32. Grunfeld C, Pang M, Shimizu L et al (1992) Resting energy expenditure, caloric intake and short-term weight change in human immunodeficiency virus infection and the acquired immunodeficiency syndrome. Am J Clin Nutr 55:455–460

33. Shevitz AH (2000) Resting energy expenditure in the HAART era. AIDS Reader 10:539–544

34. WHO (1986) Working group on the use and interpretation of anthropometric indicators of nutritional status. Bull WHO 64:929–941

35. Kotler DP, Rosenbaum K, Wang J, Pearson RN (1999) Studies of body composition and fat distribution in HIV-infected and control subjects. J Acquir Immune Defic Syndr Hum Retrovirol 20:228–237

36. Scevola D (1993) La cachessia nelle malattie infettive e neoplastiche. Edizioni Medico Scientifiche, Pavia, Italy

37. Scevola D, Giglio O, Scevola S(2006) Treatment of AIDS anorexia-cachexia syndrome and lipodystrophy. Mantovani G (ed) In: Cachexia and wasting: a modern approach. Springer, Milan, pp 429–456

38. Expert Panel on Detection, Evaluation, and Treatment of High Blood Cholesterol in Adults (2001) Executive summary of the third report of the National Cholesterol Education Program (NCEP) Expert Panel on Detection, Evaluation, and Treatment of High Blood Cholesterol in Adults (Adult Treatment Panel III). JAMA 285:2486–2497

39. Scevola D, Di Matteo A, Lanzarini P et al (2003) Effect of exercise and strength training on cardiovascular status in HIV-infected patients receiving highly active antiretroviral therapy. AIDS 17(S1):S123–S129

40. Volberding PA, Murphy RL, Barbaro G et al (2003) The Pavia consensus statement. AIDS 17(S1):S170–S179

41. Dubé MP, Stein JH, Aberg JA et al (2003) Guidelines for the evaluation and management of dyslipidemia in human immunodeficiency virus (HIV)-infected adults receiving antiretroviral therapy: recommendations of the HIV Medicine Association of the Infectious Disease Society of America and the Adult AIDS clinical trials group. Clin Inf Dis 37:613–627

42. Williams MA, Haskell WL, Ades PA et al (2007) Resistance exercise in individuals with and without cardiovascular disease: 2007 update. A scientific statement from the American Heart Association Council on Clinical Cardiology and Council on Nutrition, Physical Activity, and Metabolism. Circulation 116:572. doi:10.1161/CIRCULATIONAHA.107.185214

43. Pollock ML, Vincent KR (1996) Resistance training for health. In: The President's Council on Physical Fitness and Sports Research Digest, series 2, no. 8

44. Smit E, Crespo CJ, Semba RD et al (2006) Physical activity in a cohort of HIV-positive and HIV-negative injection drug users. AIDS Care 18:1040–1045

45. American College of Sports Medicine(2006) ACSM's guidelines for exercise testing and prescription, 7th edn., Lippincott, Baltimore, MD

46. Brochu M, Savage P, Lee M et al (2002) Effects of resistance training on physical function in older disable women with coronary heart disease. J Appl Physiol 92:672–678

47. Brown SP, Miller WC, Eason JM Exercise (2006) Physiology: basis of human movement in health and disease. Lippincott, Baltimore, MD, pp 98–124

48. Ibanez J, Izquierdo M, Arguelles I et al (2005) Twice-weekly progressive resistance training decreases abdominal fat and improves insulin sensitivity in older men with type 2 diabetes. Diabetes Care 28:662–667

49. Sax PE (2006) Strategies for management and treatment of dyslipidemia in HIV/AIDS. AIDS Care 18:149–157

50. Scevola D, Di Matteo A, Giglio O, Uberti F (2007) Starvation: social, voluntary, and involuntary causes of weight loss. In: Mantovani G (ed) Cachexia and wasting: a modern approach. Springer, Milan, pp 149–160

51. Scevola D, DiMatteo A, Giglio O, Scevola S (2006) Nutritional status assessment. In: Manto-

vani G (ed) Cachexia and wasting: a modern approach. Springer, Milan, pp 93–110

52. Barrios A, Blanco F, Garcìa-Benayas T et al (2002) Effect of dietary intervention on highly active antiretroviral therapy-related dyslipemia. AIDS 16:2079–2081

53. Von Roenn JH (1994) Management of HIV-related body weight loss. Drugs 47:774–783

54. Scevola D, Bottari G, Zambelli A et al (1992) Trattamento dietetico ed ormonale dei deficit nutrizionali nell'AIDS. Clin Dietol 19:127–140

55. Tisdale M, Beck SA (1991) Inhibition of tumour induced lipolysis in vitro and cachexia and tumour growth in vivo by eicosapentaenoic acid. Biochem Pharmacol 41:103–107

56. Kardinal CG, Loprinzi CL, Schaid DJ et al (1990) A controlled trial of cyproheptadine in cancer patients with anorexia and/or cachexia. Cancer 65:2657–2662

57. Scevola D, Zambelli A, Bottari G et al (1991) Appetite stimulation and body weight gain with medroxyprogesterone acetate in AIDS anorexia and cachexia. Farmaci Terapia 3:77–83

58. Scevola D, Parazzini F, Negri C, Moroni M (1995) Efficacy and safety of high-dose MPA treatment of AIDS cachexia: the Italian multicentre study. Fourth Congress of the European Association for Palliative Care, Barcelona, 6–9 December 1995, abstracts book, pp 443–447

59. Scevola D, Bottari G, Oberto L et al (1995) A double-blind-placebo controlled trial of megestrol acetate on caloric intake and nutritional status in AIDS cachexia. Fourth Congress of European Association for Palliative Care, Barcelona, 6–9 December 1995, abstracts book, pp 427–437

60. Rondanelli M, Solerte SB, Fioravanti M et al (1997) Circadian secretory pattern of growth hormone, insulin-like growth factor type I, cortisol, adrenocorticotropic hormone, thyroid-stimulating hormone, and prolactin during HIV infection. AIDS Res Hum Retroviruses 14:1243–1249

61. Scevola D, Bottari G, Oberto L et al (1995) Megestrol acetate (MA) and growth hormone (rHGH) as combined therapy for AIDS cachexia. Fourth Congress of European Association for Palliative Care, Barcelona, 6–9 December 1995, abstracts book, pp 438–442

62. Wanke C, Gerrior J, Kantaros J et al (1999) Recombinant human growth hormone improves the fat redistribution syndrome (lipodystrophy) in patients with HIV. AIDS 13:2099–2103

63. Saint-Marc T, Touraine JL (1999) Effects of metformin on insulin resistance and central adiposity in patients receiving effective protease inhibitor (PI). 6th Conference on Retroviruses and Opportunistic Infections, Chicago, ILL, 31 Jan–4 Feb 1999, abstract 672

64. Walli RK, Michl GM, Bogner JR et al (1999) Effects of the PPAR-Activator troglitazone on protease inhibitor associated peripheral insulin resistance. 6th Conference on Retroviruses and Opportunistic Infections, Chicago, ILL, 31 Jan–4 Feb 1999, abstract 673

65. Carr A, Workman C, Carey D, Rogers G, Martin A, Baker D et al (2004) No effect of rosiglitazone for treatment of HIV-1 lipoatrophy: randomised, double-blind, placebo-controlled trial. Lancet 363:429–38

66. Torres R, Unger K (1999) The effect of recombinant human growth hormone on protease-inhibitor- associated fat maldistribution syndrome. 6th Conference on Retroviruses and Opportunistic Infections, Chicago, ILL, 31 Jan–4 Feb 1999, abstract 675

67. Strawford A, Barbieri T, Parks E et al (1999) Resistance exercise and supraphysiologic androgen therapy in eugonadal men with HIV-related weight loss. JAMA 281:1282–1290

68. Scevola D, Oberto L, Bottari G, Faggi A (1995) Lipidi e Malattie Infettive. Abstracts Book XII Congresso Nazionale ADI. Torino, Italy, 16–18 November 1995, p 187

69. Scevola D, Bottari G, Oberto L et al (1996) Problemi nutrizionali del paziente AIDS e strategie terapeutiche. Quad Cure Palliat (S1):51–64

70. Lauretani F, Russo CR, Bandinelli S et al (2003) Age-associated changes in skeletal muscles and their effect on mobility: an operational diagnosis of sarcopenia. J Appl Physiol 95:1851–1860

71. Amsterdam EA (1997) Exercise in cardiovascular health and disease. Yorke, New York

72. Smith BA, Neidig JL, Nickel JT et al (2001) Aerobic exercise: effects on parameters related to fatigue, dyspnea, weight and body composition in HIV-infected adults. AIDS 15:693–701

73. Montoye HJ (1975) Physical activity and health: an epidemiologic study of an entire community. Prentice-Hall, Englewood Cliffs, NJ

74. Katch FI, Freedson PS, Jones CA et al (1985) Evaluation of acute cardiorespiratory responses to hydraulic resistance exercise. Med Sci Sports Exerc 17:168–173

75. Crow RS, Rantahargiu PM, Prineas RJ et al (1986) Risk factors, exercise fitness and electrocardiographic response to exercise in 12,866 men at risk of symptomatic coronary heart disease. Am J Cardiol 57:1075–1082

76. Pollock M, Gaesser G, Butcher J et al (1998) The recommended quantity and quality of exercise for developing and maintaining cardiorespiratory and muscular fitness and flexibility in healthy adults. Med Sci Sports Exerc 30:975–991

77. Stringer WW, Berezovskaya M, O'Brien WA et al (1998) The effect of exercise training on aerobic fitness, immune indices, and quality of life in HIV+ patients. Med Sci Sports Exerc 30:11–16

78. Beniamini Y, Rubenstein JJ, Faigenbaum AD et al (1999) High-intensity strength training of patients enrolled in an outpatient cardiac rehabilitation program. J Cardiopulm Rehabil 19:8–17

79. Braith RW, Stewart KJ (2006) Resistance exercise training: its role in the prevention of cardiovascular disease. Circulation 113:2642–2650

80. McCartney N, McKelvie RS, Haslam DR, Jones NL (1991) Usefulness of weightlifting training in improving strength and maximal power output in coronary artery disease Am J Cardiol 67:939–945

81. Maeda S, Miyauchi T, Iemitsu M et al (2004) Resistance exercise training reduces plasma endothelin-1 concentration in healthy young humans. J Cardiovasc Pharmacol 44(suppl1): S443–S446

82. Stewart KJ, Bacher AC, Turner K et al (2005) Exercise and risk factors associated with metabolic syndrome in older adults. Am J Prev Med 28:9–18

83. Swain DP, Franklin BA (2006) Comparison of cardioprotective benefits of vigorous versus moderate intensity aerobic exercise. Am J Cardiol 97:141–147

84. Vincent KR, Vincent HK, Braith RW et al (2002) Resistance exercise training attenuates exercise-induced lipid peroxidation in the elderly. Eur J Appl Physiol 87:416–423

Appendix 1

Cardiovascular Monitoring of HIV-Infected Subjects and Cardiovascular Risk Stratification and Prevention of Cardiovascular Disease in Patients Receiving HAART

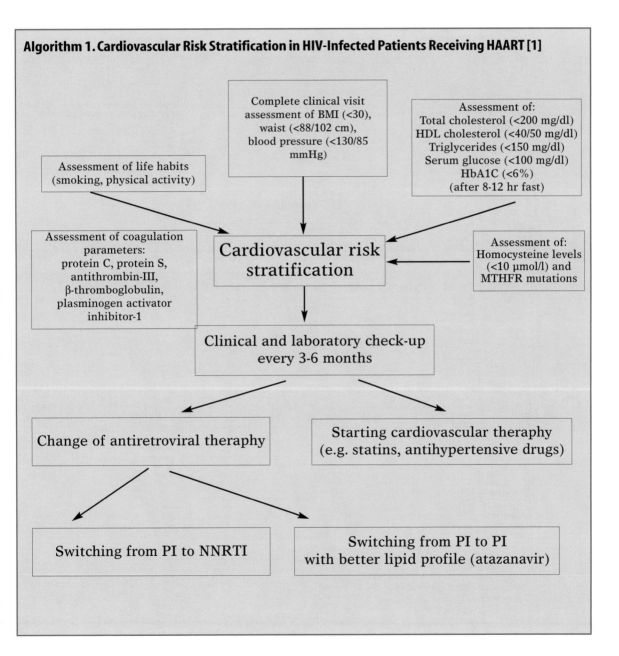

Algorithm 1. Cardiovascular Risk Stratification in HIV-Infected Patients Receiving HAART [1]

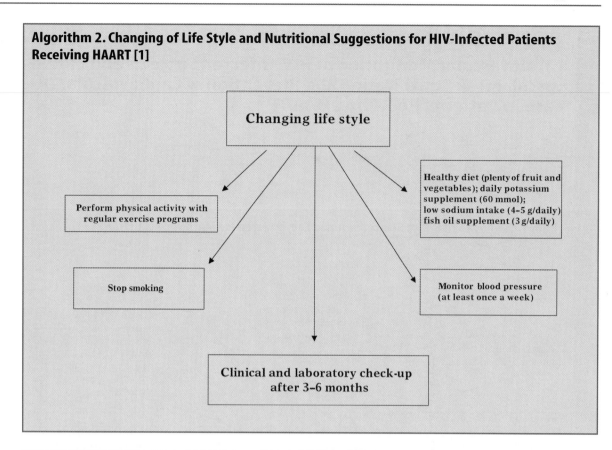

Algorithm 2. Changing of Life Style and Nutritional Suggestions for HIV-Infected Patients Receiving HAART [1]

Changing life style

Perform physical activity with regular exercise programs

Healthy diet (plenty of fruit and vegetables); daily potassium supplement (60 mmol); low sodium intake (4–5 g/daily) fish oil supplement (3 g/daily)

Stop smoking

Monitor blood pressure (at least once a week)

Clinical and laboratory check-up after 3–6 months

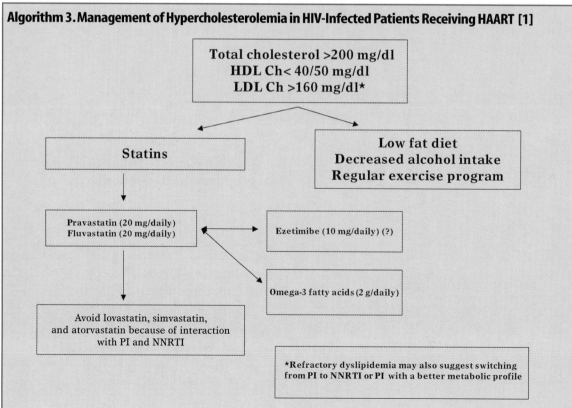

Algorithm 3. Management of Hypercholesterolemia in HIV-Infected Patients Receiving HAART [1]

Total cholesterol >200 mg/dl
HDL Ch< 40/50 mg/dl
LDL Ch >160 mg/dl*

Statins

Low fat diet
Decreased alcohol intake
Regular exercise program

Pravastatin (20 mg/daily)
Fluvastatin (20 mg/daily)

Ezetimibe (10 mg/daily) (?)

Omega-3 fatty acids (2 g/daily)

Avoid lovastatin, simvastatin, and atorvastatin because of interaction with PI and NNRTI

*Refractory dyslipidemia may also suggest switching from PI to NNRTI or PI with a better metabolic profile

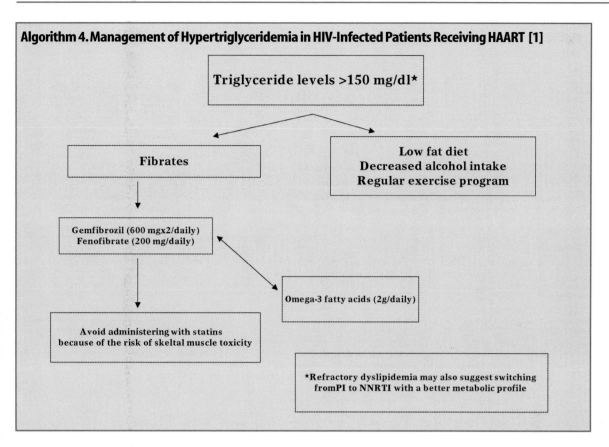

Algorithm 4. Management of Hypertriglyceridemia in HIV-Infected Patients Receiving HAART [1]

Triglyceride levels >150 mg/dl*

Fibrates

Low fat diet
Decreased alcohol intake
Regular exercise program

Gemfibrozil (600 mgx2/daily)
Fenofibrate (200 mg/daily)

Omega-3 fatty acids (2g/daily)

Avoid administering with statins
because of the risk of skeltal muscle toxicity

*Refractory dyslipidemia may also suggest switching
fromPI to NNRTI with a better metabolic profile

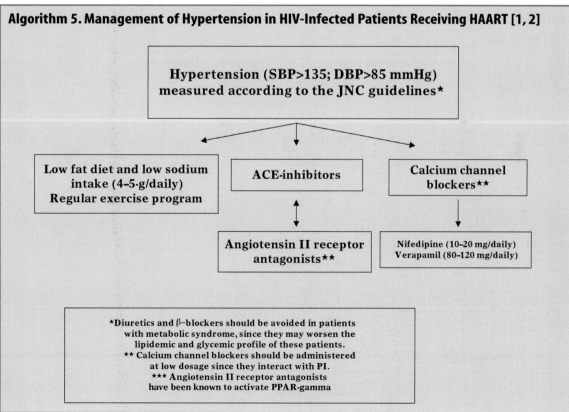

Algorithm 5. Management of Hypertension in HIV-Infected Patients Receiving HAART [1, 2]

Hypertension (SBP>135; DBP>85 mmHg)
measured according to the JNC guidelines*

Low fat diet and low sodium
intake (4–5-g/daily)
Regular exercise program

ACE-inhibitors

Calcium channel
blockers**

Angiotensin II receptor
antagonists**

Nifedipine (10–20 mg/daily)
Verapamil (80–120 mg/daily)

*Diuretics and β–blockers should be avoided in patients
with metabolic syndrome, since they may worsen the
lipidemic and glycemic profile of these patients.
** Calcium channel blockers should be administered
at low dosage since they interact with PI.
*** Angiotensin II receptor antagonists
have been known to activate PPAR-gamma

Algorithm 6. Management of Hyperglycemia in HIV-Infected Patients Receiving HAART [1,3,4]

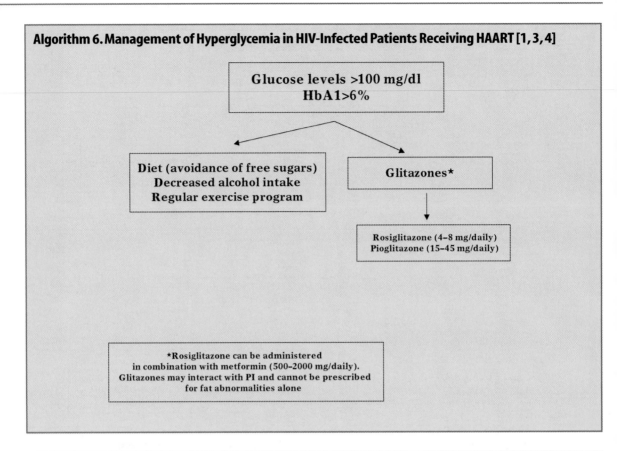

Algorithm 7. Management of HIV-Infected Patients Receiving HAART with Previous Cardiovascular Events [1]

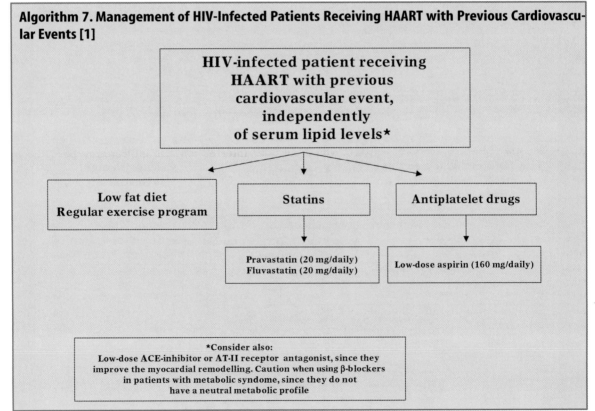

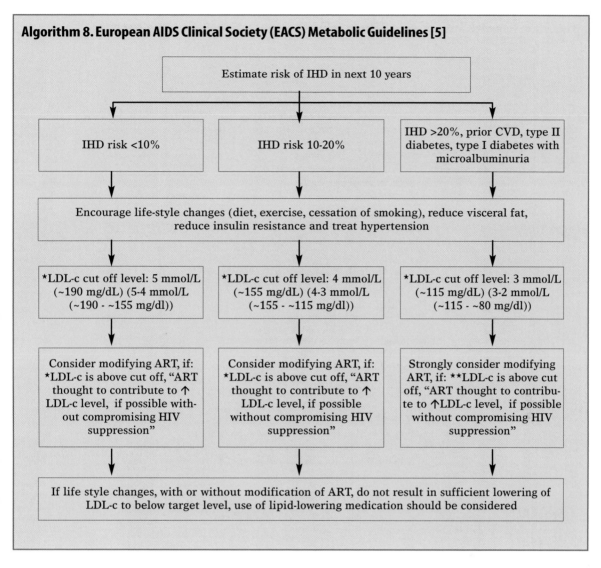

Algorithm 8. European AIDS Clinical Society (EACS) Metabolic Guidelines [5]

Estimate risk of IHD in next 10 years

| IHD risk <10% | IHD risk 10-20% | IHD >20%, prior CVD, type II diabetes, type I diabetes with microalbuminuria |

Encourage life-style changes (diet, exercise, cessation of smoking), reduce visceral fat, reduce insulin resistance and treat hypertension

| *LDL-c cut off level: 5 mmol/L (~190 mg/dL) (5-4 mmol/L (~190 - ~155 mg/dl)) | *LDL-c cut off level: 4 mmol/L (~155 mg/dL) (4-3 mmol/L (~155 - ~115 mg/dl)) | *LDL-c cut off level: 3 mmol/L (~115 mg/dL) (3-2 mmol/L (~115 - ~80 mg/dl)) |

| Consider modifying ART, if: *LDL-c is above cut off, "ART thought to contribute to ↑ LDL-c level, if possible without compromising HIV suppression" | Consider modifying ART, if: *LDL-c is above cut off, "ART thought to contribute to ↑ LDL-c level, if possible without compromising HIV suppression" | Strongly consider modifying ART, if: **LDL-c is above cut off, "ART thought to contribute to ↑LDL-c level, if possible without compromising HIV suppression" |

If life style changes, with or without modification of ART, do not result in sufficient lowering of LDL-c to below target level, use of lipid-lowering medication should be considered

*LDL-c cut off levels (unit: mmol/L (mg/dL)) are higher than in guidelines for the general population (more stringent levels where some experts would consider intervention also indicated in parenthesis below). In cases where LDL-c cannot be reliably calculated because of high triglyceride levels, the non-HDL-c target level should be used which is 0.8 mmol/L (30 mg/dl) higher than the corresponding LDL-c target

**Options for ART modification include: (1) replacing PI(/r) by NNRTI, by another PI(/r) known to cause less metabolic disturbances or by abacavir; should not be done if patient is known or suspected to harbour archived virus containing drug-related mutations against the new drug the patient is switched to (switch to abacavir should not be done in case (archived) thymidine analogue mutations are known or suspected to be present (e.g. due to prior use of suboptimal mono- or dual NRTI therapy); (2) replacing d4T or ZDV by ABC or TDF. In patients with >20% 10 year risk or with prior CVD, the risk of CVD events and cardiac death will usually be higher than risk of progression to AIDS or death and in such patients a strategy to reduce risk of CVD by switching ART is hence most appropriate

Algorithm 9. Switch Strategies of Antiretroviral Therapy: Rationale and Requirements

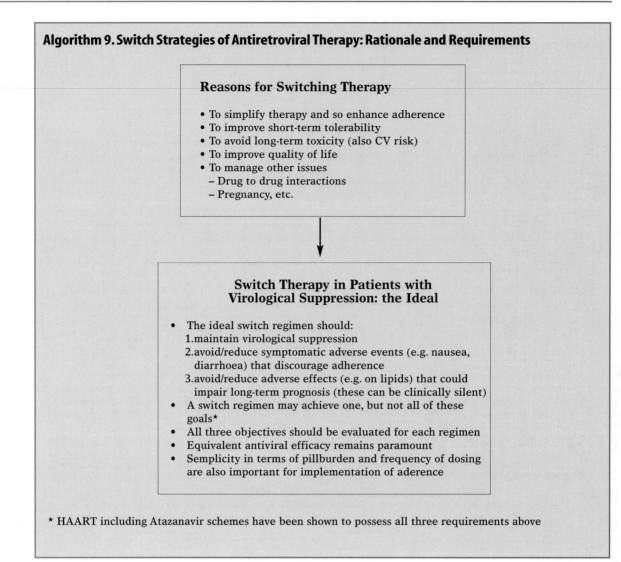

Reasons for Switching Therapy

- To simplify therapy and so enhance adherence
- To improve short-term tolerability
- To avoid long-term toxicity (also CV risk)
- To improve quality of life
- To manage other issues
  - Drug to drug interactions
  - Pregnancy, etc.

**Switch Therapy in Patients with
Virological Suppression: the Ideal**

- The ideal switch regimen should:
  1. maintain virological suppression
  2. avoid/reduce symptomatic adverse events (e.g. nausea, diarrhoea) that discourage adherence
  3. avoid/reduce adverse effects (e.g. on lipids) that could impair long-term prognosis (these can be clinically silent)
- A switch regimen may achieve one, but not all of these goals*
- All three objectives should be evaluated for each regimen
- Equivalent antiviral efficacy remains paramount
- Semplicity in terms of pillburden and frequency of dosing are also important for implementation of aderence

* HAART including Atazanavir schemes have been shown to possess all three requirements above

Table 1 Antiretroviral therapy-associated adverse effects and management recommendations [9]

Adverse effects	Causative ARVs	Onset/clinical manifestation	Estimated frequency	Risk Factors	Prevention/ monitoring	Management
Cardiovascular effects	Possibly PIs and other ARVs with unfavorable effects on lipids (e.g. EFV, d4T)	Onset: months to years after beginning of therapy. Presentation: premature coronary artery disease	3-6 per 1,000 patients-years	Other risk factors for cardiovascular disease such as smoking, age, hyperlipidemia, hypertension, diabetes mellitus, family history of premature coronary artery disease, and personal history of coronary artery disease	• Assess each patient's cardiac risk factors • Consider non-PI based regimen • Monitor & identify patients with hyperlipidemia or hyperglycemia • Counseling for life style modification: smoking cessation, diet, and exercise	• Early diagnosis, prevention, and pharmacologic management of other cardiovascular risk factors such as hyperlipidemia, hypertension, and insulin resistance/diabetes mellitus • Assess cardiac risk factors • Lifestyle modifications: diet, exercise, and/or smoking cessation • Switch to agents with less propensity for increasing cardiovascular risk factors, i.e., NNRTI- or ATV-based regimen & avoid d4T use
Hyperlipidemia	All PIs (except ATV); d4T; EFV (to a lesser extent)	Onset: weeks to months after beginning of therapy. Presentation: • all PIs except ATV: $\uparrow$ in LDL & total cholesterol (TC) & triglyceride (TG), $\downarrow$ in HDL • LPV/r & RTV: disproportionate $\uparrow$ in TG • d4T: mostly $\uparrow$ in TG; may also have $\uparrow$ in LDL & total cholesterol (TC) • EFV or NVP: $\uparrow$ in HDL, slight $\uparrow$ TG	Varies with different agents. Swiss cohort: $\uparrow$TC & TG – 1.7-2.3x higher in patients receiving (non-ATV) PI	Underlying hyperlipidemia. Risk based on ARV therapy • PI: LPV/r & RTV-boosted PIs> NFV & APV > mv > ATV; • NNRTI: EFV more common than NVP • NRTI: d4T most common	• Use non-PI, non-d4T based regimen • Use ATV-based regimen • Fasting lipid profile at baseline, 3-6 months after starting new regimen, then annually or more frequently if indicated (in high-risk patients, or patients with abnormal baseline levels)	• Follow HIVMA/ACTG guidelines for management • Assess cardiac risk factor • Lifestyle modification: diet, exercise, and/or smoking cessation • Switching to agents with less propensity for causing hyperlipidemia. Pharmacologic management: • $\uparrow$ total cholesterol, LDL, TG 200-500 mg/dL: "statins" – pravastatin or atorvastatin • TG >500 mg/dL: gemfibrozil or micronized fenofibrate
Insulin resistance/ Diabetes mellitus	All PIs	Onset: weeks to months after beginning of therapy. Presentation: polyuria, polydipsia, polyphagia, fatigue, weakness; exacerbation of hyperglycemia in patients with underlying diabetes	Up to 3%-5% of patients developed diabetes in some series	Underlying hyperglycemia family history of diabetes mellitus	• Use PI-sparing regimens • Fasting blood glucose 1-3 months after starting new regimen, then at least every 3-6 months	• Diet and exercise • Consider switching to an NNRTI-based regimen • Metformin • "Glitazones" • Sulfonylurea • Insulin
Osteonecrosis	All PIs	Clinical presentation (generally similar to non-HIV population): • insidious in onset, with subtle symptoms of mild to moderate periarticular pain • 85% of the cases involving one or both femoral heads, but other bones may also be affected • pain may be triggered by weight bearing or movement	Reported incidence on the rise. Symptomatic osteonecrosis: 0.08%-1.33%; Asymptomatic osteonecrosis: 4% from MRI reports	• Diabetes • Prior steroid use • Old age • Alcohol use • Hyperlipidemia • Role of ARVs and osteonecrosis – still controversial	• Risk reduction (e.g., limit steroid and alcohol use) • Asymptomatic cases w/ <15% bony head involvement – follow with MRI every 3-6 months x 1 yr, then every 6 months x 1 yr, then annually – to assess for disease progression	Conservative management: • $\downarrow$ weight bearing on affected joint; • Remove or reduce risk factors • Analgesics as needed. Surgical intervention: • Core decompression +/- bone grafting – for early stages of disease • For more severe and debilitating disease – total joint arthroplasty

References

1. Volberding P, Murphy R, Barbaro G et al (2003) The Pavia Consensus Statement. AIDS 17(S1):S170–S179

2. Chobanian AV, Bakris GL, Black HR et al (2003) The Seventh Report of the Joint National Committee on Prevention, Detection, Evaluation, and Treatment of High Blood Pressure: the JNC 7 report. JAMA 289:2560–2572

3. Hadigan C, Yawetz S, Thomas A, Havers F, Sax PE, Grinspoon S (2004) Metabolic effects of rosiglitazone in HIV lipodystrophy: a randomized, controlled trial. Ann Intern Med 140:786–794

4. Carr A, Workman C, Carey D et al (2004) No effect of rosiglitazone for treatment of HIV-1 lipoatrophy: randomised, double-blind, placebo-controlled trial. Lancet 363:429–438

5. European AIDS Clinical Society (EACS). Guidelines on the prevention and management of metabolic diseases in HIV. http://www.eacs.eu/c_acceuil.htm

6. Gatell J, Salmon-Ceron D, Lazzarin A et al (2007) Efficacy and safety of atazanavir-based highly active antiretroviral therapy in patients with virologic suppression switched from a stable, boosted or unboosted protease inhibitor treatment regimen: the SWAN study (AI424-097) 48-week results. CID 44 (1 June)

7. Mallolas J, Podzamczer D, Domingo P et al (2007) Efficacy and safety of switching from boosted lopinavir to boosted atazanavir in patients with virologic suppression receiving a LPV/r-containing HAART: the ATAZIP study, - IAS - Poster WEPEB117LB

8. Rubio R, Carmena J, Asensi et al (2007) Effect of simplification from protease inhibitor to boosted atazanavir -based regimens in real-life conditions: Preliminary results of GESIDA 44/04 SIMPATAZ study EACS Poster P7.5/03

9. Panel on Antiretroviral Guidelines for Adult and Adolescents. Guidelines for the use of antiretroviral agents in HIV-1-infected adults and adolescents. Department of Health and Human Services. January 29, 2008; 1-128. Available at http://www.aidsinfo.nih.gov/ContentFiles/AdultandAdolescentGL.pdf. Accessed 18/02/2008 [page 82, table 18b]

Appendix 2

Interactions Between Antiretrovirals and Drugs Commonly Used to Treat Cardiovascular Diseases

Interactions among protease inhibitors (PIs) and drugs used to treat cardiovascular diseases

PIs	Amprenavir	Indinavir	Lopinavir/ ritonavir	Atazanavir ritonavir	Ritonavir	Saquinavir/ ritonavir
Ca++ channel blocker						
Bepridil	Yes	None	Yes?	Yes?	Yes	Yes?
Diltiazem				AUC ↑ 125% ↓ diltiazem dose by 50%; ECG monitoring is recommended	Yes	Yes?
Other Ca+ channel blocker	For all: potential interaction that may require close monitoring, alteration of drug dosage or timing of administration, potential increased levels and toxicity					
Antiarrhythmics						
Amiodarone	None	None	None	None	*Affected drug*: Amiodarone *Interacting drug*: Ritonavir *Mechanism*: Inhibition of metabolism – potential for increased levels and toxicity. *Recommendation*: Use with caution or avoid concomitant use	None
Flecainide	None	None	*Affected drug:* Flecainide *Interacting drug:* Lopinavir/ritonavir *Mechanism:* Potential for increased levels due to inhibition of metabolism *Recommendation:* Avoid concomitant use	None	*Affected drug*: Flecainide *Interacting drug*: Ritonavir *Mechanism*: Inhibition of metabolism – potential for increased levels and toxicity *Recommendation*: Use with caution or avoid concomitant use	None
Propafenone	None	None	*Affected drug:* Propafenone *Interacting drug*: Lopinavir/ritonavir *Mechanism:* Potential for increased levels due to inhibition of metabolism *Recommendation:* Avoid concomitant use	None	*Affected drug*: Propafenone *Interacting drug*: Ritonavir *Mechanism*: Inhibition of metabolism – potential for increased levels and toxicity *Recommendation*: Use with caution or avoid concomitant use	None

cont. →

cont.

Quinidine	None	None	None	None	*Affected drug*: Quinidine *Interacting drug*: Ritonavir *Mechanism*: Inhibition of metabolism – potential for increased levels and toxicity *Recommendation*: Use with caution or avoid concomitant use	None

Statins

Fluvastatin	*Affected drug*: Fluvastatin *Interacting drug*: Amprenavir *Mechanism*: Inhibition of metabolism – potential for increased levels and toxicity *Recommendation*: Potential for hypolipidemic toxicity (dizziness, headache, GI side effects). Monitor patient closely and consider dose reduction	*Affected drug*: Fluvastatin *Interacting drug*: Indinavir *Mechanism*: Inhibition of metabolism – potential for increased levels and toxicity *Recommendation*: Potential for hypolipidemic toxicity (dizziness, headache, GI side effects). Monitor patient closely and consider dose reduction	None	None	*Affected drug*: Fluvastatin *Interacting drug*: Ritonavir *Mechanism*: Inhibition of metabolism – potential for increased levels and toxicity *Recommendation*: Potential for hypolipidemic toxicity (dizziness, headache, GI side effects). Monitor patient closely and consider dose reduction	None
Lovastatin	*Affected drug*: Lovastatin *Interacting drug*: Amprenavir *Mechanism*: Inhibition of metabolism – potential for increased levels and toxicity *Recommendation*: Potential for hypolipidemic toxicity (dizziness, headache, GI side effects). Monitor patient closely and consider dose reduction	*Affected drug*: Lovastatin *Interacting drug*: Indinavir *Mechanism*: Inhibition of metabolism – potential for increased levels and toxicity *Recommendation*: Potential for hypolipidemic toxicity (dizziness, headache, GI side effects). Monitor patient closely and consider dose reduction	*Affected drug*: Lovastatin *Interacting drug*: Lopinavir/ritonavir *Mechanism*: Potential for increased levels due to inhibition of metabolism *Recommendation*: Avoid concomitant use	*Affected drug*: Lovastatin *Interacting drug*: Atazanavir *Mechanism*: Inhibition of metabolism – potential for increased levels and toxicity *Recommendation*: Potential for hypolipidemic toxicity (dizziness, headache, GI side effects). Monitor patient closely and consider dose reduction	*Affected drug*: Lovastatin *Interacting drug*: Ritonavir *Mechanism*: Inhibition of metabolism – potential for increased levels and toxicity *Recommendation*: Potential for hypolipidemic toxicity (dizziness, headache, GI side effects). Monitor patient closely and consider dose reduction	None
Pravastatin	None	*Affected drug*: Pravastatin *Interacting drug*: Indinavir *Mechanism*: Inhibition of metabolism – potential for increased levels and toxicity *Recommendation*: Potential for hypolipidemic toxicity (dizziness, headache, GI side effects). Monitor patient closely and consider dose reduction	*Affected drug*: Pravastatin *Interacting drug*: Lopinavir/ritonavir *Mechanism*: Inhibition of metabolism – atorvastatin AUC increased 33% *Recommendation*: No dose adjustment necessary	None	*Affected drug*: Pravastatin *Interacting drug*: Ritonavir *Mechanism*: Pravastatin AUC decreased by median 0.5-fold in patients receiving RTV/SQV *Recommendation*: No dosage change necessary	None

cont. →

cont.

						None
Simvastatin	*Affected drug*: Simvastatin *Interacting drug*: Aprenavir *Mechanism*: Inhibition of metabolism – potential for increased levels and toxicity *Recommendation*: Potential for hypolipidemic toxicity (dizziness, headache, GI side effects). Monitor patient closely and consider dose reduction	*Affected drug*: Simvastatin *Interacting drug*: Indinavir *Mechanism*: Inhibition of metabolism – potential for increased levels and toxicity *Recommendation*: Potential for hypolipidemic toxicity (dizziness, headache, GI side effects). Monitor patient closely and consider dose reduction	*Affected drug*: Simvastatin *Interacting drug*: Lopinavir/ritonavir *Mechanism*: Potential for increased levels due to inhibition of metabolism *Recommendation*: Avoid concomitant use	*Affected drug*: Simvastatin *Interacting drug*: Atazanavir *Mechanism*: Inhibition of metabolism – AUC increased 5-fold *Recommendation*: Avoid concomitant use	*Affected drug*: Simvastatin *Interacting drug*: Ritonavir *Mechanism*: Inhibition of metabolism – simvastatin AUC increased 31.6-fold in patients receiving RTV/SQV *Recommendation*: Avoid simvastatin in patients on ritonavir/saquinavir	None
Atorvastatin	*Affected drug*: Atorvastatin *Interacting drug*: Aprenavir *Mechanism*: Inhibition of metabolism – potential for increased levels and toxicity *Recommendation*: Potential for hypolipidemic toxicity (dizziness, headache, GI side effects). Monitor patient closely and consider dose reduction	*Affected drug*: Atorvastatin *Interacting drug*: Indinavir *Mechanism*: Inhibition of metabolism – potential for increased levels and toxicity *Recommendation*: Potential for hypolipidemic toxicity (dizziness, headache, GI side effects). Monitor patient closely and consider dose reduction	*Affected drug*: Atorvastatin *Interacting drug*: Lopinavir/ritonavir *Mechanism*: Inhibition of metabolism – atorvastatin AUC increased 5.8-fold *Recommendation*: Use with caution - start at low doses and monitor	*Affected drug*: Atorvastatin levels have potential for large increase. Use lowest possible starting dose of atorvastatin with careful monitoring	*Affected drug*: Atorvastatin *Interacting drug*: Ritonavir *Mechanism*: Inhibition of metabolism – atorvastatin AUC increased 4.5-fold in patients receiving RTV/SQV *Recommendation*: Use atorvastatin with caution in patients on ritonavir/saquinavir	None

Anticoagulants

						None
Warfarin	*Affected drug*: Warfarin *Interacting drug*: Amprenavir *Mechanism*: Inhibition of metabolism – potential for increased risk of bleeding *Recommendation*: Monitor INR closely or avoid concomitant use	None	None	None	*Affected drug*: Warfarin *Interacting drug*: Ritonavir *Mechanism*: Induction of metabolism – decreased anticoagulation and risk of blood clot or embolus *Recommendation*: Monitor INR closely or avoid concomitant use	None

Light red shadowing indicates major interactions; *yellow shadowing* indicates moderate interactions; *light blue shadowing* indicates minor interactions.
AUC, area under the curve; *INR*, international normalized ratio

Interactions among nucleoside reverse transcriptase inhibitors (NRTI) and nucleotide reverse transcriptase inhibitors (NtRTI) and drugs used to treat cardiovascular diseases

NRTI	Abacavir	Zidovudine	Lamivudine	Zalcitabine	Stavudine	Didanosine	Tanofovir
Ca++ channel blocker							None
Antiarrhythmics							
Amiodarone	None	None	None	None	None	None	None
Flecainide	None	None	None	None	None	None	None
Propafenone	None	None	None	None	None	None	None
Quinidine	None	None	None	None	None	None	None
Statins							
Quinidine	None	None	None	None	None	None	None
Lovastatin	None	None	None	None	None	None	None
Pravastatin	None	None	None	None	None	None	None
Simvastatin	None	None	None	None	None	None	None
Atorvarstatin	None	None	None	None	None	None	None
Anticoagulants							
Warfarin	None	None	None	None	None	None	None

Interactions among non-nucleoside reverse transcriptase inhibitors (NNRTI) and drugs used to treat cardiovascular diseases

NNRTI	Delavirdine	Nevirapine	Efavirenz
Ca++ channel blocker	None	None	None
Antiarrhythmics			
Amiodarone	None	None	None
Flecainide	None	None	None
Propafenone	None	None	None
Quinidine	None	None	None
Statins			
Fluvastatin	*Affected drug*: Fluvastatin *Interacting drug*: Delavirdine *Mechanism*: Inhibition of metabolism – potential for increased levels and toxicity *Recommendation*: Potential for hypolipidemic toxicity (dizziness, headache, GI side effects). Monitor patient closely and consider dose reduction	None	None

Lovastatin	*Affected drug*: Lovastatin *Interacting drug*: Delavirdine *Mechanism*: Inhibition of metabolism – potential for increased levels and toxicity *Recommendation*: Potential for hypolipidemic toxicity (dizziness, headache, GI side effects). Monitor patient closely and consider dose reduction	None	None
Pravastatin	*Affected drug*: Pravastatin *Interacting drug*: Delavirdine *Mechanism*: Inhibition of metabolism – potential for increased levels and toxicity *Recommendation*: Potential for hypolipidemic toxicity (dizziness, headache, GI side effects). Monitor patient closely and consider dose reduction	None	None
Simvastatin	*Affected drug*: Simvastatin *Interacting drug*: Delavirdine *Mechanism*: Inhibition of metabolism – potential for increased levels and toxicity *Recommendation*: Potential for hypolipidemic toxicity (dizziness, headache, GI side effects). Monitor patient closely and consider dose reduction	None	None
Atorvastatin	*Affected drug*: Atorvastatin *Interacting drug*: Delavirdine *Mechanism*: Inhibition of metabolism – potential for increased levels and toxicity *Recommendation*: Potential for hypolipidemic toxicity (dizziness, headache, GI side effects). Monitor patient closely and consider dose reduction	None	None
Anticoagulants			
Warfarin	*Affected drug*: Warfarin *Interacting drug*: Delavirdine *Mechanism*: Inhibition of metabolism – potential for increased risk of bleeding *Recommendation*: Monitor INR closely or avoid concomitant use	*Affected drug*: Warfarin *Interacting drug*: Nevirapine *Mechanism*: Induction of metabolism – decreased anticoagulation and risk of blood clot or embolus *Recommendation*: Monitor INR closely or avoid concomitant use	*Affected drug*: Warfarin *Interacting drug*: Efavirenz *Mechanism*: Induction of metabolism – decreased anticoagulation and risk of blood clot or embolus *Recommendation*: Monitor INR closely or avoid concomitant use

Light red shadowing indicates major interactions; *yellow shadowing* indicates moderate interactions; *light blue shadowing* indicates minor interactions.

AUC, area under the curve; *INR*, international normalized ratio

Reference

1. Volberding P, Murphy R, Barbaro G et al (2003) The Pavia Consensus Statement. AIDS 17(S1):S170–S179

Subject Index

Printed in September 2008